# MANUAL of GLAUCOMA
Diagnosis and Management

# MANUAL of GLAUCOMA
## Diagnosis and Management

---


**Theodore Krupin, M.D.**
Chief, Glaucoma Service, Scheie Eye Institute
Professor, Department of Ophthalmology
University of Pennsylvania School of Medicine

Andrew J. Adelson, M.D.
Sylvia Beck, M.D.
Neil Dorfman, M.D.
Marianne E. Feitl, M.D.
J. Charles Henry, M.D.
David M. Kozart, M.D.
Charles W. Nichols, M.D.
Jeffrey Schultz, M.D.
Scott M. Spector, M.D.
Richard A. Stone, M.D.
Martin B. Wax, M.D.
Elliott B. Werner, M.D.

The Glaucoma Service, Scheie Eye Institute
Department of Ophthalmology
University of Pennsylvania School of Medicine
Philadelphia, Pennsylvania

*Illustrated by Timothy Hengst, M.A., A.M.I.*


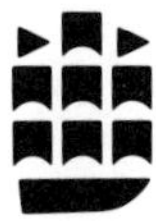


**CHURCHILL LIVINGSTONE**
New York, Edinburgh, London, Melbourne 1988

**Library of Congress Cataloging-in-Publication Data**

Manual of Glaucoma : diagnosis and management /
Theodore Krupin . . . [et al.] ; illustrated by Timothy
Hengst.
p. cm.
Includes bibliographies and index.
ISBN 0-443-08510-2
1. Glaucoma. I. Krupin, Theodore, 1942–
[DNLM: 1. Glaucoma—diagnosis. 2. Glaucoma—
therapy. WW 290 M294]
RE871.M36 1988
617.7'41—dc19
DNLM/DLC
for Library of Congress 88-20321
CIP



Distributed in the United Kingdom by Churchill Livingstone, Robert Stevenson House, 1–3 Baxter's Place, Leith Walk, Edinburgh EH1 3AF, and by associated companies, branches, and representatives throughout the world.

Accurate indications, adverse reactions, and dosage schedules for drugs are provided in this book, but it is possible that they may change. The reader is urged to review the package information data of the manufacturers of the medications mentioned.

The Publishers have made every effort to trace the copyright holders for borrowed material. If they have inadvertently overlooked any, they will be pleased to make the necessary arrangements at the first opportunity.

Acquisitions Editor: *Kim Loretucci*
Copy Editor: *David Terry*
Production Designer: *Jill Little*
Production Supervisor: *Jocelyn Eckstein*

Printed in the United States of America

First published in 1988

# PREFACE

This manual provides a practical source of information for the clinical management of glaucoma patients. The manual is not intended as a comprehensive glaucoma textbook. However, details necessary for performing and interpreting glaucoma diagnostic techniques (intraocular pressure, tonography, and gonioscopy) and glaucomatous pathologic changes (optic disc cupping and visual field loss) are presented. This information is integrated into an overall approach to the medical, laser, and conventional surgical management of the glaucoma patient.

The manual has evolved through resident and postgraduate teaching by the members of the Glaucoma Service of the Department of Ophthalmology, the University of Pennsylvania School of Medicine and Scheie Eye Institute. It is written for both the resident and the practicing ophthalmologist in a step-by-step approach for the diagnosis and management of glaucoma. Many of the preferences presented in this manual are intended as a guide to the ophthalmologist for the development of his own individual approach to glaucoma therapy. We apologize to those readers who find our "steps" either trite or contrary to their belief. Glaucoma therapy has many different approaches that are based on an individual's clinical experiences, highlighting the "art" and not only the "science" in the management of the glaucomas.

Glaucoma management is constantly evolving and improving. The basis for our education in the field is credited to our teachers: Bernard Becker, Allan E. Kolker, Stephen M. Drance, and Harold G. Scheie. Enhancements in our approach to glaucoma have been influenced by the inquisitive and challenging minds of colleagues, fellows, and residents. To all of them go credit and a thank you.

*Theodore Krupin, M.D.*
*David M. Kozart, M.D.*
*Richard A. Stone, M.D.*
*Martin B. Wax, M.D.*
*Elliott B. Werner, M.D.*

# CONTENTS

# 1

# Aqueous Dynamics

## AQUEOUS HUMOR DYNAMICS

Knowledge of aqueous humor dynamics is necessary to understand the pathophysiology of glaucoma and its medical therapy. Under steady-state conditions with a constant intraocular pressure, aqueous humor inflow equals aqueous humor outflow by conventional and uveal routes. This relationship is described by the classical mathematical formulation:

$$F = (Po - Pv)\,C + U$$

or

$$Po = \frac{F - U}{C} + Pv$$

where

F = aqueous humor flow rate in μl/min; Po = intraocular pressure in mmHg; Pv = episcleral venous pressure in mmHg; C = outflow facility in μl/min/mmHg; U = uveoscleral outflow in μl/min.

All parameters in the flow equation can be measured clinically except for uveoscleral outflow. From this formulation, the following relationships are evident:

1. Intraocular pressure is directly related to the rate of aqueous humor formation: the greater the rate, the higher the intraocular pressure.
2. Intraocular pressure is inversely related to the outflow facility: the lower the facility, the higher the intraocular pressure.
3. Intraocular pressure is directly dependent on the episcleral venous pressure: for each mmHg change in venous pressure, there is a corresponding change in intraocular pressure.
4. Intraocular pressure negatively correlates with the uveoscleral outflow: the lower the outflow, the higher the intraocular pressure.

## AQUEOUS HUMOR

### Production

I. Active secretion

Active secretion takes place in the double-layered ciliary epithelium (outer pigmented, inner nonpigmented). Active, energy-dependent transport of ions by the enzymes carbonic anhydrase, sodium–potassium ATPase, and others results in the net movement of fluid into the posterior chamber.

II. Ultrafiltration

Energy-independent flow of water across the ciliary epithelium in response to the osmotic gradient or the hydrostatic pressure difference between the blood vessels of the ciliary processes and the posterior chamber.

III. Diffusion

Energy-independent movement of substances across the membranes of the ciliary epithelium in response to a concentration gradient.

### Composition (Table 1-1)

I. Aqueous humor composition differs from the composition of plasma. Its composition varies among species. In humans, aqueous humor has an excess of hydrogen and chloride ions, an excess

**Table 1-1.** Composition of Plasma and Aqueous Humor of Humans (mmole/kg$H_2O$)

| Substance | Anterior Aqueous | Plasma |
|---|---|---|
| Sodium | 145 | 146 |
| Chloride | 126 | 117 |
| Bicarbonate | 22 | 26 |
| pH | 7.21 | 7.40 |
| Ascorbate | 0.92 | 0.06 |

of ascorbate, and a deficit of protein and bicarbonate.

II. The composition of aqueous humor is altered as it flows from the posterior chamber through the pupil and into the anterior chamber. Aqueous humor alterations occur across the hyaloid face of the vitreous, the blood vessels of the iris, and the corneal endothelium, and are secondary to dilutional exchanges and active transport processes.

### Rate of Formation (Inflow)

I. Aqueous humor formation is approximately 2.0–2.5 μl/min.

II. Inflow is generally unaffected in open-angle glaucoma, except in the rare entity of "hypersecretory glaucoma."

III. Measurement techniques

A. Tonography (see Chap. 3) using the Goldmann equation and measured intraocular pressure, episcleral venous pressure, and outflow facility. If one ignores uveal flow, the previous equation reduces to:

$$\text{Calculated flow} = (Po - Pv)\,C$$

This method is useful and easy to apply clinically. However, it is indirect and ignores the contribution of uveal outflow.

B. Anterior chamber fluorophotometry involving instillation of fluorescein into the cornea and anterior chamber by systemic, topical, or iontophoretic administration with subsequent measurement of the change in the fluorescein concentration in the cornea and anterior chamber aqueous humor over time. While this is a direct measurement and useful clinically, it requires expensive equipment.

C. Invasive laboratory techniques using the decay of intracamerally injected radioisotopes, the aqueous accumulation of intravenously administered radioisotopes, or by constant pressure perfusion of the cannulated anterior chamber. These methods are generally applicable only in experimental animals.

IV. Factors influencing aqueous inflow

A. Increased intraocular pressure is associated with decreased aqueous production (pseudofacility), because of the dependence of ultrafiltration on intraocular pressure.

B. Aqueous production decreases with increasing age.

C. Aqueous production decreases during sleep.

D. Aqueous production decreases with physical exercise.

E. Aqueous production decreases with ciliary body inflammation (uveitis) and choroidal detachment.

F. Aqueous production decreases following the administration of many pharmacologic agents. These include not only antiglaucoma medications, but also general anesthetics. For this reason, intraocular pressure measurements under general anesthesia may be artifactually low.

## AQUEOUS HUMOR OUTFLOW

### Pressure-Dependent Outflow (see Chapter 3)

The flow of aqueous humor out of the eye is dependent upon the magnitude of the intraocular pressure.

### Trabecular Meshwork

I. The trabecular meshwork is composed of multiple layers, each of which consists of a collagenous connective tissue core covered by a continuous endothelial layer covering. The endothelial cells are phagocytic.

II. The trabecular meshwork is divided into three portions.

A. Uveal meshwork

The innermost tissues adjacent to the anterior chamber are arranged in bands that extend from the iris root and ciliary body to the peripheral cornea. It contains irregular openings varying in size from 25 to 75 μm.

B. Corneoscleral meshwork

Sheets of trabeculum extend from the scleral spur to the lateral wall of the scleral sulcus. It contains elliptical openings, 5–50 μm in diameter, which become progressively smaller as Schlemm's canal is approached.

C. Juxtacanalicular meshwork

The outermost meshwork is adjacent to Schlemm's canal and forms its inner wall.

### Schlemm's Canal

I. Lined with endothelium, the canal is a single or branched channel with an average diameter of 370 μm.

II. Inner wall intercellular spaces are between 150 and 200 Å wide.

III. Inner wall openings consist of pores and giant vacuoles that have a direct communication with the intertrabecular spaces.

IV. The outer wall is a single layer of endothelial cells that does not contain pores.

### Intrascleral Aqueous Veins (Collector Channels)

I. Complex system of vessels that connect Schlemm's canal to the episcleral and conjunctival veins.

### Episcleral Veins

I. Drain into the anterior ciliary and superior ophthalmic veins, which drain into the cavernous sinus.

## Resistance to Aqueous Humor Outflow

### Trabecular Meshwork

I. Accounts for 60–65% of the resistance with the major site at the juxtacanicular trabecular tissue.

### Schlemm's Canal

I. Normally there is a free flow of aqueous humor within the canal.

II. Collapse of the canal occurs with an elevated intraocular pressure. This collapse is associated with increased resistance to aqueous humor flow.

### Inner Half of the Sclera

I. Accounts for approximately 25% of the resistance.

### Outer Half of the Sclera

I. Accounts for approximately 15% of the resistance.

## Pressure-Independent (Uveoscleral) Outflow

I. Aqueous humor enters the stroma and vessels of the iris root and the ciliary body and flows posteriorly to leave the eye via the suprachoroidal vessels or a transcleral exit.

II. Flow of aqueous humor out of the eye is through nontrabecular routes. This flow is independent of intraocular pressure.

III. Accounts for 5–15% of the total aqueous outflow under normal circumstances; pressure-dependent trabecular outflow accounts for the remaining 85–95%.

IV. Uveoscleral outflow increases after the administration of topical atropine and decreases following the topical administration of miotics.

## EPISCLERAL VENOUS PRESSURE

I. Episcleral venous pressure is normally a mean of 9.0 mmHg with a standard deviation of 1.6 mmHg. Episcleral venous pressure does not usually affect aqueous outflow resistance.
II. Abnormally elevated episcleral venous pressure contributes to the intraocular pressure, approximately 1 mmHg increase in intraocular pressure for each 1 mmHg increase in episcleral venous pressure.
III. Abnormally elevated episcleral venous pressure can cause collapse of Schlemm's canal and an increased aqueous outflow resistance.
IV. Measurement techniques
   A. Laboratory methods are based on the direct cannulation of an episcleral vein and pressure measurement by manometric means.
   B. Clinical methods are based on the principle of applying a measurable pressure external to the vein until the wall of the vein collapses. It is assumed that the wall of the vein has little inherent rigidity, so that as soon as the external pressure exceeds the intraluminal pressure, the wall of the vein will begin to collapse. External pressure is applied via:
      1. A pressure chamber consisting of a hollow viewing chamber covered with a transparent membrane attached to an air- or fluid-containing manometric system.

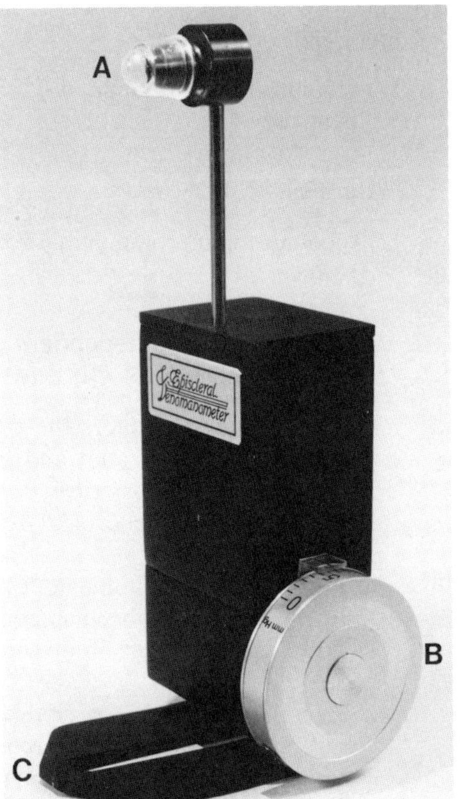


**Figure 1-1** The episcleral venomanometer based on the pressure chamber method. A, membrane; B, dial graduated in mmHg; C, footplate for mounting on the slit-lamp.

2. A torsion balance consisting of a transparent applanating window through which the vein is viewed and a force is applied to collapse the vein. A commercial device is available (Fig. 1-1).

## SUGGESTED READINGS

Kolker, AE, Hetherington J, Jr.: Becker-Shaffer's Diagnosis and Therapy of the Glaucomas. 5th Ed. CV Mosby, St. Louis, 1983.

Moses, R, Hart W: Adler's Physiology of the Eye. 8th Ed. CV Mosby, St. Louis, 1986.

Shields MB: Textbook of Glaucoma. 2nd Ed. Williams and Wilkins, Baltimore, 1986.

# 2

# Methods of Measuring Intraocular Pressure

## STERILIZATION OF OPHTHALMIC INSTRUMENTS

The spread of acquired immune deficiency syndrome (AIDS) has renewed the need for adequate sterilization of ophthalmic instruments including tonometers and gonioprisms. In fact, all devices that come into contact with the eye or tears, should not be reused prior to sterilization. Such devices include scleral depressors and ocular occluders. The Center for Infectious Diseases in Atlanta currently recommends the use of gloves during the ophthalmologic examination.

I. The Center for Infectious Diseases in Atlanta and the American Academy of Ophthalmology recommend the following methods for disinfection of office ophthalmic instruments:
   A. Wipe the tip or soak the instrument in 70% ethanol.
   B. Soak the instrument in 3% hydrogen peroxide.
   C. Soak the instrument in 0.5% sodium hypochlorite (diluted household bleach).

II. Ethanol wiping with air drying or soaking for 5–10 min with the other agents produces effective viral deactivation.

III. Care must be taken to rinse the disinfectant completely from the instrument to prevent possible injury to the cornea.

## INTRAOCULAR PRESSURE MEASUREMENT

The techniques available for clinical measurement of intraocular pressure depend on altering the eye in a predictable manner and measuring the results of that alteration. The two basic types of tonometry, applanation and indentation, differ in the shape of the deformation they induce on the globe.

## APPLANATION TONOMETRY

I. Performed either by flattening the cornea to a predetermined area and measuring the required applanating force or by using a constant applanating force to flatten the cornea to a variable area.

II. Theoretical basis is the Imbert-Fick principle (Fig. 2-1). For a dry, perfectly flexible sphere, the pressure within the sphere is equal to the force necessary to flatten (or applanate) a region of the surface, divided by the flattened area.

   If $P$ = the pressure within the sphere after applanation, $F$ = the applanating force, and $A$ = the area of flattening, then $P = F/A$

III. The eye has properties that alter the validity of the Imbert-Fick principle.
   A. The eye is not a perfect sphere.
   B. The cornea is not infinitely thin.
   C. The eye is not perfectly dry: capil-

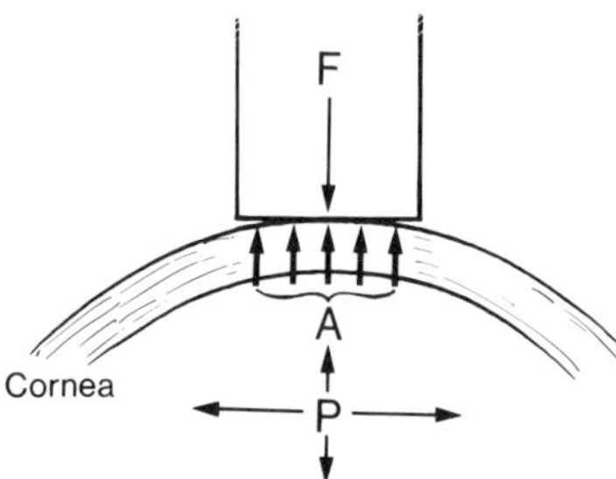


**Fig. 2-1** Imbert-Fick law: F = P × A or P = F/A where F = applanating force; P = the pressure within the eye after applanation; A = the area of corneal flattening.

lary attraction of the tear film adds to the applanating force.

D. The eye is not perfectly flexible: corneal resistance to flattening opposes the applanating force.

IV. If the applanated area has a diameter of 3–4 mm, the additive forces relating to capillary attraction and the subtractive forces due to the resistance of the cornea to flattening approximately cancel each other and can be eliminated.

## Goldmann Applanation Tonometer (Fig. 2-2)

### Description of Mechanism

I. The diameter of the external area of applanation is 3.06 mm. With the use of this diameter, the applanation force applied to the eye (the reading on the dial) times 10 equals the intraocular pressure in mmHg.

II. The degree of corneal flattening results in minimal displacement of aqueous humor, so that the resulting ocular pressure after applying the tonometer is insignificantly different from the resting intraocular pressure (approximately 0.5 g applied to the eye).

III. The use of topical fluorescein allows visualization of the tear film around the applanating head, which contains an image-splitting prism (biprism) and, therefore, allows for accurate adjustment of the applanating force.

### Technique

Steps 1. Topical anesthetic is instilled and fluorescein applied to the eye either as a fluorescein-impregnated paper strip or as a solution. Fluress, a commercial solution containing an anesthetic (0.4% benoxinate), 0.25% fluorescein, and a preservative to prevent bacterial contamination, especially the bacteria *Pseudomonas*, can be used. Failure to use fluorescein results in a significant underestimation of the intraocular pressure. Excessive fluorescein may result in overestimation of the intraocular pressure.

2. The adjustment knob is set at 10 mmHg (a scale reading of 1.0) or higher and the biprism is brought into contact with the cornea.

3. The fluorescent semicircles are viewed through the biprism attached to the slit-lamp (Fig. 2-3).
   a. The semicircles are adjusted using the slit-lamp so that they are horizontally centered in the prism.
   b. The semicircles are adjusted using the slit-lamp so that they are vertically aligned until each semicircle is of the same size.
   c. The prism is rotated from the horizontal position if the semicircles are elliptical, indicating marked corneal astigmatism, so the red axis mark on the biprism is 45 degrees between the major axes of the corneal astigmatism. For example, if corneal astigmatism is 4 diopters at 175 degrees, the red axis mark is placed at 130 degrees midway between 175 degrees and 85 degrees.
   d. The knob is rotated so that the inner edges of the two semicircles overlap (Fig. 2-3).
      1. Overlapping semicircles indicate excess applanating force (knob reading too high).
      2. Separated semicircles indicate insufficient applanating force (knob reading too low).
   e. The influence of ocular pulsations are observed when the instrument is

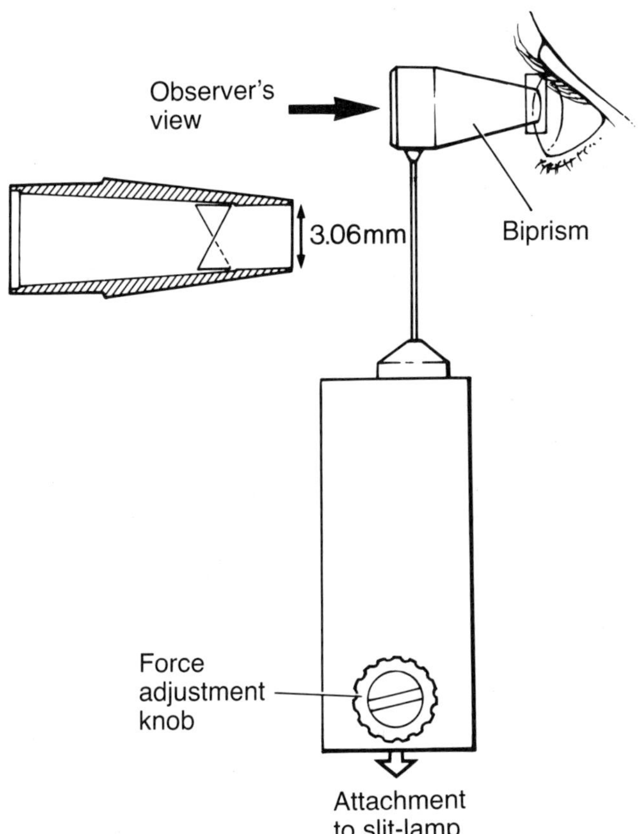


**Fig. 2-2** Goldmann applanation tonometer and prism.

properly positioned and the excursions are averaged to provide the desired endpoint.

**Sources of Error**

I. Meniscus width (amount of applied fluorescein): too wide a meniscus may cause false high readings.
II. Improper vertical alignment will lead to false high readings.
III. A high degree of corneal curvature will result in elevated pressure readings: 1 mmHg increase for each 3 diopters of increased corneal power.
IV. Corneal thickness affects the pressure readings: thin corneas give a false low reading and thick corneas a false high reading.
V. An irregular cornea will distort the applanation mires and interfere with the accuracy of the reading.
VI. Corneal edema results in irregular mires and a false low pressure reading.
VII. Corneal epithelial defects with fluorescein staining result in poor applanation mires and a poor pressure reading.
VIII. External pressure on the globe, either squeezing by the patient or pressure by the examiner, results in a false high pressure reading.
IX. Valsalva maneuver or compression of the jugular veins will increase epis-

cleral venous pressure and result in a high intraocular pressure.

## Complications

I. Corneal abrasion
II. Allergy to the topical anesthetics or to fluorescein
III. Transfer of bacterial or viral contamination. Cleaning the prism as described above is effective in destroying most infectious agents including deactivation of HTLV-III virus associated with AIDS.

## Tonometer Check (Fig. 2-4)

Steps 1. Force adjustment of the tonometer should be checked monthly.
2. The balance bar provided with the instrument is clipped over the main pivot on the body of the instrument.
3. The force adjustment knob is set to zero.
4. The bar is decentered to index at one of the black lines, which results in movement of the prism arm backward.
5. The adjustment knob is rotated until the prism moves
   a. At a scale reading of 2 (or 20 mmHg) if the bar is decentered to the first black line.
   b. At a scale reading of 6 (or 60 mmHg) if the bar is decentered to the black line near the end of the bar.
6. The force adjustment is performed for both marks on the bar.
7. The zero force-applied position is checked by rotating the adjustment knob (without the balance bar) to zero, which should result in free movement of the prism arm.
8. The check of the tonometer ensures proper calibration of the force adjustment mechanism. An inaccurate instru-

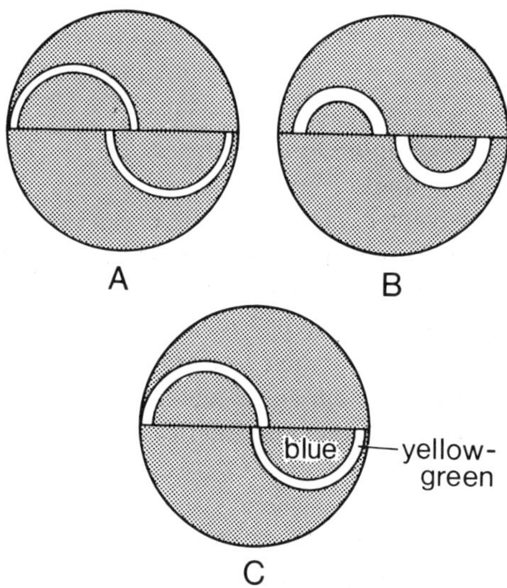


**Fig. 2-3** Goldmann applanation semicircles. **(A)** Excess applanating force: pressure reading too high. **(B)** Insufficient applanating force; pressure reading too low. **(C)** Proper endpoint: overlapping of inner edges.

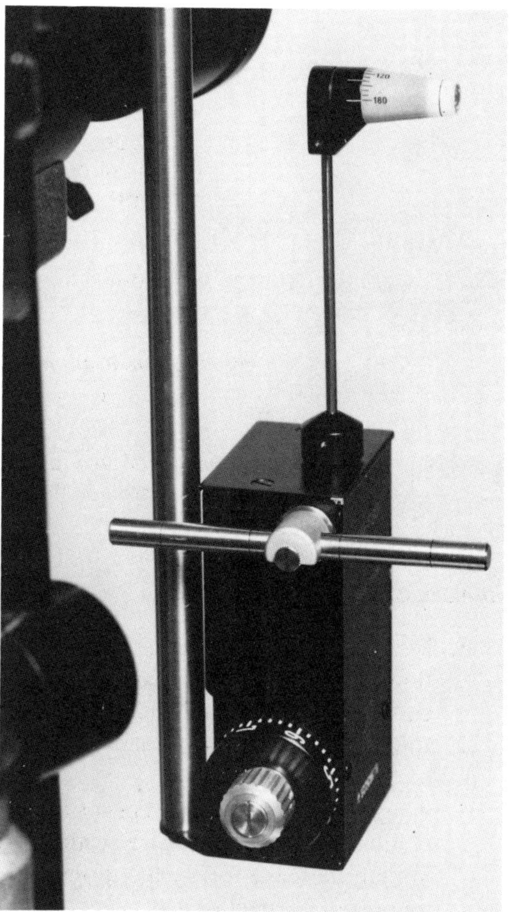

**Fig. 2-4** Goldmann applanation tonometer with balancebar attached to check instrument force adjustment.

ment must be returned to the manufacturer for adjustment.

## Other Applanation Tonometers

### Hand-Held Goldmann-Type Tonometers

Portable units are available that allow accurate measurement of the intraocular pressure without requiring a slit-lamp. These instruments have a counterbalanced prism-arm that permits one to use the instrument in the vertical and horizontal position. These instruments are ideal for operating room measurement of intraocular pressure in patients with congenital glaucoma.

#### Perkins Applanation Tonometer (Fig. 2-5)

I. Utilizes the same biprism as the Goldman instrument.
II. Battery-powered light source with a cobalt blue filter.
III. Applanation force is varied manually via a rotating dial.

#### Draeger Applanation Tonometer

I. Utilizes a specialized prism that maintains the Goldmann 3.06 mm applanating diameter.
II. Electrically powered light source.
III. Applanation force is varied by an electric motor connected to the prism-arm via a rotating switch.

### Mackay-Marg Tonometer

I. Probe tip consists of a hollow probe with an inner 1.5 mm diameter movable plunger.
II. The probe is brought into contact with the anesthetized cornea and flattens the cornea.
III. The force required to align the flat-plate of the plunger flush with the surrounding probe is recorded.
IV. The recording (Fig. 2-6) represents the pressure required to bend the cornea so that the plunger is flush with the probe.
V. The instrument is a combined applanation and indentation tonometer.
VI. The instrument tends to overestimate the actual intraocular pressure.
VII. Accurate intraocular pressure measurements are obtained with this instrument in eyes with corneal edema.

### Pneumatonometer (Fig. 2-7)

I. The pneumatonometer, which is more of an applanation device than the Mackay-Marg tonometer, has an air-pressure-sensitive probe that contacts the cornea.
II. The sensing tip has an outer diameter of 0.25 inches and is covered by a plastic diaphragm with pressurized air filling the central chamber and the diaphragm.
III. The tip is applied to an anesthetized cornea and force is applied to bend the cornea.
IV. The force required to deflect the cornea is converted by a transducer to a pressure reading.
V. Intraocular pressure is a combined applanation and indentation measurement.
VI. Each instrument and probe requires a calibration check against Goldmann applanation readings, since probes and transducers vary. The intraocular pressure tends to be higher with the pneumatonometer than with Goldmann applanation tonometry.

## Noncontact Tonometer

### Theory of Measurement

I. Intraocular pressure is measured without direct contact to the eye.
II. A puff of room air is directed to the cornea and momentarily deforms (flattens) the cornea.
III. The time from an internal reference point to the moment of presumed corneal flattening is measured and con-

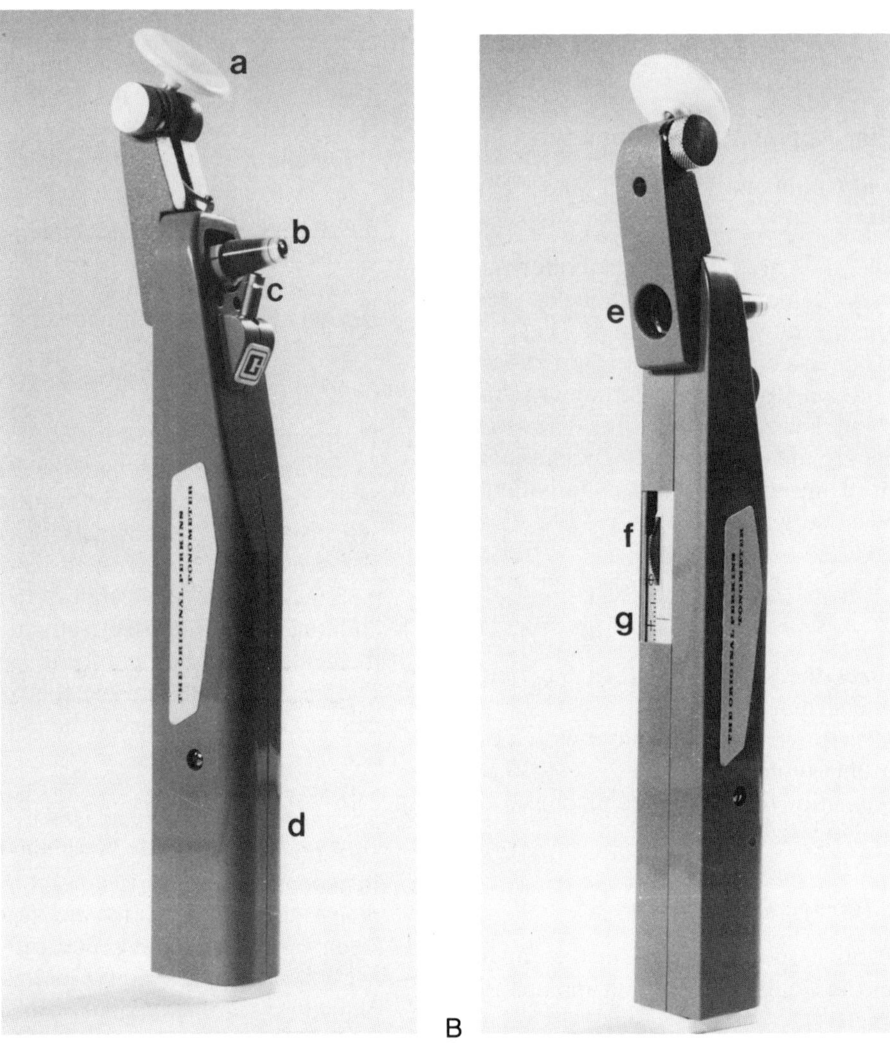


**Fig. 2-5** Perkins applanation tonometer: **(A)** Front view withh forehead support bracket (a), biprism (b), and light source (c). Batteries are housed in the base of the instrument (d). **(B)** Rear view with observing port (e), adjustment knob (f), and intraocular pressure scale (g).

verted to an internally calibrated intraocular pressure.

## Technique

Steps
1. The cornea is aligned by superimposing a reflected target on a stationary ring within the viewing system.
2. A trigger releases a puff of air directed at the cornea, which induces flattening and an increase in the reflected light which is recorded.
3. A digital readout converts the moment of maximum light detection to intraocular pressure.
4. A minimum of three readings is taken to average for the effect of the ocular pulse.
5. Topical anesthesia is recommended since the air puff can be uncomfortable.
6. Repeat readings should be within 3 mmHg to ensure an accurate pressure estimate.
7. Intraocular pressure tends to be higher than Goldmann applanation readings.

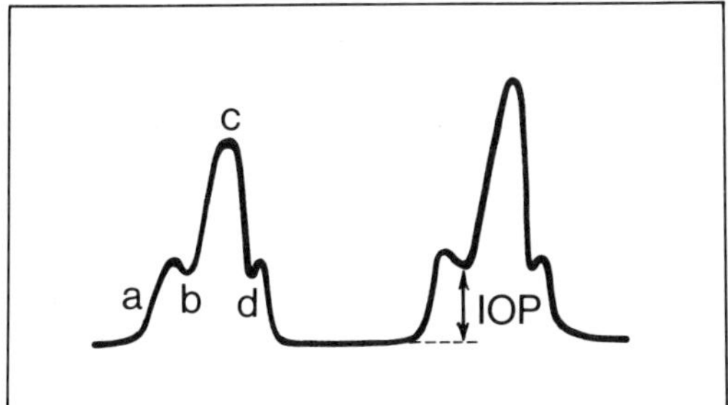


**Fig. 2-6** Mackay-Marg tonographic tracing. (a) Increasing tracing as plate contacts and begins to indent the cornea. (b) Diameter of contact equals the diameter of the footplate surface with the corneal bend transferred to the footplate. (c) Additional corneal flattening results in artificial increase in intraocular pressure. (d) Point of equal corneal–footplate contact as the probe is removed. Point d is lower than point b due to expression of aqueous humor by the instrument, which lowers intraocular pressure (IOP). The area within the arrow is the IOP.

## Constant Weight Applanation Tonometry

Intraocular pressure is measured by applying a known weight to the cornea and measuring the area of corneal flattening. Since the area of flattening depends upon the intraocular pressure, resistance to flattening and the capillary attraction of the tear film are important factors. The original concept was introduced by Maklakov in 1885 and several variable area tonometers are available with the technique very popular in some European countries. However, measurement of the applanated area may be cumbersome.

### Maklakov Tonometer (Fig. 2-8)

Instrument

I. It consists of a dumbell-shaped metal cylinder with polished glass flat endplates with a diameter of 10 mm.
II. The instrument has a set of weights: 5, 7.5, 10, or 15 g.
III. The instrument is supported by a cross-action wire holder.

Technique

Steps 1. Dye (suspension of argyrol, glycerin, and water) is applied to footplate.
2. The instrument is placed in a vertical position on the anesthetized cornea for 1 sec.
3. A circular white imprint is created on the endplate, which corresponds to the area of corneal flattening.
4. A transparent plastic scale (0.1 mm divisions) is used to measure the white area. The area is converted to intraocular pressure from a table, according to the weight used.
5. Conversion tables are available to compensate for scleral rigidity.

## INDENTATION (SCHIOTZ) TONOMETRY

This technique applies a known weight to the cornea, causing a variable indentation that is proportional to the intraocular pressure.

### Schiotz Tonometer (Fig. 2-9)

I. Instrument has a body with a handle and numerical scale.
II. A footplate with a movable plunger comes into contact with the anesthetized cornea.
III. The degree to which the plunger indents the cornea is indicated by movement of the needle on the scale.
IV. A 5.5 g weight is permanently fixed to the plunger.
V. Additional weights (7.5, 10, or 15 g) can be added to the plunger to increase the weight of the indentation.

### Basic Concept (Fig. 2-10)

I. The plunger indents the cornea resulting in an artificial elevation of the baseline intraocular pressure (Po) to a new value (Pt).
II. Pt with the Schiotz tonometer often is very much higher than Po (See Appendix, Table 2A-1), meaning that large cor-

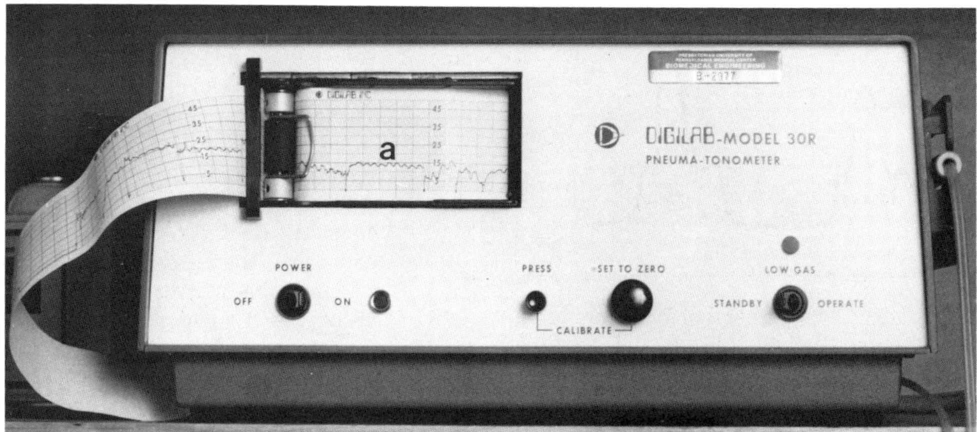


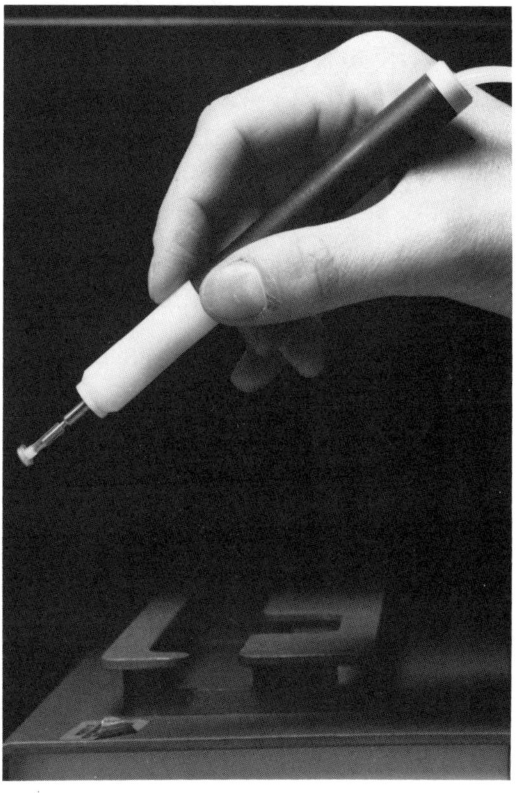


**Figure 2-7** Pneumatonometer. (**A**) Instrument with patient tracings indicating a pressure of 14 mmHg (a). (**B**) Probe tip.

rections are required in calibration curves for intraocular pressure.

III. One of the main advantages of applanation tonometry is the small displacement of aqueous so that Pt is only approximately 3% greater than Po.

IV. Po is estimated from calibration tables obtained from experiments on enucleated eyes in which the intraocular pressure was set and the Schiotz value (scale reading and weight) determined.

## Friedenwald Calibration Tables

I. The change between Po and Pt relates to the resistance of the eye to displacement of a volume of fluid.

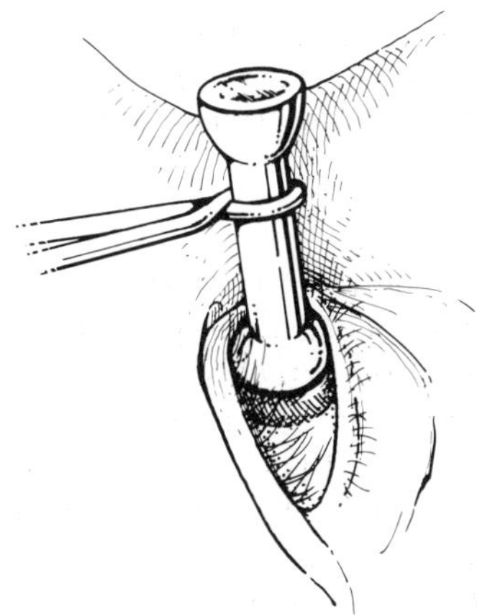

**Fig. 2-8** Maklakov-type tonometer.

II. The relationship between pressure and the volume change can be expressed as a numerical constant, the coefficient of ocular rigidity. Ocular rigidity is an expression of the distensibility of the eye.

III. The Friedenwald nomogram for estimating the coefficient of ocular rigidity is based on two tonometric readings with different Schiotz weights (See Appendix, Figs. 2A-1, 2A-3, 2A-4.)

IV. The coefficient of ocular rigidity can also be estimated from the difference between applanation and Schiotz indentation pressure readings (See Appendix, Figs. 2A-1, 2A-2.)

V. The 1948 tables for conversion of a Schiotz scale reading to intraocular pressure are based on an average ocular rigidity of 0.0245.

VI. The 1955 tables for conversion of a Schiotz scale reading to introcular pressure are revised for a mean coefficient of ocular rigidity of 0.0215.

VII. While the 1955 tables are currently used (See Appendix, Table 2A-2), the 1948 tables may more closely agree with Goldmann applanation measurements.

VIII. Both the 1948 and 1955 tables are based on a mean coefficient of ocular rigidity and not the individual patient's value.

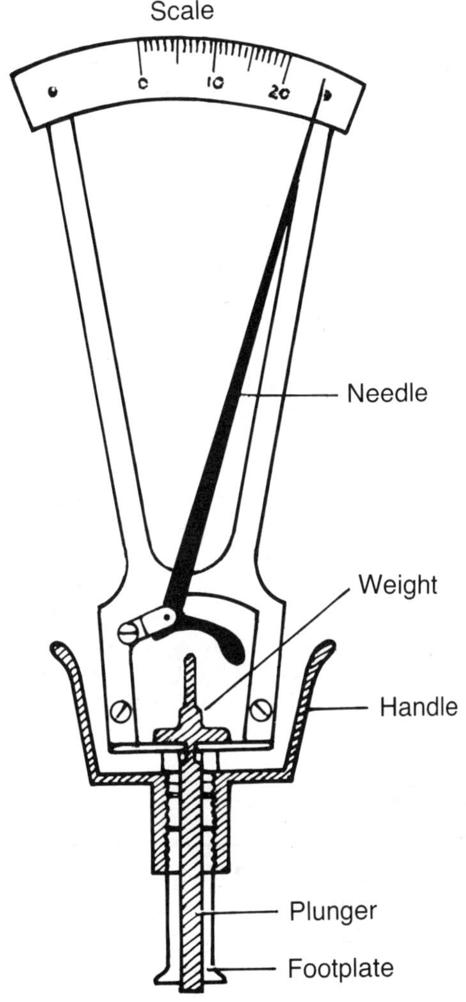


**Fig. 2-9** Schiotz tonometer. The weight either snaps or screws onto the footplate bar. Additional weights are added as needed.

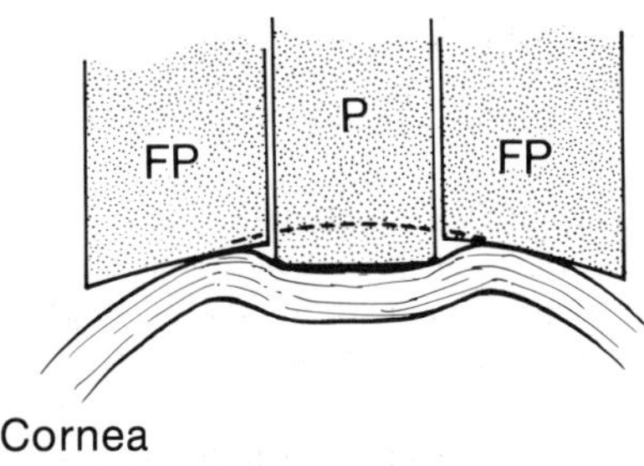


**Fig. 2-10** Schiotz tonometer footplate (FP) with the plunger (P) indenting the cornea.

### Technique

Steps
1. The patient is placed in a supine position and instructed to fixate on an overhead target with the eye not undergoing measurement.
2. The eyelids are gently separated without pressure applied on the globe.
3. The footplate of the tonometer with the 5.5 g weight is placed on the anesthetized cornea.
4. Proper vertical positioning of the instrument allows free movement of the plunger and the indicator needle in response to ocular pulsations.
5. If the scale reading is 4.0 or less, additional weights are added to the tonometer so that the measured scale reading is in a more accurate area of the calibration curve.
6. The scale reading and weight used are recorded (e.g., 5.5 scale/7.5 g). The intraocular pressure is obtained from the conversion tables (e.g., 23.8 mmHg) (1955 table) (see Appendix Table 2A-2).

### Cleaning the Tonometer

I. The tonometer must be disassembled and cleaned after each use.

II. The weight is either unsnapped or unscrewed from the plunger, which is removed.

III. The plunger and barrel are rinsed with distilled water and wiped dry with a lint-free tissue and the instrument is reassembled. Sterilization is performed as described above.

### Tonometer Check

Steps
1. The zero-check disc is placed on a flat surface.
2. The clean tonometer with the 5.5 g weight is placed perpendicular on the metal disc, with the entire weight of the instrument resting on the disc without any support by the handle.
3. The scale reading should be zero.
4. Repeat checks with the other Schiotz weights should also be zero.
5. An instrument that does not read a zero scale during this check must be returned to the manufacturer for repair.

### Sources of Error

I. Patient variation from the average coefficient of ocular rigidity used to generate the conversion tables will result in an incorrect intraocular pressure.

A. A higher than "average" rigidity results in a false low intraocular pressure reading.

B. Rigidity may be increased
1. in high hyperopia.
2. with long-standing glaucoma.
3. with vasoconstrictors.

C. A lower than "average" rigidity will result in a false low intraocular pressure.

D. Rigidity may be decreased
1. in myopia.
2. during a water provocative test.
3. by miotics, especially cholinesterase inhibitors.
4. following ocular surgery including retinal detachment repair and cataract removal.

II. A steeper or thicker than normal cornea will result in a greater displacement of fluid and a falsely low intraocular pressure.

## STATISTICAL CONSIDERATIONS OF INTRAOCULAR PRESSURE

### Normal Population

I. Mean intraocular pressure is 15.4 mmHg with a standard deviation of 2.5 mmHg.

II. Distribution in the population is non-Gaussian, with a skew towards higher pressure levels.

III. Despite these statistics, two standard deviations are often used to estimate upper limits of normal, and frequently 21 mmHg is considered the division between normal and elevated intraocular pressure.

IV. Mean intraocular pressure rises with increasing age, the mean approaching 22 to 23 mmHg by the sixth decade.

V. Intraocular pressure is slightly higher in women than men, particularly after menopause.

VI. Intraocular pressure tends to be symmetrical between the two eyes (within 2 mmHg).

VII. Intraocular pressure has a significant diurnal variation, with the maximum intraocular pressure occurring in the early morning hours. However, the time of this peak may vary widely in any given patient. Diurnal fluctuation is exaggerated in patients with glaucoma.

VIII. Intraocular pressure may follow a seasonal variation, with higher pressures occurring in the winter months and lower pressures in the summer months.

## Factors Affecting Intraocular Pressure

I. Acutely or chronically elevated episcleral venous pressure is reflected in the intraocular pressure: a tight collar, a Valsalva maneuver, change in body position from the erect to the horizontal position, elevated central venous pressure, or elevated ophthalmic vein pressure will increase intraocular pressure.

II. External pressure on the eye, including patient squeezing, increases intraocular pressure.

III. Acute and prolonged periods of physical exercise may reduce aqueous humor production and intraocular pressure.

IV. Elevated body temperature may be associated with an increase in aqueous humor production and increased intraocular pressure.

V. General anesthesia is usually associated with a reduction in aqueous production and reduced intraocular pressure.

VI. Ketamine dissociative anesthesia may cause an increase in intraocular pressure.

VII. Depolarizing muscle relaxants (e.g., succinylcholine and suxamethonium) cause a transient rise in intraocular pressure due to contraction of extraocular muscles.

VIII. Systemic acidosis, either metabolic or respiratory, results in reduced aqueous humor production and decreased intraocular pressure.

IX. A number of hormonal influences can affect intraocular pressure.
   A. Intraocular pressure decreases at the time of ovulation and is lower during pregnancy.
   B. Intraocular pressure may be higher in patients with hypothyroidism and lower in patients with hyperthyroidism.
   C. Thyroid exophthalmos and limitation of upward gaze may result in marked elevation in intraocular pressure upon attempted upward gaze.

X. A number of drugs, excluding antiglaucoma therapy, alter intraocular pressure.
   A. Alcohol lowers intraocular pressure.
   B. Heroin and marijuana may lower intraocular pressure.
   C. LSD increases intraocular pressure.
   D. Corticosteroids, topical or systemic, can elevate intraocular pressure in susceptible patients (see Ch. 7).
   E. A number of cholinergic drugs can elevate intraocular pressure by dilating the pupil and precipitating acute closed-angle glaucoma in susceptible patients.

## SUGGESTED READINGS

Kolker, AE, Hetherington J, Jr: Becker-Shaffer's Diagnosis and Therapy of the Glaucomas. 5th Ed. C V Mosby, St. Louis, 1983

Moses R, Hart W: Adler's Physiology of the Eye. 8th Ed. C V Mosby, St. Louis, 1986

Shields MB: Textbook of Glaucoma. 2nd Ed. Williams & Wilkins, Baltimore, 1986

Recommendations for preventing possible transmission of human T-lymphocyic virus type III/lymphadenopathy-associated virus from tears. MMWR 34:533, 1985

Van Buskirk EM: Disinfectant receptacle for applanation tonometers. Am J Ophthalmol 104: 307, 1987

# Appendix

Friedenwald nomogram for estimation of true intraocular pressure and scleral rigidity (Fig. 2A-1).

I. Tonometry is performed with two different weights of the Schiotz tonometer or with both the applanation and the Schiotz tonometers.

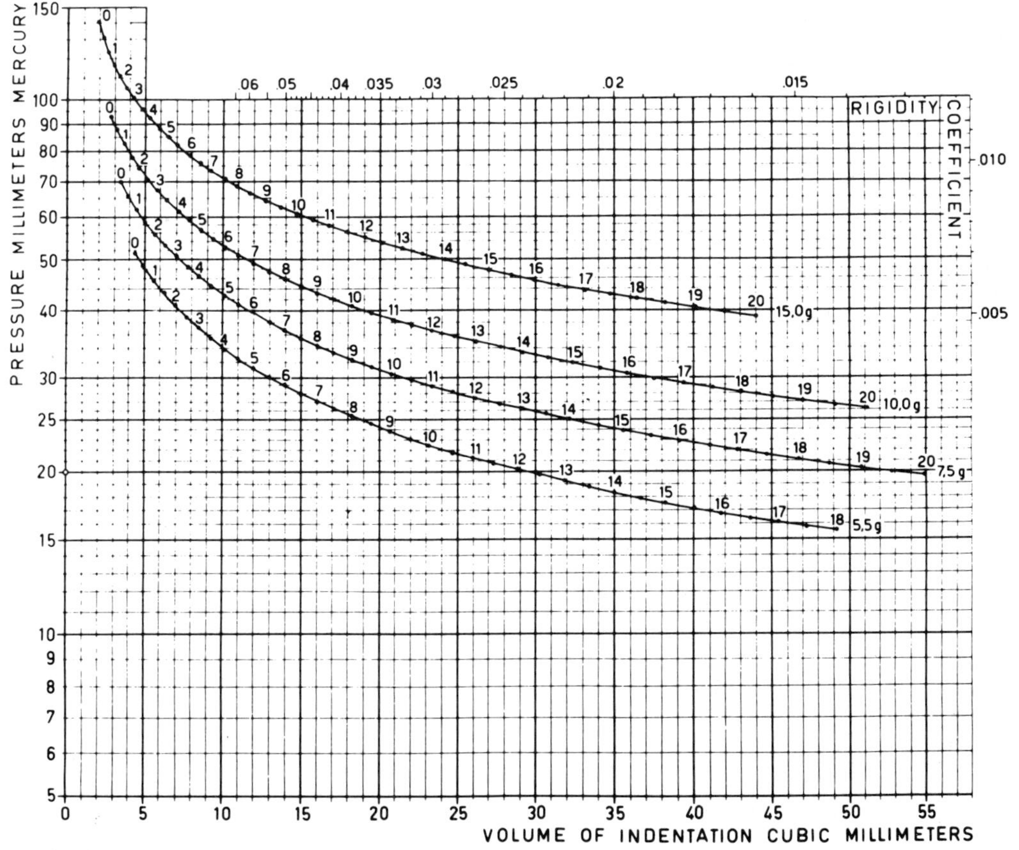


Fig. 2A-1

II. These results are plotted on the nomogram: the applanation pressure is plotted at a 0.5 volume of indentation and the Schiotz scale reading for a given weight on the appropriately labeled curved line.

III. By drawing a line through these two points, the true intraocular pressure is determined by the intercept of the line on the Y axis (pressure mmHg).

IV. To determine scleral rigidity, a second line is drawn through "20" on the pressure scale, parallel to the line determined in step 3. Scleral rigidity is read where the second line crosses the top or upper right margins of the nomogram.

**Examples using the Friedenwald nomogram.**

I. Line A connects the points representing an applanation pressure of 24 mmHg and a Schiotz scale reading of 5 with the 7.5 g weight. Line A crosses the Y axis at 23 mmHg, the true intraocular pressure. Line B, which is parallel to Line A and drawn through "20" on the Y axis, crosses the top of the nomogram at 0.026, the scleral rigidity determination (Fig. 2A-2A).

II. Line A connects the points representing a Schiotz scale reading of 3.5 with the 5.5 g weight (a pressure of 22.4 mmHg, see Table 2A-2) and a Schiotz scale reading of 9.5 with the 10.0 g weight (a pressure of 18.0 mmHg, Table 2A-2). Line A crosses the Y axis at 27 mmHg, the true intraocular pressure, which is higher than the Schiotz scale conversions from Table 2A-2. Line B, which is parallel to Line A and drawn through "20" on the Y axis, crosses the top of the nomogram at approximately 0.012, the scleral rigidity determination, which is an extremely low value (Fig. 2A-2B).

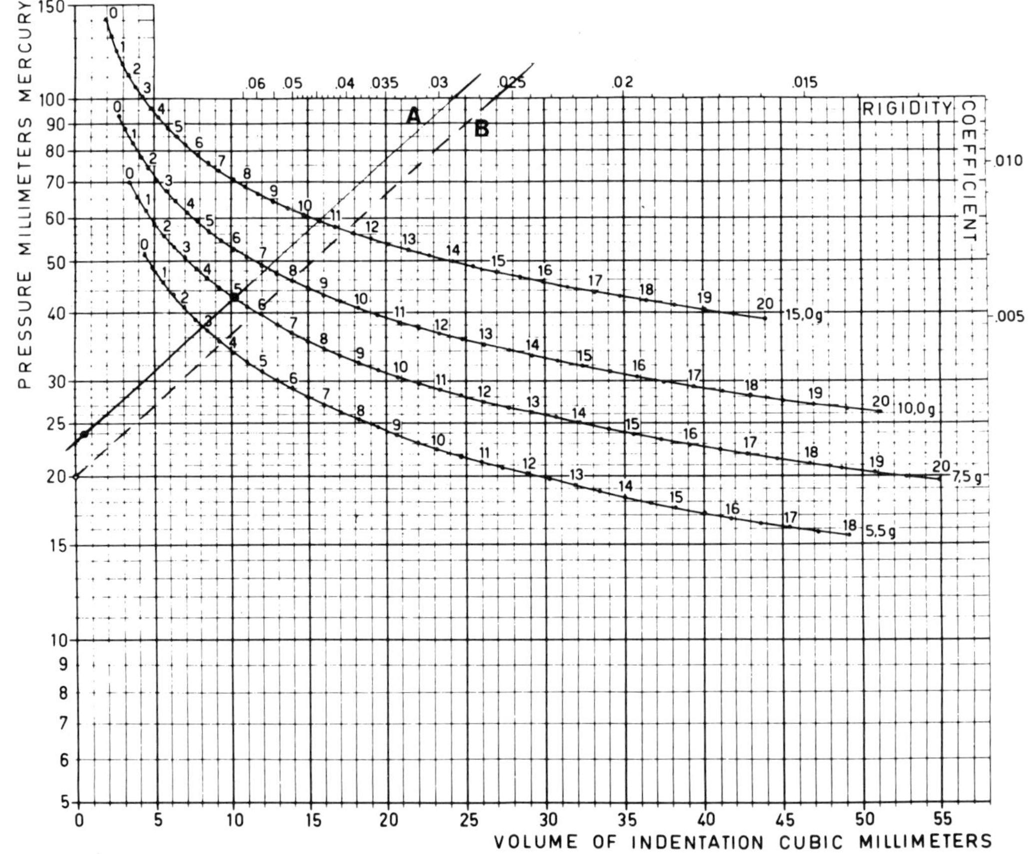


Fig. 2A-2(A)

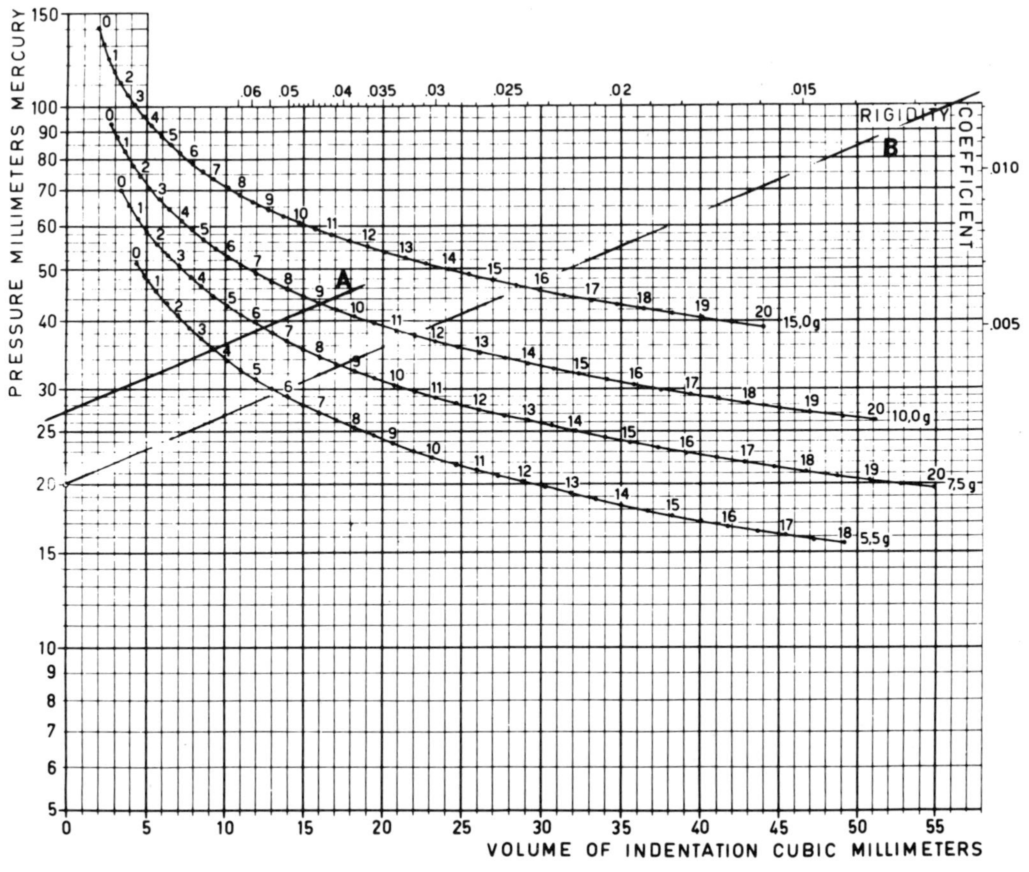
FRIEDENWALD 1955 NOMOGRAM FOR SCHIOTZ TONOMETER
PRESSURE MILLIMETERS MERCURY
VOLUME OF INDENTATION CUBIC MILLIMETERS
RIGIDITY COEFFICIENT
15,0 g
10,0 g
7,5 g
5,5 g
A
B
.06 .05 .04 .035 .03 .025 .02 .015
.010
.005

**Fig. 2A-2(B)**

**Table 2A-1.** Intraocular Pressure during Schiotz Tonometry

| | Plunger Load | | | |
|---|---|---|---|---|
| Scale Reading | 5.5 g | 7.5 g | 10 g | 15 g |
| 3.0 | 37.1 | 50.5 | 67.4 | 101.1 |
| 3.5 | 35.4 | 48.3 | 64.6 | 96.6 |
| 4.0 | 33.9 | 46.2 | 61.7 | 92.5 |
| 4.5 | 32.5 | 44.4 | 59.1 | 88.7 |
| 5.0 | 31.5 | 42.6 | 56.8 | 85.2 |
| 5.5 | 30.1 | 41.0 | 54.7 | 82.0 |
| 6.0 | 29.0 | 39.5 | 52.7 | 79.0 |
| 6.5 | 28.0 | 38.1 | 50.8 | 76.3 |
| 7.0 | 27.0 | 36.8 | 49.1 | 73.7 |
| 7.5 | 26.1 | 35.6 | 47.5 | 71.3 |
| 8.0 | 25.3 | 34.5 | 46.0 | 69.0 |
| 8.5 | 24.5 | 33.4 | 44.6 | 66.9 |
| 9.0 | 23.8 | 32.4 | 43.3 | 64.9 |
| 9.5 | 23.1 | 31.5 | 42.0 | 63.0 |
| 10.0 | 22.5 | 30.6 | 40.8 | 61.2 |
| 10.5 | 21.8 | 29.8 | 39.7 | 59.6 |
| 11.0 | 21.3 | 29.0 | 38.6 | 58.0 |
| 11.5 | 20.7 | 28.2 | 37.6 | 56.5 |
| 12.0 | 20.2 | 27.5 | 36.7 | 55.0 |
| 12.5 | 19.7 | 26.8 | 35.8 | 53.7 |
| 13.0 | 19.2 | 26.2 | 34.9 | 52.4 |
| 13.5 | 18.8 | 25.6 | 34.1 | 51.1 |
| 14.0 | 18.3 | 25.0 | 33.3 | 50.0 |
| 14.5 | 17.9 | 24.4 | 32.6 | 48.8 |
| 15.0 | 17.5 | 23.9 | 31.9 | 47.8 |

**Table 2A-2.** 1955 Calibration Scale for the Schiotz Tonometer

| | Plunger Load | | | |
|---|---|---|---|---|
| Scale Reading | 5.5 g | 7.5 g | 10 g | 15 g |
| 3.0 | 24.4 | 35.8 | 50.6 | 81.8 |
| 3.5 | 22.4 | 33.0 | 46.9 | 76.2 |
| 4.0 | 20.6 | 30.4 | 43.4 | 71.0 |
| 4.5 | 18.9 | 28.0 | 40.2 | 66.2 |
| 5.0 | 17.3 | 25.8 | 37.2 | 61.8 |
| 5.5 | 15.9 | 23.8 | 34.4 | 57.6 |
| 6.0 | 14.6 | 21.9 | 31.8 | 53.6 |
| 6.5 | 13.4 | 20.1 | 29.4 | 49.9 |
| 7.0 | 12.2 | 18.5 | 27.2 | 46.5 |
| 7.5 | 11.2 | 17.0 | 25.1 | 43.2 |
| 8.0 | 10.2 | 15.6 | 23.1 | 40.2 |
| 8.5 | 9.4 | 14.3 | 21.3 | 38.1 |
| 9.0 | 8.5 | 13.1 | 19.6 | 34.6 |
| 9.5 | 7.8 | 12.0 | 18.0 | 32.0 |
| 10.0 | 7.1 | 10.9 | 16.5 | 29.6 |

| Reading with 5.5-g weight | Reading with 10.0-g weight | | | | | | | | | | | | | | | | | | |
|---|---|---|---|---|---|---|---|---|---|---|---|---|---|---|---|---|---|---|---|
| | 6.0 | 6.5 | 7.0 | 7.5 | 8.0 | 8.5 | 9.0 | 9.5 | 10.0 | 10.5 | 11.0 | 11.5 | 12.0 | 12.5 | 13.0 | 13.5 | 14.0 | 14.5 | 15.0 |
| 3.0 | .0904 | .0536 | .0353 | .0244 | .0173 | .0124 | .0088 | .0063 | .0049 | .0027 | .0015 | | | | | | | | |
| | 6 | 13 | 19 | 23 | 26 | 29 | 31 | 33 | 34 | 35 | 36 | | | | | | | | |
| 3.5 | | .0877 | .0526 | .0350 | .0244 | .0176 | .0127 | .0094 | .0068 | .0048 | .0033 | .0021 | .0011 | | | | | | |
| | | 7 | 12 | 17 | 21 | 24 | 27 | 29 | 31 | 32 | 33 | 34 | 35 | | | | | | |
| 4.0 | | | .0870 | .0523 | .0349 | .0245 | .0177 | .0132 | .0098 | .0073 | .0053 | .0038 | .0026 | .0016 | | | | | |
| | | | 5 | 10 | 15 | 19 | 22 | 25 | 27 | 29 | 30 | 31 | 32 | 33 | | | | | |
| 4.5 | | | | | .0517 | .0346 | .0244 | .0180 | .0135 | .0102 | .0076 | .0057 | .0042 | .0030 | .0020 | .0012 | | | |
| | | | | | 9 | 14 | 18 | 21 | 23 | 25 | 27 | 28 | 29 | 30 | 31 | 32 | | | |
| 5.0 | | | | | | .0511 | .0342 | .0246 | .0182 | .0137 | .0104 | .0080 | .0061 | .0046 | .0034 | .0024 | .0016 | | |
| | | | | | | 8 | 12 | 16 | 19 | 21 | 24 | 25 | 26 | 28 | 29 | 29 | 30 | | |
| 5.5 | | | | | | | .0498 | .0341 | .0245 | .0182 | .0138 | .0106 | .0082 | .0063 | .0049 | .0037 | .0027 | .0019 | .0013 |
| | | | | | | | 7 | 11 | 15 | 18 | 20 | 22 | 24 | 25 | 26 | 27 | 28 | 28 | 29 |
| 6.0 | | | | | | | | .0493 | .0336 | .0242 | .0181 | .0139 | .0107 | .0084 | .0066 | .0051 | .0039 | .0030 | .0022 |
| | | | | | | | | 6 | 10 | 13 | 16 | 19 | 21 | 22 | 24 | 25 | 26 | 26 | 27 |
| 6.5 | | | | | | | | | .0486 | .0332 | .0240 | .0181 | .0139 | .0109 | .0085 | .0067 | .0053 | .0042 | .0032 |
| | | | | | | | | | 5 | 9 | 12 | 15 | 17 | 19 | 21 | 22 | 23 | 24 | 25 |
| 7.0 | | | | | | | | | | .0475 | .0325 | .0237 | .0179 | .0139 | .0109 | .0086 | .0069 | .0055 | .0044 |
| | | | | | | | | | | 5 | 8 | 11 | 14 | 16 | 18 | 20 | 21 | 22 | 23 |
| 7.5 | | | | | | | | | | | | .0320 | .0233 | .0178 | .0138 | .0109 | .0086 | .0070 | .0056 |
| | | | | | | | | | | | | 7 | 10 | 13 | 15 | 17 | 19 | 20 | 21 |
| 8.0 | | | | | | | | | | | | | .0313 | .0230 | .0176 | .0137 | .0109 | .0087 | .0071 |
| | | | | | | | | | | | | | 7 | 10 | 12 | 14 | 16 | 18 | 19 |
| 8.5 | | | | | | | | | | | | | | .0307 | .0226 | .0173 | .0136 | .0108 | .0088 |
| | | | | | | | | | | | | | | 6 | 9 | 11 | 13 | 15 | 17 |
| 9.0 | | | | | | | | | | | | | | | .0300 | .0222 | .0171 | .0135 | .0108 |
| | | | | | | | | | | | | | | | 6 | 8 | 11 | 13 | 14 |

**Fig. 2A-3** Pressure and rigidity table for paired Schiotz readings with 5.5 g and 10 g weights.

| Reading with 7.5-g weight | Reading with 15.0-g weight | | | | | | | | | | | | | | | | | |
|---|---|---|---|---|---|---|---|---|---|---|---|---|---|---|---|---|---|---|
| | 6.5 | 7.0 | 7.5 | 8.0 | 8.5 | 9.0 | 9.5 | 10.0 | 10.5 | 11.0 | 11.5 | 12.0 | 12.5 | 13.0 | 13.5 | 14.0 | 14.5 | 15.0 |
| 3.0 | .1145 | .0705 | .0480 | .0343 | .0252 | .0189 | .0143 | .0108 | .0082 | .0061 | .0044 | .0031 | .0020 | .0011 | | | | |
| | 8 | 16 | 23 | 29 | 34 | 37 | 40 | 43 | 44 | 46 | 47 | 48 | 49 | 50 | | | | |
| 3.5 | | .1146 | .0707 | .0481 | .0345 | .0256 | .0194 | .0148 | .0114 | .0087 | .0067 | .0050 | .0037 | .0026 | .0016 | | | |
| | | 6 | 14 | 21 | 26 | 31 | 34 | 37 | 39 | 41 | 43 | 44 | 45 | 46 | 49 | | | |
| 4.0 | | | | .0710 | .0481 | .0347 | .0259 | .0197 | .0152 | .0118 | .0092 | .0071 | .0055 | .0041 | .0031 | .0021 | .0014 | |
| | | | | 12 | 18 | 24 | 28 | 32 | 34 | 37 | 39 | 40 | 42 | 43 | 44 | 44 | 45 | |
| 4.5 | | | | | .0705 | .0482 | .0347 | .0260 | .0199 | .0155 | .0122 | .0096 | .0075 | .0059 | .0046 | .0035 | .0026 | .0018 |
| | | | | | 10 | 16 | 21 | 25 | 29 | 32 | 34 | 36 | 38 | 39 | 40 | 41 | 42 | 43 |
| 5.0 | | | | | | .0705 | .0480 | .0347 | .0261 | .0201 | .0157 | .0124 | .0099 | .0079 | .0063 | .0049 | .0038 | .0029 |
| | | | | | | 8 | 14 | 19 | 23 | 27 | 30 | 32 | 34 | 35 | 37 | 38 | 39 | 40 |
| 5.5 | | | | | | | .0701 | .0475 | .0345 | .0260 | .0201 | .0159 | .0126 | .0101 | .0082 | .0065 | .0052 | .0042 |
| | | | | | | | 7 | 12 | 17 | 21 | 24 | 27 | 30 | 32 | 33 | 35 | 36 | 37 |
| 6.0 | | | | | | | | .0694 | .0472 | .0343 | .0259 | .0202 | .0160 | .0127 | .0102 | .0083 | .0068 | .0055 |
| | | | | | | | | 6 | 11 | 15 | 19 | 23 | 26 | 28 | 30 | 32 | 33 | 34 |
| 6.5 | | | | | | | | | | .0479 | .0346 | .0262 | .0204 | .0161 | .0130 | .0105 | .0086 | .0070 |
| | | | | | | | | | | 9 | 14 | 17 | 21 | 24 | 26 | 28 | 30 | 38 |
| 7.0 | | | | | | | | | | | .0462 | .0337 | .0257 | .0200 | .0160 | .0129 | .0105 | .0086 |
| | | | | | | | | | | | 8 | 13 | 16 | 19 | 22 | 24 | 26 | 25 |
| 7.5 | | | | | | | | | | | | .0458 | .0334 | .0254 | .0199 | .0159 | .0129 | .0109 |
| | | | | | | | | | | | | 7 | 11 | 15 | 18 | 21 | 23 | 21 |
| 8.0 | | | | | | | | | | | | | .0453 | .0330 | .0252 | .0198 | .0159 | .0126 |
| | | | | | | | | | | | | | 6 | 10 | 14 | 17 | 19 | 21 |
| 8.5 | | | | | | | | | | | | | | .0446 | .0326 | .0249 | .0196 | .0158 |
| | | | | | | | | | | | | | | 6 | 9 | 13 | 15 | 18 |
| 9.0 | | | | | | | | | | | | | | | .0440 | .0322 | .0248 | .0194 |
| | | | | | | | | | | | | | | | 5 | 8 | 12 | 14 |

**Fig. 2A-4** Pressure and rigidity table for paired Schiotz readings with 7.5 g and 15 g weights.

# 3

# Tonography

Tonography is a clinical technique used to measure aqueous humor outflow facility noninvasively. The clinical value of tonography in managing individual glaucoma patients is limited. When applied to population studies, however, the technique has provided much information about the underlying pathophysiology of glaucoma and the mechanism of action of antiglaucoma medications.

In 1949, Goldmann applied to the eye the mathematical work of Poiseuille for the flow of liquids in small-diameter rigid tubes. Poiseuille's law states that the velocity of flow of fluid in a rigid tube is equal to the pressure drop per length of the tube times the product of the tube radius to the fourth power times pi divided by eight times the coefficient of the fluid's viscosity.

The Goldmann relationship is expressed in the following equation:

$$F = (Po - Pv) \times C$$

where F = flow of aqueous humor in μl/min; Po = intraocular pressure in mmHg; Pv = episcleral venous pressure in mmHg; C = outflow facility in μl/min/mmHg (C = 1/R where R = outflow resistance).

## BASIS FOR TONOGRAPHY

I. Tonography is based on the observation that external pressure on the eye (either massage or the weight of a Schiotz tonometer), with time causes a lowering in intraocular pressure.

II. Tonography quantitates this effect by utilizing electronic techniques to measure intraocular pressure continuously and the subsequent decrease in intraocular pressure secondary to the weight of the Schiotz tonometer. However, tonography can also be performed by recording manually the change in scale readings over time using a handheld Schiotz tonometer.

## ESTIMATION OF OUTFLOW FACILITY

I. Tonography yields an estimation of outflow facility (a "C-value"), the total facility that consists of both true facility and pseudofacility.

II. Pseudofacility represents the decrease in ultrafiltration of aqueous humor arising from the intraocular pressure elevation induced by the weight of the tonometer.

III. True facility represents the flow of aqueous humor through the pressure-sensitive (trabecular pathways) and the pressure-insensitive (uveoscleral pathways) routes.

IV. Outflow facility is estimated by raising the intraocular pressure with the weight of the Schiotz tonometer and observing the subsequent decay curve in the intraocular pressure.

   A. Baseline intraocular pressure (Po) is increased to a new, higher level (Pt) secondary to the total weight of the tonometer (16.5 g with the 5.5 g weight).

B. The increased pressure results in an increased rate of aqueous outflow, which causes a change in aqueous volume.

C. Tables by Friedenwald relate the volume change to the Schiotz scale readings.

D. If we assume that the elevated pressure does not alter other ocular parameters (i.e., steady state is unchanged), the rate of volume decrease over time equals the rate of outflow.

V. Standard tonographic technique involves measuring the intraocular pressure for 4 min with the change in pressure during this time computed as a mean of pressure increments for successive half-minute intervals (mean Pt − Po).

VI. The C-value is derived from Grant's formula:

$$C = \text{change in volume} \div [\text{time} \times (\text{mean Pt} - \text{Po})]$$

## CLINICAL MEASUREMENT

### Instrumentation

I. Electronic tonometer (Fig. 3-1) is connected to a recorder.

II. To ensure minimal variation secondary to changes in line voltage, a voltage regulator should be incorporated in the set up.

III. The clean tonometer is calibrated daily for scale divisions and the calibration recording used for reading the tonography curve (Fig. 3-2).

### Technique

Steps 1. Applanation tonometry is performed before tonography to provide data for estimation of ocular rigidity and to determine the Schiotz weight to be used during tonography:

| Schiotz weight | Applanation pressure |
|---|---|
| 5.5 g | < 20 mmHg |
| 7.5 g | 20 to 29 mmHg |
| 10.0 g | > 30 mmHg |

2. The patient is comfortably positioned in the supine position on a stretcher in an isolated and quiet room. Topical anesthetic is instilled into the eye.
3. The nontested eye fixates on an overhead target.
4. The tonometer is held over the eye to be tested with gentle separation of the eyelids to expose the globe without pressure on the eye. The tonometer's footplate is placed perpendicularly on the cornea with the full weight of the instrument resting on the globe. The scale indicator should show pulsations (ocular pulse), indicating free movement of the plunger within the footplate assembly.
5. The tonometer is maintained on the eye for 4 min. If the eye moves or the tonometer slips off, the instrument is repositioned. A new 4 min period is not started but the tracing is continued to maintain the 4 min of recording.

### Calculations from the Tonographic Tracing (See Appendix, Figs. 3A-1, 3A-2)

I. The tracing is not a straight line. The best smooth curve through the tracing is determined.

II. The Schiotz scale reading and weight at the start of the tracing and the scale reading after 4 min of the tracing are determined.

III. The start and end (4 min) scale readings are determined. The C-value is determined from tables (See Appendix, Tables 3A-1, 3A-2, 3A-3) using the beginning Schiotz scale reading for the appropriate weight and the difference in scale readings between the start and end of the tracing (See Appendix, Figs. 3A-1, 3A-2).

IV. The initial Schiotz intraocular pressure, the pretonogram applanation intraocular

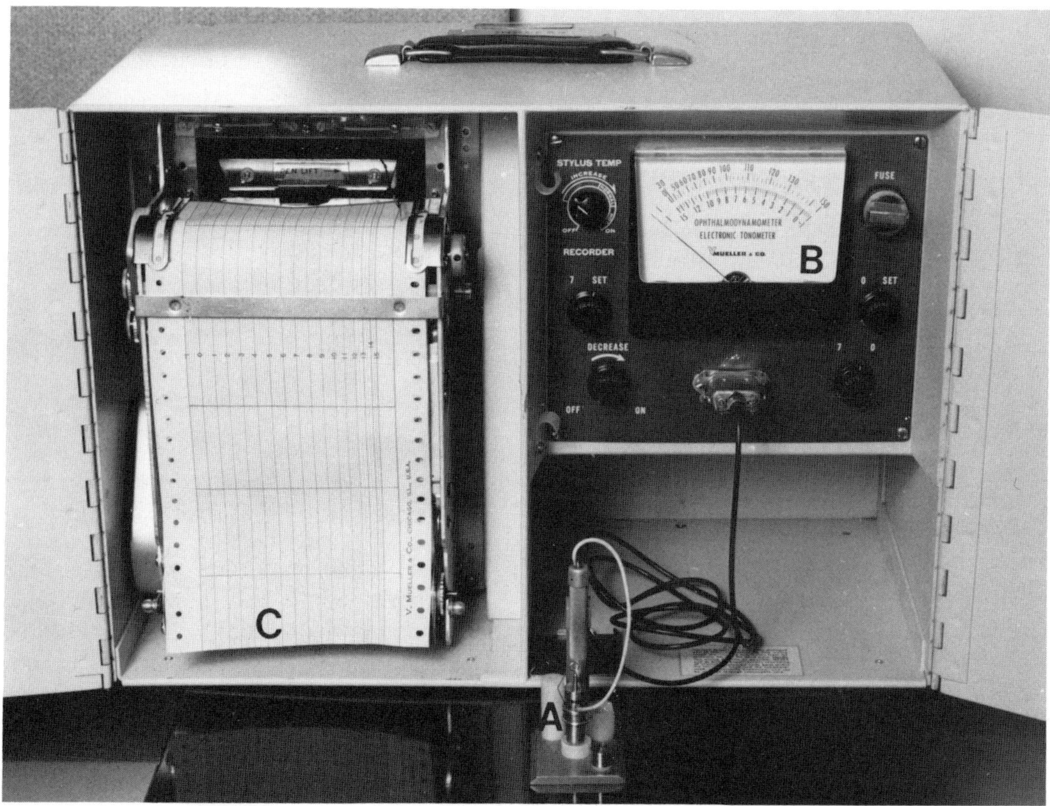


**Fig. 3-1** Tonography instrumentation: **(A)** Electronic Schiotz tonometer connected to **(B)** amplifier with **(C)** graft recorder.

pressure, and the outflow facility are marked on the tracing.

V. Ocular rigidity can be determined using the Friedenwald nomogram, as previously described (See Ch. 2 Appendix, Fig. 2A-2).

## Sources of Error

I. Any variation in curvature of the cornea (assumed to be 7.8 mm for the Schiotz tonometer) will affect the intraocular pressure measurements.

II. External pressure on the globe will artificially elevate intraocular pressure and act as an additional "weight" on the eye. This expresses additional fluid from the eye and artificially increases outflow facility.

III. Sticking of the plunger within the footplate will result in a flat tracing. Electronic tonometers have a larger footplate hole to prevent this problem.

IV. At low intraocular pressures, the cornea can mold and extend into the space between the plunger and the hole. This can push the plunger up and result in a false high outflow facility.

V. Patient-related factors, such as squeezing, blinking, lack or loss of fixation, or excessive eye movements, can cause a poor tracing.

VI. Improper operator-related actions, such as a dirty instrument, poor calibration of the instrument, or poor positioning of the instrument on the eye, can cause a poor tracing.

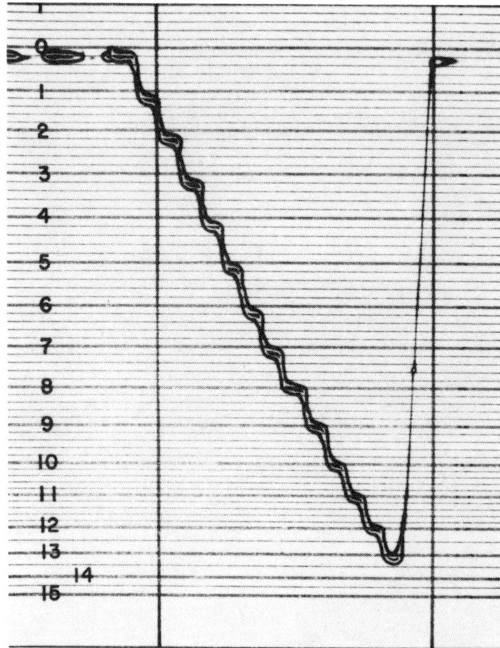


**Fig. 3-2** Calibration curve for the electronic Schiotz tonometer. The numbers on the left are the markings on the chart paper. The tonometer is calibrated for each scale division using a micrometer gauge. Each plateau represents the appropriate scale reading location on the graph paper.

VII. If intraocular pressure is normal and outflow facility is low in an eye not receiving glaucoma therapy, consider the following possibilities:
   A. Low ocular rigidity
   B. Aqueous humor hyposecretion
   C. A sticky tonometer plunger

VIII. If intraocular pressure is elevated and outflow facility is high, consider the following possibilities:
   A. High ocular rigidity
   B. Aqueous humor hypersecretion
   C. An artificially elevated intraocular pressure
   D. Elevated episcleral venous pressure
   E. Elevated pseudofacility
   F. Closed-angle glaucoma with the weight of the tonometer opening the iridocorneal angle resulting in a rapid decrease in intraocular pressure

## Wave Components of the Tonographic Tracing

I. Cardiac pulse is reflected as fine oscillations.

II. Large, irregular waves of the tracing reflect periodic changes in systemic blood pressure.

III. Irregularities may relate to cardiac irregularities (e.g., extrasystole).

## Interpretation of Outflow Facility

I. Mean value in normal patients is 0.28 with a standard deviation of 0.05.

II. Among normal patients, 2.5% will have an outflow facility <0.18 (2 standard deviations from the mean). Among glaucoma patients, 65–70% have an outflow facility <0.18 and 45–50% have an outflow facility <0.13.

III. The ratio of Po divided by C (Po/C) has been used to evaluate aqueous humor dynamics. The mean Po/C for a normal population is 56. Patients with glaucoma have an increased Po/C : 75% > 100, 50% > 140.

## Water Loading Tonography

The effects of water loading and the use of tonography as a provocative test for open-angle glaucoma are presented for historical value and not as a currently recommended procedure.

I. Drinking 1L of water in the fasting state elevates intraocular pressure. While the actual mechanism for this response is uncertain, outflow facility is reduced. The maximal increase in intraocular pressure and decrease in outflow facility occur 45 min after water consumption.

II. The response is greater in eyes with open-angle glaucoma.

III. To maximize the effects of water loading, the ratio Po/C is used. A Po/C ratio $> 100$ after water drinking occurs in 95% of eyes with untreated glaucoma and in less than 2.5% of normal eyes. A ratio $> 138$ occurs in 73% of glaucoma eyes and in only 0.15% of normal eyes.

IV. Water loading tonography was used as a provocative test to make the diagnosis of open-angle glaucoma. While altered aqueous humor dynamic changes occur following water drinking, it is erroneous to assume that this parameter should represent the basis for diagnosis and the initiation of glaucoma therapy.

## CLINICAL VALUE

In spite of the limitations and difficulties associated with tonography, useful clinical information regarding outflow facility can be obtained. Tonography provides an additional measurement, which, when taken in conjunction with other data, can be important in the management of patients with glaucoma. However, abnormal tonographic (and tonometric) results do not make the diagnosis of glaucoma.

I. A low outflow facility may correlate with a wide diurnal fluctuation in intraocular pressure. An eye with a low outflow facility will show a marked increase in intraocular pressure if aqueous secretion increases. This information can be helpful in the evaluation and therapy of patients with low-tension glaucoma.

II. Outflow facility can be helpful in identifying a low rate of aqueous humor secretion in face of a low intraocular pressure, for example, ocular inflammation secondary to surgery, trauma, uveitis, etc. In these conditions, a low pressure with a low outflow facility indicates aqueous hyposecretion.

III. In an eye with low intraocular pressure after filtration surgery, a very steep tonographic tracing indicates a functioning bleb but a flat tracing implies aqueous hyposecretion.

IV. Tonography can be an adjunct to the diagnosis of myasthenia gravis. Intravenous administration of Tensilon (edrophonium chloride) during tonography is associated with an increased intraocular pressure (2–5 mmHg) in patients with this condition secondary to Tension-induced contractions of the extraocular muscles.

V. Electronic or manual tonography can be informative during examination under anesthesia for the diagnosis of congenital glaucoma. General anesthesia lowers the rate of aqueous humor production and therefore can lower intraocular pressure. Outflow facility is not altered by general anesthesia. Therefore, a low intraocular pressure with a low outflow facility under general anesthesia indicates an abnormal outflow system. For similar reasons, tonography can be useful for postoperative follow-up examinations in patients with this condition.

## SUGGESTED READINGS

Kolker AE, Hetherington J, Jr: Becker-Shaffer's Diagnosis and Therapy of the Glaucomas, 5th Ed. CV Mosby Company, St Louis, 1984

Moses RA: Intraocular pressure. In Moses RA, Hart WM (eds): Adler's Physiology of the Eye: Clinical Applications, CV Mosby Company, St Louis, 1987

Podos SM: Tonography. In Glaucoma Symposium, New Orleans Academy of Ophthalmology. CV Mosby Company, St Louis, 1975

# Appendix

I. Normal tonographic tracing. With the 5.5 g Schiotz weight (Fig. 3A-1), the tonogram has a start scale reading of 7.50 (a) and an end scale reading of 10.50 (b), a difference of 3.00. Table 3A-1 shows the initial scale reading of 7.50 located on column R (an intraocular pressure of 11 mmHg). One reads across this line until the column Δ R 3.00 is reached, which indicates the outflow facility of 0.24. If the applanation pressure was measured at 12 mmHg, one would record the results as follows: Ta = 12 mmHg; Po(5.5 g) = 11 mmHg; C = 0.24 μm/min/mmHg

II. Glaucoma tonographic tracings. With the 7.5 g Schiotz weight (Fig. 3A-2), the tonogram has a start scale reading of 7.00 (a) and an end scale reading of 8.00 (b), a difference of 1.00. Table 3A-2 shows the initial scale reading of 7.00 located on column R (an intraocular pressure of 18 mmHg). One reads across this line until the column Δ R 1.00 is reached, which indicates the outflow facility of 0.05. If the applanation pressure was measured at 20 mmHg, one would record the results as follows: Ta = 20 mmHg; Po(7.5 g) = 18 mmHg; C = 0.05 μm/min/mmHg

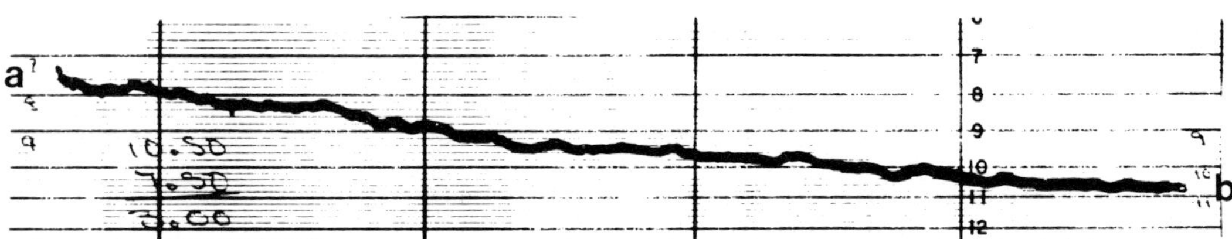


Fig. 3A-1

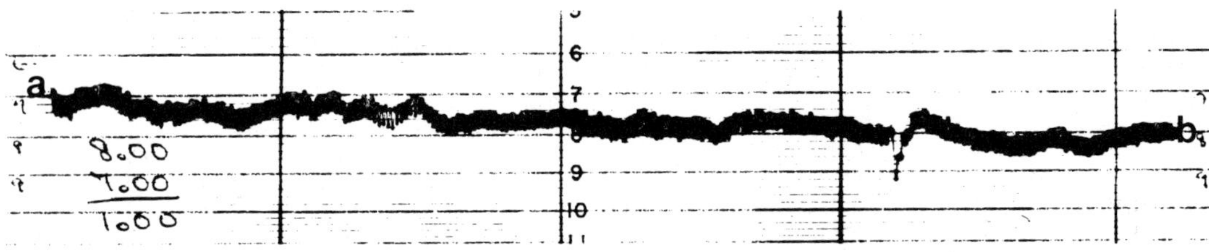


Fig. 3A-2

III. Tonography tables for 5.5 g, 7.5 g, and 10.0 g weights (Tables 3A-1, 3A-2, 3A-3). The initial Schiotz intraocular pressure is determined from the initial Schiotz scale reading. The difference (Δ R) between the start and the scale readings is determined. Outflow facility is determined by reading down the Δ R column and across the start pressure line to the point of crossing.

**Table 3A-1.** Tonography Table for a 5.5 g Schiotz Weight

| Initial Reading | | ΔR (Change in Scale Reading) | | | | | | | | | | |
|---|---|---|---|---|---|---|---|---|---|---|---|---|
| $P_0$ | R | 0 | 0.50 | 1.00 | 1.50 | 2.00 | 2.50 | 3.00 | 3.50 | 4.00 | 4.50 | 5.00 |
| 21 | 4.00 | 0 | 0.04 | 0.08 | 0.13 | 0.18 | 0.24 | 0.30 | 0.37 | 0.45 | 0.54 | 0.63 |
| 20 | 4.25 | 0 | 0.04 | 0.08 | 0.13 | 0.18 | 0.24 | 0.30 | 0.36 | 0.43 | 0.52 | 0.60 |
| 19 | 4.50 | 0 | 0.04 | 0.08 | 0.12 | 0.17 | 0.23 | 0.29 | 0.35 | 0.42 | 0.50 | 0.58 |
| 18 | 4.75 | 0 | 0.04 | 0.08 | 0.12 | 0.17 | 0.23 | 0.28 | 0.34 | 0.41 | 0.48 | 0.56 |
| 17 | 5.00 | 0 | 0.04 | 0.08 | 0.12 | 0.17 | 0.22 | 0.27 | 0.33 | 0.40 | 0.47 | 0.54 |
| 17 | 5.25 | 0 | 0.04 | 0.08 | 0.12 | 0.17 | 0.22 | 0.27 | 0.33 | 0.39 | 0.46 | 0.53 |
| 16 | 5.50 | 0 | 0.04 | 0.08 | 0.12 | 0.16 | 0.21 | 0.26 | 0.32 | 0.38 | 0.45 | 0.52 |
| 15 | 5.75 | 0 | 0.04 | 0.08 | 0.12 | 0.16 | 0.21 | 0.26 | 0.32 | 0.38 | 0.44 | 0.50 |
| 15 | 6.00 | 0 | 0.03 | 0.07 | 0.11 | 0.15 | 0.20 | 0.25 | 0.31 | 0.37 | 0.43 | 0.49 |
| 14 | 6.25 | 0 | 0.03 | 0.07 | 0.11 | 0.15 | 0.20 | 0.25 | 0.31 | 0.37 | 0.43 | 0.49 |
| 13 | 6.50 | 0 | 0.03 | 0.07 | 0.11 | 0.15 | 0.20 | 0.25 | 0.30 | 0.36 | 0.42 | 0.48 |
| 13 | 6.75 | 0 | 0.03 | 0.07 | 0.11 | 0.15 | 0.20 | 0.24 | 0.30 | 0.36 | 0.41 | 0.47 |
| 12 | 7.00 | 0 | 0.03 | 0.07 | 0.11 | 0.15 | 0.20 | 0.24 | 0.29 | 0.35 | 0.40 | 0.46 |
| 11 | 7.50 | 0 | 0.03 | 0.07 | 0.11 | 0.15 | 0.19 | 0.24 | 0.29 | 0.34 | 0.39 | 0.45 |
| 10 | 8.00 | 0 | 0.03 | 0.07 | 0.11 | 0.15 | 0.19 | 0.24 | 0.29 | 0.34 | 0.39 | 0.45 |
| 9 | 8.50 | 0 | 0.03 | 0.07 | 0.11 | 0.15 | 0.19 | 0.23 | 0.28 | 0.33 | 0.39 | 0.44 |
| 9 | 9.00 | 0 | 0.03 | 0.07 | 0.11 | 0.15 | 0.19 | 0.23 | 0.28 | 0.33 | 0.38 | 0.44 |

**Table 3A-2.** Tonography Table for a 7.5 g Schiotz Weight

| Initial Reading | | ΔR (Change in Scale Reading) | | | | | | | | | | |
|---|---|---|---|---|---|---|---|---|---|---|---|---|
| $P_0$ | R | 0 | 0.50 | 1.00 | 1.50 | 2.00 | 2.50 | 3.00 | 3.50 | 4.00 | 4.50 | 5.00 |
| 30 | 4.00 | 0 | 0.03 | 0.06 | 0.10 | 0.15 | 0.20 | 0.25 | 0.32 | 0.39 | 0.46 | 0.55 |
| 29 | 4.25 | 0 | 0.03 | 0.06 | 0.10 | 0.15 | 0.19 | 0.25 | 0.30 | 0.37 | 0.44 | 0.52 |
| 28 | 4.50 | 0 | 0.03 | 0.06 | 0.10 | 0.14 | 0.18 | 0.24 | 0.29 | 0.35 | 0.42 | 0.50 |
| 27 | 4.75 | 0 | 0.03 | 0.06 | 0.10 | 0.14 | 0.18 | 0.23 | 0.28 | 0.34 | 0.40 | 0.47 |
| 26 | 5.00 | 0 | 0.03 | 0.06 | 0.10 | 0.13 | 0.17 | 0.22 | 0.27 | 0.33 | 0.39 | 0.45 |
| 25 | 5.25 | 0 | 0.03 | 0.06 | 0.10 | 0.13 | 0.17 | 0.22 | 0.27 | 0.32 | 0.38 | 0.43 |
| 24 | 5.50 | 0 | 0.03 | 0.06 | 0.09 | 0.13 | 0.16 | 0.21 | 0.26 | 0.31 | 0.37 | 0.42 |
| 23 | 5.75 | 0 | 0.03 | 0.06 | 0.09 | 0.13 | 0.16 | 0.21 | 0.26 | 0.31 | 0.36 | 0.41 |
| 22 | 6.00 | 0 | 0.03 | 0.06 | 0.09 | 0.12 | 0.16 | 0.20 | 0.25 | 0.30 | 0.35 | 0.40 |
| 21 | 6.25 | 0 | 0.03 | 0.06 | 0.09 | 0.12 | 0.16 | 0.20 | 0.25 | 0.29 | 0.34 | 0.39 |
| 20 | 6.50 | 0 | 0.03 | 0.05 | 0.09 | 0.12 | 0.15 | 0.19 | 0.24 | 0.28 | 0.33 | 0.38 |
| 19 | 6.75 | 0 | 0.03 | 0.05 | 0.09 | 0.12 | 0.15 | 0.19 | 0.24 | 0.28 | 0.33 | 0.38 |
| 18 | 7.00 | 0 | 0.03 | 0.05 | 0.08 | 0.12 | 0.15 | 0.19 | 0.23 | 0.27 | 0.32 | 0.37 |
| 17 | 7.50 | 0 | 0.03 | 0.05 | 0.08 | 0.12 | 0.15 | 0.19 | 0.23 | 0.27 | 0.31 | 0.36 |
| 16 | 8.00 | 0 | 0.03 | 0.05 | 0.08 | 0.11 | 0.15 | 0.18 | 0.22 | 0.26 | 0.30 | 0.35 |
| 14 | 8.50 | 0 | 0.03 | 0.05 | 0.08 | 0.11 | 0.15 | 0.18 | 0.22 | 0.26 | 0.30 | 0.35 |
| 13 | 9.00 | 0 | 0.03 | 0.05 | 0.08 | 0.11 | 0.15 | 0.18 | 0.22 | 0.25 | 0.29 | 0.34 |
| 12 | 9.50 | 0 | 0.03 | 0.05 | 0.08 | 0.11 | 0.15 | 0.18 | 0.22 | 0.25 | 0.29 | 0.34 |

**Table 3A-3.** Tonography Table for a 10.0 g Schiotz Weight

| Initial Reading | | ΔR (Change in Scale Reading) | | | | | | | | | | |
|---|---|---|---|---|---|---|---|---|---|---|---|---|
| $P_0$ | R | 0 | 0.50 | 1.00 | 1.50 | 2.00 | 2.50 | 3.00 | 3.50 | 4.00 | 4.50 | 5.00 |
| 43 | 4.00 | 0 | 0.02 | 0.05 | 0.08 | 0.12 | 0.17 | 0.22 | 0.28 | 0.35 | 0.43 | 0.52 |
| 42 | 4.25 | 0 | 0.02 | 0.05 | 0.08 | 0.12 | 0.17 | 0.21 | 0.26 | 0.33 | 0.40 | 0.48 |
| 40 | 4.50 | 0 | 0.02 | 0.05 | 0.07 | 0.11 | 0.16 | 0.20 | 0.25 | 0.31 | 0.38 | 0.44 |
| 38 | 4.75 | 0 | 0.02 | 0.05 | 0.07 | 0.11 | 0.16 | 0.20 | 0.24 | 0.29 | 0.36 | 0.42 |
| 37 | 5.00 | 0 | 0.02 | 0.05 | 0.07 | 0.10 | 0.15 | 0.19 | 0.23 | 0.28 | 0.34 | 0.40 |
| 36 | 5.25 | 0 | 0.02 | 0.05 | 0.07 | 0.10 | 0.15 | 0.19 | 0.23 | 0.27 | 0.32 | 0.38 |
| 34 | 5.50 | 0 | 0.02 | 0.05 | 0.07 | 0.10 | 0.14 | 0.18 | 0.22 | 0.26 | 0.31 | 0.36 |
| 33 | 5.75 | 0 | 0.02 | 0.05 | 0.07 | 0.10 | 0.14 | 0.18 | 0.22 | 0.25 | 0.30 | 0.34 |
| 32 | 6.00 | 0 | 0.02 | 0.04 | 0.07 | 0.10 | 0.13 | 0.17 | 0.21 | 0.24 | 0.29 | 0.33 |
| 31 | 6.25 | 0 | 0.02 | 0.04 | 0.07 | 0.10 | 0.13 | 0.17 | 0.21 | 0.24 | 0.28 | 0.32 |
| 29 | 6.50 | 0 | 0.02 | 0.04 | 0.07 | 0.10 | 0.13 | 0.16 | 0.20 | 0.23 | 0.27 | 0.31 |
| 28 | 6.75 | 0 | 0.02 | 0.04 | 0.07 | 0.10 | 0.13 | 0.16 | 0.20 | 0.23 | 0.27 | 0.31 |
| 27 | 7.00 | 0 | 0.02 | 0.04 | 0.07 | 0.09 | 0.12 | 0.15 | 0.19 | 0.22 | 0.26 | 0.30 |
| 26 | 7.25 | 0 | 0.02 | 0.04 | 0.07 | 0.09 | 0.12 | 0.15 | 0.19 | 0.22 | 0.26 | 0.30 |
| 25 | 7.50 | 0 | 0.02 | 0.04 | 0.07 | 0.09 | 0.12 | 0.15 | 0.18 | 0.21 | 0.25 | 0.29 |
| 24 | 7.75 | 0 | 0.02 | 0.04 | 0.07 | 0.09 | 0.12 | 0.15 | 0.18 | 0.21 | 0.25 | 0.29 |
| 23 | 8.00 | 0 | 0.02 | 0.04 | 0.06 | 0.09 | 0.12 | 0.14 | 0.18 | 0.21 | 0.24 | 0.28 |
| 21 | 8.50 | 0 | 0.02 | 0.04 | 0.06 | 0.09 | 0.11 | 0.14 | 0.18 | 0.20 | 0.23 | 0.27 |
| 20 | 9.00 | 0 | 0.02 | 0.04 | 0.06 | 0.09 | 0.11 | 0.14 | 0.17 | 0.20 | 0.23 | 0.26 |
| 18 | 9.50 | 0 | 0.02 | 0.04 | 0.06 | 0.09 | 0.11 | 0.14 | 0.17 | 0.20 | 0.23 | 0.26 |
| 16 | 10.00 | 0 | 0.02 | 0.04 | 0.06 | 0.09 | 0.11 | 0.14 | 0.17 | 0.19 | 0.22 | 0.26 |
| 14 | 11.00 | 0 | 0.02 | 0.04 | 0.06 | 0.09 | 0.11 | 0.14 | 0.17 | 0.19 | 0.22 | 0.25 |

# 4

# Gonioscopy

Gonioscopy is the clinical technique that allows visualization of the anterior chamber iridocorneal angle by overcoming internal reflection of light by the curved corneal surface. Light rays coming from the anterior chamber angle exceed the critical angle of refraction at the cornea–air interface with the light rays reflected back into the eye, preventing visualization of the angle (Fig. 4-1). Gonioscopy eliminates the front corneal surface (the air–cornea interface) by using a contact lens with an index of refraction similar to the cornea. This results in minimal refraction at the cornea–contact lens interface and allows the light rays from the anterior chamber to pass through the contact lens–air interface, where they can be visualized.

## GONIOSCOPIC ANATOMY (FIG. 4-2)

Gonioscopy of an open iridocorneal angle reveals the following structures: cornea and Schwalbe's line, the trabecular meshwork, the scleral spur, the ciliary band, and the iris root. Often three divisions of the trabecular meshwork are evident. Just anterior to the scleral spur is the effective filtering portion of the meshwork lying in front of Schlemm's canal; a middle trabecular pigmented band also has filtration properties; and an anterior nonpigmented area, between Schwalbe's line and the pigmented band, which has limited filtration properties.

### Schwalbe's Line

I. Located at the termination of Descemet's membrane. It consists of a circumferential ring of collagenous fibers and basement membrane material.
II. Marks the forward limit of the anterior chamber angle structures.
III. Serves as the anterior attachment site for the trabecular meshwork.
IV. The line may be pigmented, especially inferiorly.
V. The ring may be prominent and visible at the slit-lamp, especially at the temporal limbus, when it is called a "posterior embryotoxin."
VI. Schwalbe's line may be identified due to its transition between the transparent corneal tissue and the off-white, translucent tissue of the trabecular meshwork as well as its transition from the steeper curvature of the cornea to the flatter curvature of the angle recess and sclera. Identification is enhanced, especially if the landmarks are not clear, by using the slit-lamp parallelepiped (Fig. 4-3):
    A. A thin slit-beam is projected onto the iridocorneal angle at an oblique incident angle through the goniolens.
    B. Above Schwalbe's line the slit-beam forms a three-dimensional parallelepiped of light in the transparent corneal tissue.
    C. At Schwalbe's line the figure of light collapses to a two-dimensional tape of light on the trabecular surface.

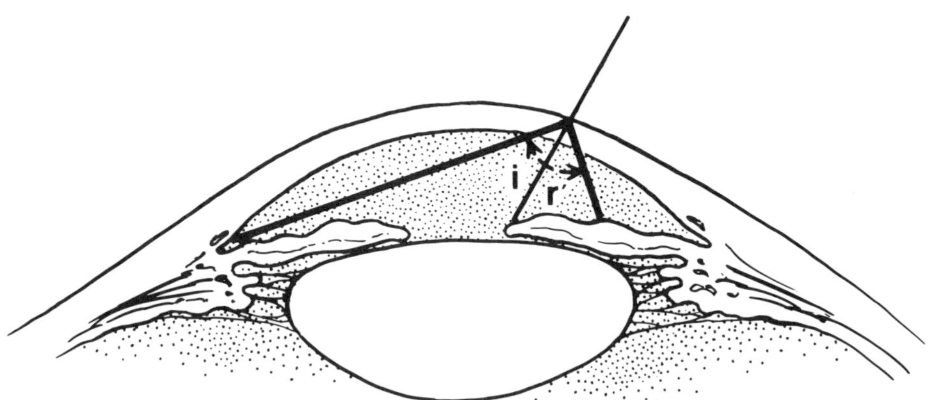


**Fig. 4-1** The critical angle at the cornea–air interface is exceeded by light originating from the anterior chamber: the angle of incidence (i) equals the angle of refraction (r). This results in internal reflection of the light rays back into the eye.

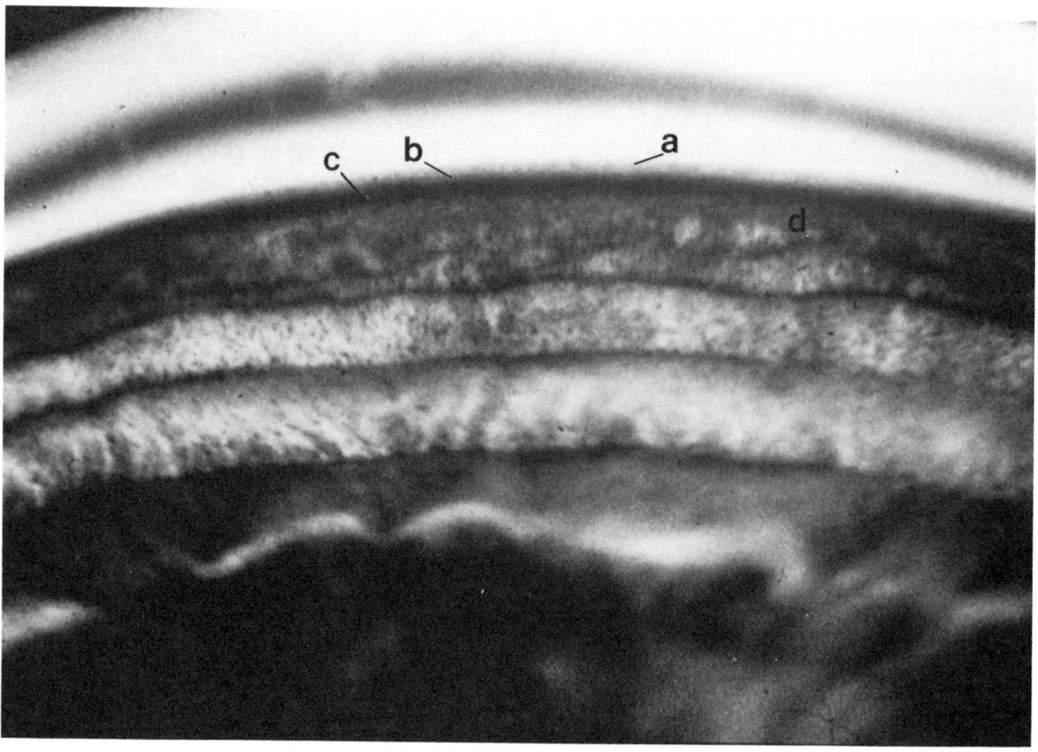


**Fig. 4-2** Goniophotograph of an eye with pigmentary glaucoma. (a) Schwalbe's line. (b) Junction of nonpigmented and pigmented trabecular meshwork. (c) Location of the iris root/ciliary body, which is highly pigmented in this eye. (d) Iris surface.

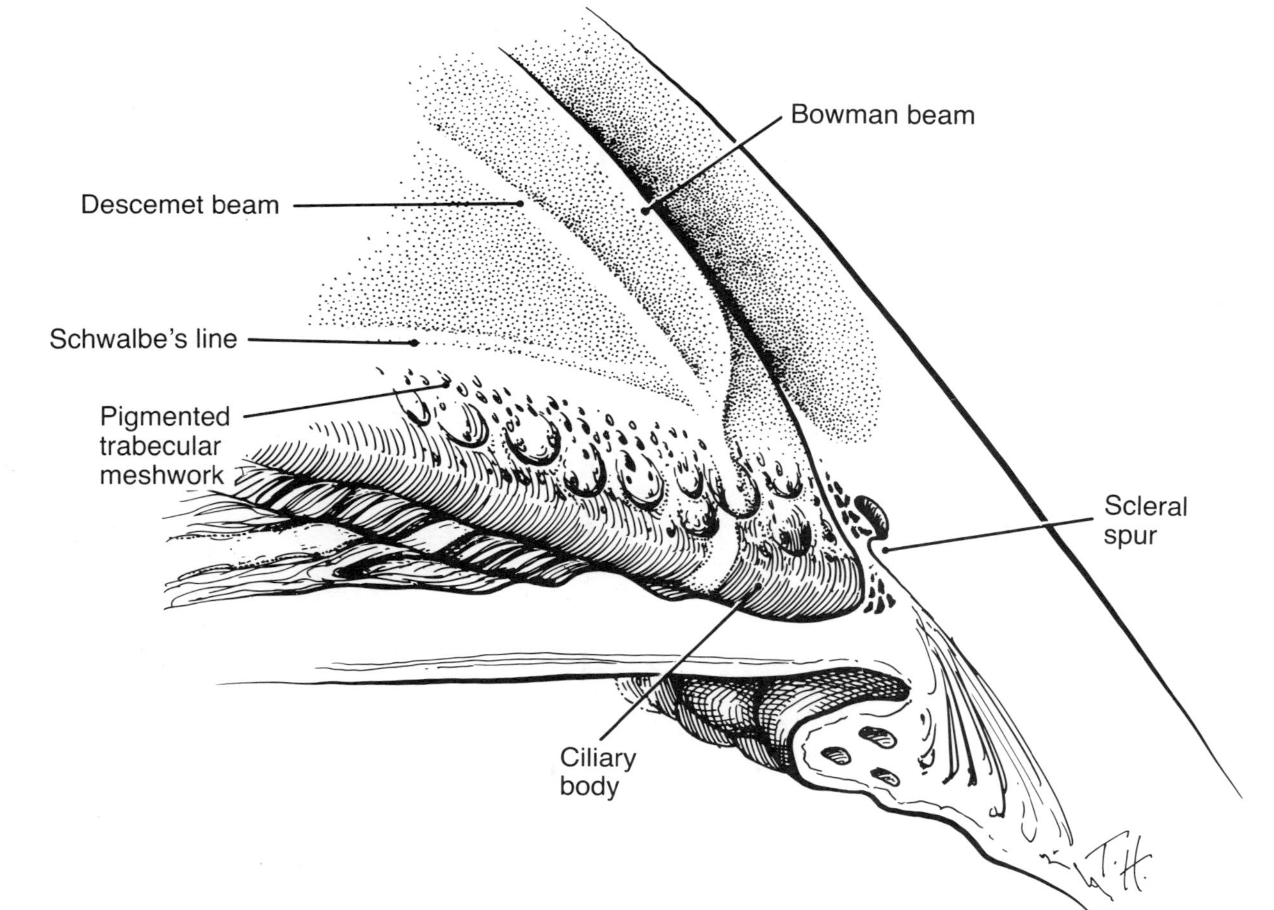


**Fig. 4-3** Anatomic view of iridocorneal angle structures. The junction of the parallelepiped formed by the beam from Descemet's membrane and the beam from Bowman's membrane meet at Schwalbe's line and mark the anterior limits of the iridocorneal angle.

D. This method to define Schwalbe's line is extremely important when looking at iridocorneal angles that have no trabecular pigmentation or at angles that are closed.

E. Pigment can settle at the ridge created by the transition of curvatures from cornea to angle recess. The pigment line is known as a Sampaolesi line and can mimic the trabecular meshwork. Definition of Schwalbe's line eliminates this confusion.

### Trabecular Meshwork

I. A band of tissue extending posterior from Schwalbe's line to the scleral spur.

II. The meshwork has a variable amount of pigment deposition, from a faint tan color to a dark brown. Pigmentation tends to be greater in the lower angle.

III. The central one-third corresponds to the site of Schlemm's canal. When filled with blood, Schlemm's canal can sometimes be seen as a red band.

IV. Blood reflux into Schlemm's canal is rare in glaucoma, except if episcleral venous pressure is elevated. Blood in the canal is observed in the following conditions:

   A. In normal eyes
   B. Intraocular inflammation, especially if the intraocular pressure is not increased
   C. States of increased episcleral venous pressure including jugular compression, a Valsalva's maneuver, or pathologic conditions
   D. Sudden lowering in intraocular pressure, such as following a paracentesis or an injury

V. The effective filtering portion of the meshwork lies in front of Schlemm's canal.

### Scleral Spur

I. A thin, prominent white line that is the posterior portion of the scleral sulcus.

II. May be obscured from view by dense uveal meshwork or excessive pigment dispersion.

III. Represents the location for attachment of the corneoscleral meshwork anteriorly and the ciliary body posteriorly.

### Ciliary Body Band

I. Visible in the iridocorneal angle where the iris inserts into the ciliary body.

II. The band is pale gray to dark brown. The width of the ciliary body band varies with the level of the iris insertion, tending to be wider in myopia and narrower in hyperopia.

### Angle Recess

The angle recess is not an anatomically defined structure but is the area where the iris dips posteriorly to insert into the ciliary body.

## DIRECT GONIOSCOPY

Direct gonioscopy uses the front curve of the contact lens to refract the light rays at the contact lens–air interface (Fig. 4-4). Visualization is achieved using a handheld binocular magnifier and an illumination source. The examination may be done by using a direct ophthalmoscope as an illuminated magnifier. The prototype direct goniolens is the Koeppe lens, which is available in various diameters and radii of contact lens curvature.

### Technique

Steps
1. The patient is placed in a reclined position with the head extended.
2. Topical anesthetic is applied.
3. The contact lens is positioned on the cornea with the space between the inner surface of the lens and the cornea filled with saline or a more viscous solution, such as methylcellulose.
4. The Koeppe contact lens may need to be stabilized by an assistant while the examiner holds the illuminator and the binocular magnifier. A gonioscope with a mounted light source can be used, thus

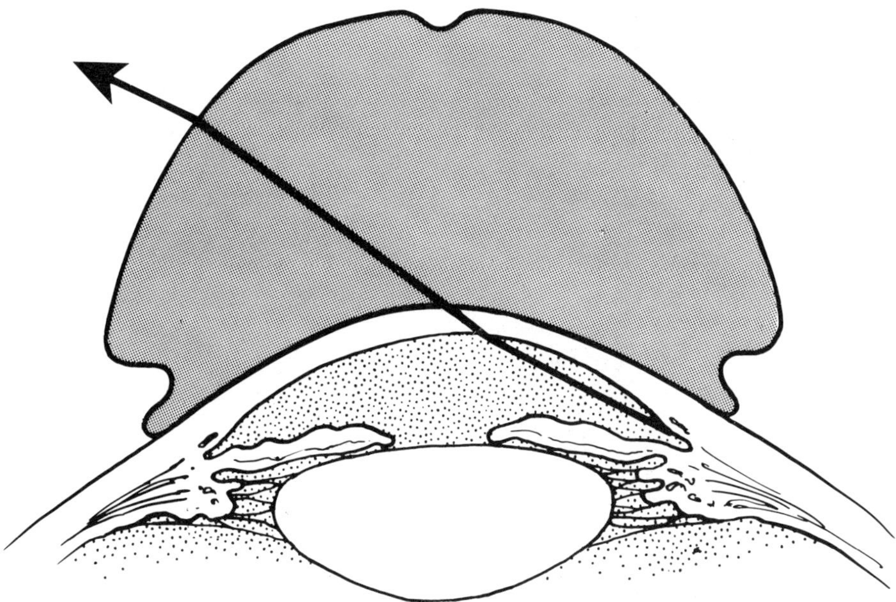

**Fig. 4-4** Direct gonioscopy. Light rays exiting from a Koeppe goniolens.

allowing the examiner a free hand to manipulate the goniolens.

5. The iridocorneal angle is viewed for 360° by shifting the positions of the magnifier, light source, and contact lens. Rapid comparison of the two eyes can be achieved by placing a contact lens on each eye. Having the patient look in various directions facilitates evaluation of the iridocorneal angle in an eye with a prominent peripheral iris roll.

## INDIRECT GONIOSCOPY

Indirect gonioscopy uses a contact lens that contains a mirror to reflect the light rays to leave the lens approximately perpendicular to the contact lens–air interface (Fig. 4-5). The major types of goniolens are the Goldmann and Zeiss lenses. Illumination and viewing of the anterior chamber are achieved with a slit-lamp while the contact lens is held by the examiner. Proper positioning of the patient and examiner at the slit-lamp is critical when performing indirect gonioscopy for either diagnosis or laser treatment. This section presents our current methods for instructing residents in performing indirect gonioscopy.

### Positioning of the Patient

I. The patient is comfortably positioned at the slit-lamp, sitting erect, by adjustment of the table height and chair.
II. The patient's head is centered using the chin rest to allow full excursion of the center of the slit-beam from the 12 to 6 o'clock positions.
III. The patient is instructed to keep the chin in the rest and to press the forehead against the instrument.
IV. If the slip-lamp is restricted from sliding forward by the patient's chest, the patient's chair is moved back from the slit-lamp and the patient is instructed to lean forward to insert his or her head in the rest.

### Positioning of the Examiner

I. The height and position of the examiner's stool are adjusted to have the examiner sit comfortably erect at the slit-lamp.

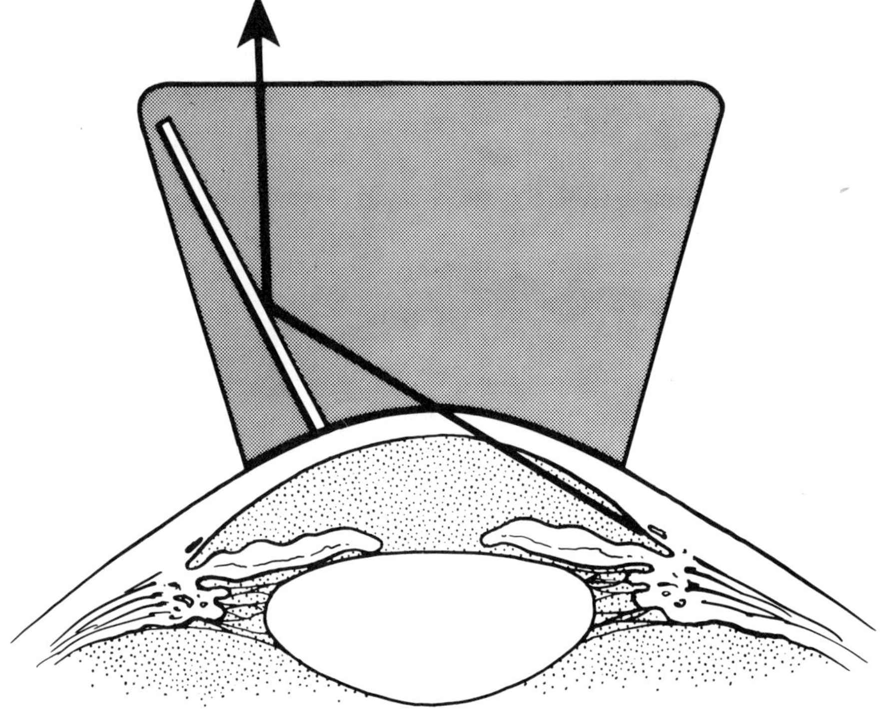

**Fig. 4-5** Indirect goniocopy. Light rays exiting from a Goldmann goniolens.

II. The goniolens is held in the examiner's left hand for examination of the patient's right eye, and in the right hand for examination of the patient's left eye.

III. The goniolens is held in the examiner's thumb and first two fingers, with the other two fingers placed gently on the patients cheek. The wrist should be held straight and the forearm as vertical as possible.

IV. The elbow should rest either on the slit-lamp table or on an elbow support to provide stability of the goniolens against the eye and to avoid fatigue-related tremor.

## Indirect Gonioprisms

### Goldmann Contact Lens (Fig. 4-6)

I. The prototype indirect goniolens.

II. Various lenses are available with different numbers, heights, and angles of mirrors.

III. This type of goniolens requires a viscous methylcellulose solution as the interface between the contact lens and cornea.

IV. The single-mirror Goldmann lens has a corneal contact diameter of 11 mm and a flatter peripheral section, extending to 14 mm, that rests on the sclera. The radius of curvature of the inner surface is 7.4 mm, so that the lens is steeper than the patient's cornea.

V. Technique

Steps 1. Topical anesthetic is applied.

2. The goniolens is filled with a viscous methylcellulose solution (air bubbles can be reduced by storing the solution inverted and avoiding shaking of the bottle).
3. The eye lids are held open and the goniolens brought near the patient's eye.
4. The goniolens is tipped so that contact is made with the globe at 6 o'clock. The goniolens holds, and may even be used

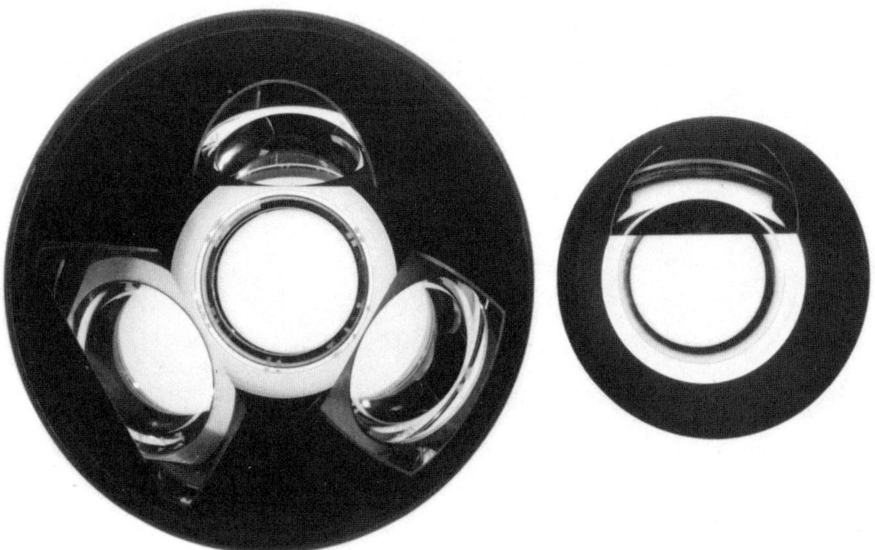

**Fig. 4-6** Goldmann-type goniolens: three mirror (left) and single mirror (right).

to retract, the palpebral margin of the lower eye lid. The goniolens is rotated forward against the cornea in a quick motion to capture the methylcellulose solution.

5. The goniolens is pressed against the eye creating a "suction cup" effect, which keeps the lens centered on the cornea. Pressure should be relaxed to avoid distortion of the chamber angle structures during routine examination (see pressure gonioscopy below).
6. The Goldmann goniolens can be viewed with a direct ophthalmoscope (at +10–+20 diopters) if a slit-lamp is not available.

### Zeiss Four-Mirror Contact Lens (Fig. 4-7)

I. The lens is designed to use the tear layer as the interface between the contact lens and cornea.

II. This lens has a holding fork to facilitate application of the goniolens to the eye.

III. The lens has a 9 mm corneal segment, and thus rests solely on the cornea. The 7.72 mm radius of curvature closely matches that of the average cornea.

IV. Technique

Steps 1. Topical anesthesia is applied.

2. The patient is positioned at the slit-lamp so that the head is centered to allow full excursion of the slit-beam.
3. The lens is applied to the cornea, using the fork handle
   a. In a "square" configuration by holding the handle at a 45° angle to the eye
   b. In a "diamond" configuration by holding the handle horizontally
   c. The square configuration is preferable since the goniolens better fits the palpebral fissure, avoiding contact of the corner of the lens with the patient's eyelid. This configuration also allows the examiner to keep the wrist straight and the forearm vertical for better support and control of the goniolens.
4. A plastic cup can be attached to the Zeiss goniolens to facilitate retraction of the upper and lower eyelids.
5. The handle is held with the thumb and first two fingers while the examiner's fourth and fifth fingers rest on the patient's cheek.

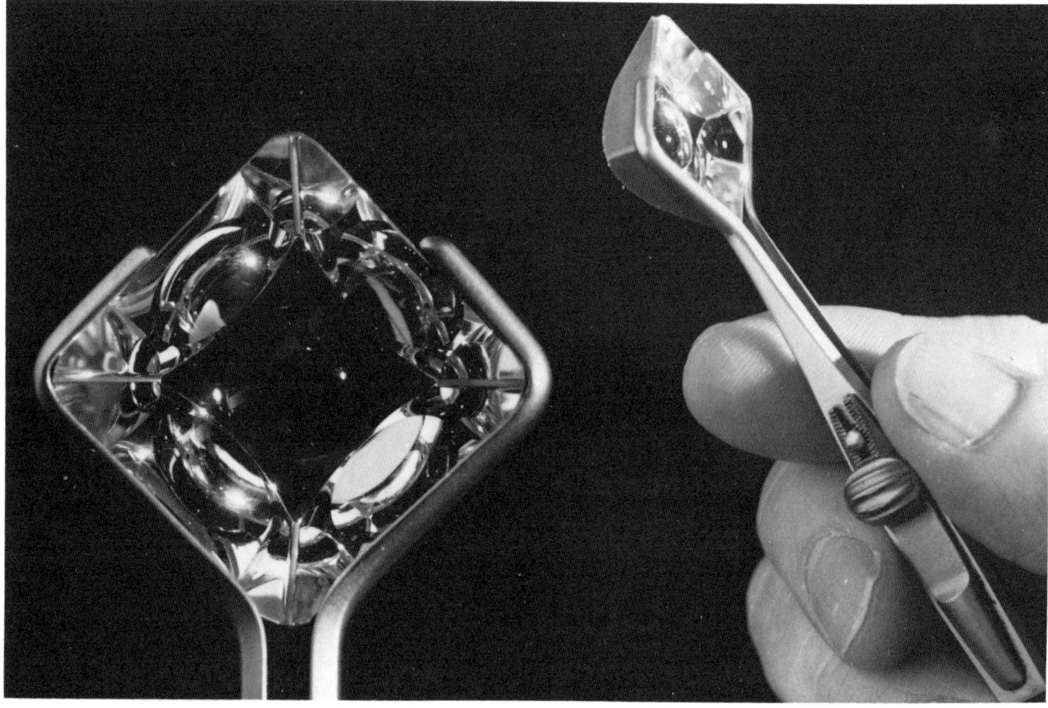

**Fig. 4-7** Zeiss goniolens with four-mirror prism and holding fork: top (left) and side (right) views.

6. The position of the goniolens is maintained on the center of the cornea by the kinesthetic guidance of the two fingers on the patient's cheek.
7. The Zeiss lens is allowed to touch the cornea just barely to view the undistorted angle structures. This is accomplished by a slight rocking forward of the wrist of the hand holding the goniolens.

## Indirect Viewing of the Iridocorneal Angle

I. The hand not holding the goniolens is used to adjust the slit-lamp microscope so that it is focused on the image of the iridocorneal angle reflected by the mirror of the goniolens.

II. The sector of the iridocorneal angle across the anterior chamber from the mirror is viewed; for example, the superior angle when the mirror is at the bottom of the goniolens. While the view in the mirror is always of the angle across the anterior chamber, this may not be 180°. For example, if the center of the mirror is at 6 o'clock, the opposite angle view is 12 o'clock; however, if the goniolens is not rotated the view from the 7 o'clock mirror is of the 11 o'clock angle, not the corresponding 180° angle at 1 o'clock.

III. The slit-beam is placed either directly coaxial or 15° to either side.

IV. The entire 360° of the iridocorneal angle is visualized with the Goldmann goniolens by a combination of rotating the contact lens and movement of the slit-lamp and with the Zeiss goniolens by moving the beam of the slit-lamp to the different mirrors.

V. Viewing of a narrow irodocorneal angle obscured by a convex iris can be achieved by

A. having the patient look in the direction of the mirror, thereby moving the view to a higher position relative to the plane of the iris. This technique maintains the perpendicular light path from the mirror to the examiner and does not induce distortion.

B. moving the goniolens along the corneal surface toward the angle under view. This technique results in tilting of the goniomirror and can induce a prismatic distortion (an important consideration when performing gonioscopy during an argon laser trabeculoplasty, see Chapter 11).

C. Goniolens-induced endothelial folds are a useful guide to possible artifactual distortion.

## COMPARISON OF GONIOSCOPIC TECHNIQUES

### Direct Gonioscopy

I. Provides an excellent and natural panoramic view of the iridocorneal angle with the ability to adjust the angle of viewing entirely by movement of the examiner. The technique does not require the use of viscous material.

II. Enables the examiner to compare rapidly the iridocorneal angles of the two eyes by placing a gonioscopy lens on each eye.

III. The direct view is necessary for direct iridocorneal angle surgery (e.g., goniotomy).

IV. The major disadvantages of direct gonioscopy include the inability to perform indentation gonioscopy (see below), low magnification, the need for an assistant to support the lens on the cornea, and the possible inconvenience of having the patient lie down for the examination.

### Indirect Gonioscopy

I. The slit-lamp provides excellent optics, illumination, and a high-magnification view of the iridocorneal angle.

II. The ease of instrumentation and examination allows the technique to be a routine part of the examination.

### Goldmann vs. Zeiss Indirect Gonioscopy

I. The Goldmann lens requires the use of a viscous material while the Zeiss lens uses the natural tear film to rest on the cornea.

II. The Goldmann lens "suction cup" effect keeps the goniolens centered on the cornea, in contrast to the Zeiss lens, which requires continued effort to correct for lens drift. This allows fine focusing of the slit-lamp beam, which is extremely important during anterior segment laser treatment.

III. The Goldman lens "suction cup" effect may distort the anatomic relationships of the iridocorneal angle, and can open a closed angle causing the examiner to miss the diagnosis of angle-closure glaucoma. Angle distortion is markedly reduced, and is under the control of the examiner, with the Zeiss lens.

IV. The Goldmann lens has a higher mirror at a steeper angle, which may be a distinct advantage in narrow-angled eyes.

## RECORDING THE APPEARANCE OF THE IRIDOCORNEAL ANGLE

Description of the gonioscopic appearance of the iridocorneal angle includes recording the configuration of the angle, the degree of trabecular pigmentation, and the presence of abnormal structures such as peripheral anterior synechiae or neovascularization. Grading systems or descriptive words and drawings are used to classify the iridocorneal angle.

### Scheie Classification (Fig. 4-8)

I. Based on the extent of the anterior chamber angle structures that can be visualized.

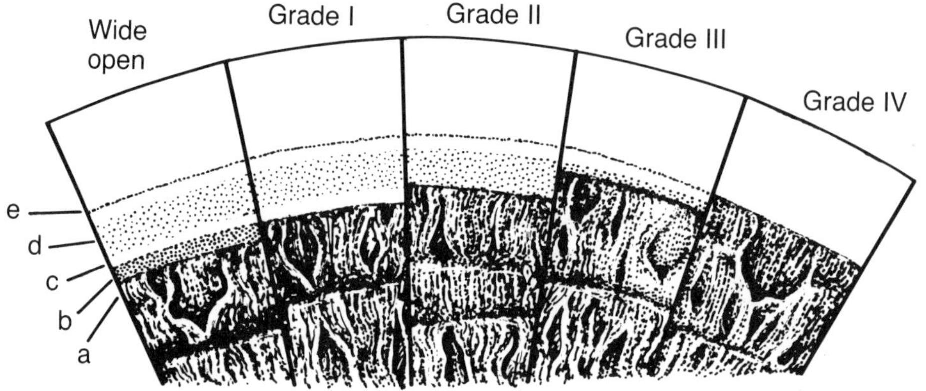


**Fig. 4-8** Scheie gonioscopic classification of the anterior chamber angle which is dependent upon the extent of visible structures. Grade IV is the most narrow grade. (a) Iris root. (b) Ciliary body. (c) Scleral spur. (d) Trabecular meshwork. (e) Schwalbe's line.[1] (From Blake RL, Sr., Shields MB: A Study Guide for Glaucoma. Williams & Wilkins, Baltimore, 1982.)

II. A high risk of angle-closure is associated with grade III or IV iridocorneal angles.

| Grading | Gonioscopic Appearance |
|---|---|
| Wide open | All structures visible |
| Grade I narrow | Hard to see over the iris root into recess |
| Grade II narrow | Ciliary band and scleral spur are obscured |
| Grade III narrow | Posterior trabeculum obscured |
| Grade IV (closed angle) | Only Schwalbe's line visible |

## Shaffer Classification (Fig. 4-9)

I. Based on the angular width of the angle recess (the angle formed by the plane of the trabecular meshwork–cornea and the plane of the iris root–iris surface in the angle recess) as the criterion for grading the angle.
II. A high risk of angle-closure is associated with grade II or I iridocorneal angles.

| Grading | Gonioscopic Appearance |
|---|---|
| Grade 0 | Complete or partial closure |
| Grade I narrow | 10° angle at recess |
| Grade II narrow | 20° angle at recess |
| Grade III narrow | 30° angle at recess |
| Grade IV open | 40° or more angle at recess |

## Spaeth Classification

I. Based on the configuration of the angle recess.
II. A three-variable classification with appropriate coding (e.g., E, 40°, b see below)

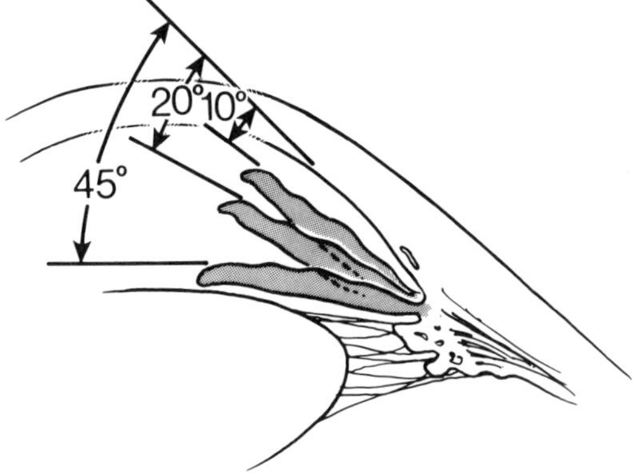


**Fig. 4-9** Shaffer gonioscopic classification of the anterior chamber angle, which is based upon the angular width (angle formed by iris plane and inner corneal plane) of the angle recess. Grades IV–III, 45°–20°; grade II, 20°; grade I, 10°; grade 0, angle closure.

| Classification | Gonioscopic Appearance |
|---|---|
| 1. Insertion of iris root | |
| code A | Anterior to Schwalbe's line |
| code B | Behind Schwalbe's line |
| code C | on the scleral spur |
| code D | Deep |
| code E | Extremely deep |
| 2. Angular width of angle recess | |
| Numbered from 0° to 40 (see Shaffer's classification) | |
| 3. Peripheral iris configuration | |
| code q | queer configuration |
| code r | regular configuration |
| code s | steep configuration |

### Grading Trabecular Pigmentation

Trabecular pigmentation is arbitrarily graded from 0 to IV with grade IV representing dense pigmentation.

### Abnormal Angle Structures

In addition to grading the width of the iridocorneal angle and separating glaucoma into primary open-angle or primary closed-angle types, gonioscopy provides the opportunity to visualize iridocorneal angle abnormalities that can be associated with various secondary glaucomas. Description of the gonioscopic examination should include the following findings:

I. Angle recession
II. Peripheral anterior synechiae
III. Angle neovascularization
IV. Angle membranes
V. Iris processes
VI. Iridodonesis

## SLIT-LAMP METHOD FOR ESTIMATING PERIPHERAL ANTERIOR CHAMBER DEPTH

I. The depth of the peripheral chamber can be estimated by the slit-lamp technique of van Herick, Shaffer, and Schwartz (Fig. 4-10). However, the technique does not replace gonioscopic grading of the iridocorneal angle.
II. A thin slit-lamp beam is focused on the cornea and anterior chamber at the temporal limbus and the depth of the peripheral anterior chamber is compared to the thickness of the peripheral cornea.
III. The technique can be compared to the Shaffer Classification.

| van Herick Finding | Shaffer Classification |
|---|---|
| AC depth = corneal thickness | Grade IV open |
| AC depth = ¼ to ½ corneal thickness | Grade III angle |
| AC depth = ¼ corneal thickness | Grade II angle |
| AC depth = less than ¼ corneal thickness | Grade I angle |
| AC depth = slitlike (extremely narrow) | Slit angle |
| AC depth absent | Closed-angle |

## INDENTATION GONIOSCOPY

I. A technique that enables the examiner to alter the position of the iris relative to the trabecular meshwork in a dynamic fashion.
II. The technique determines what portion of a closed iridocorneal angle is appositionally or synechially closed.
III. Requires use of the Zeiss four-mirror goniolens for controlled application of pressure to the globe.
IV. Technique

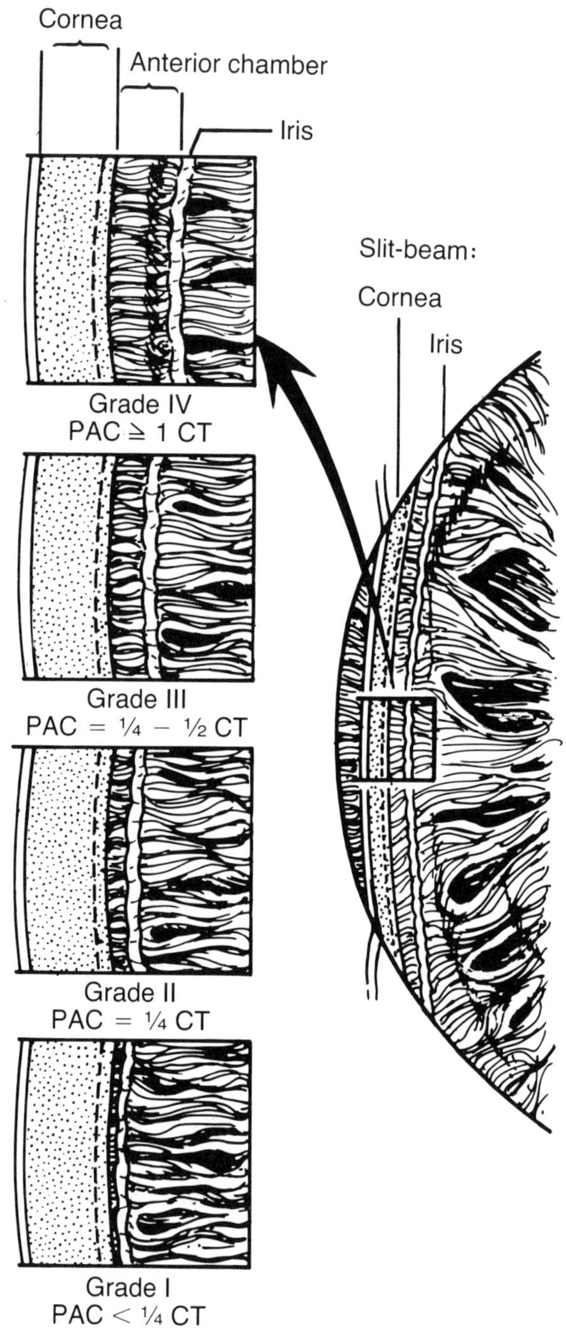


**Figure 4-10** Slit-lamp estimation of peripheral anterior chamber depth by the method of van Herick et al. The peripheral corneal thickness (CT) is used to estimate the peripheral anterior chamber depth (PAC). The PAC is related to the Shaffer gonioscopic classification (see Fig. 4-9): Grade IV, PAC ≥ 1 CT; grade III, PAC = 1/4–1/2 CT; grade II, PAC = 1/4 CT; grade I, PAC < 1/4 CT; grade O, peripheral iris in contact with the cornea. (From Blake RL, Sr., Shields MB: A Study Guide for Glaucoma. Williams & Wilkins, Baltimore, 1982.)

Steps 1. The angle quadrant to be assessed is examined using a narrow, short slit-beam with the Zeiss goniolens and no pressure on the cornea.

2. Pressure is applied to the Zeiss lens directly towards the center of the eye.

3. If the iridocorneal angle is appositionally closed, the pressure will result in deepening of the anterior chamber in the angle recess. As the iris bows backward, one can see progressively deeper iridocorneal angle structures including a previously hidden pigmented portion of the trabecular meshwork or possible peripheral anterior synechiae.

4. The technique can be used to open a closed angle during an attack of acute closed-angle glaucoma.

5. A closed angle by synechiae will not open during indentation gonioscopy.

## SUGGESTED READINGS

Kolker AE, Hetherington J., Jr: Becker-Shaffer's Diagnosis and Therapy of the Glaucomas. 5th Ed. CV Mosby, St. Louis, 1983

Moses R, Hart W: Adler's Physiology of the Eye. 8th Ed. CV Mosby, St. Louis, 1986

Scheie HG: Width and pigmentation of the angle of the anterior chamber. A system of grading by gonioscopy. Arch Ophthalmol 58:510, 1957

Shaffer RN: Symposium: primary Glaucomas. III. Gonioscopy, Ophthalmoscopy and perimetry. Trans Am Acad Ophthal Otol 62:112, 1960

Shields MB: Textbook of Glaucoma. 2nd Ed. Williams & Wilkins, Baltimore, 1986

Spaeth, GL: The normal development of the human anterior chamber angle. A new system of descriptive grading. Trans Ophthalmol Soc UK 91:709, 1971

van Herick W, Shaffer RN, Schwartz A: Estimation of width of angle of anterior chamber. Incidence and significance of the narrow angle. Am J Ophthalmol 68:626, 1969

# 5

# Optic Nerve in Glaucoma

## ANATOMY AND HISTOLOGY

### Overall Structure

The optic nerve head is composed of four types of tissue: neural, glial, vascular, and connective.

I. The normal optic disc (Fig. 5-1) is between 1.1 and 1.8 mm in diameter. The vertical diameter is normally larger than the horizontal diameter. The size of the optic disc is highly variable in the normal population.

II. The area occupied by the visible rim of neurovascular tissue (disc rim) is normally between 1.2 $mm^2$ and 1.6 $mm^2$ and does not vary a great deal in the normal population.

III. The optic nerve head can be divided into four anatomic regions: surface layer, prelaminar portion, lamina cribrosa region, and retrolaminar portion (Fig. 5-2).

#### Neural

Axons arising from the ganglion cells of the retina form the retinal nerve fiber layer and converge at the optic disc, where they leave the eye to form the optic nerve.

I. The normal optic nerve has between 1,000,000 and 1,500,000 axons. There is a steady decline in the number of optic nerve axons with age.

II. The nerve fibers are normally unmyelinated until they pass through the lamina cribrosa. Myelin sheaths are acquired in the retrolaminar portion of the nerve.

III. The nerve fibers from the ganglion cells in the retina temporal to the optic disc are above and below the macula (Fig. 5-3). Fibers from the nasal retina run in a direct radial fashion to the optic disc.

IV. The retina is divided into two vertical halves by the horizontal raphe. Ganglion cells located above the raphe generally send their axons into the superior portion of the disc while those below the raphe send their axons into the inferior portion. Fibers from the macula form the maculopapillary bundle and enter the optic nerve on the temporal side. The fovea is located slightly below the horizontal and most of the foveal fibers enter the optic disc on the temporal side just below the horizontal meridian (Fig. 5-3). The anatomy of the nerve fibers in

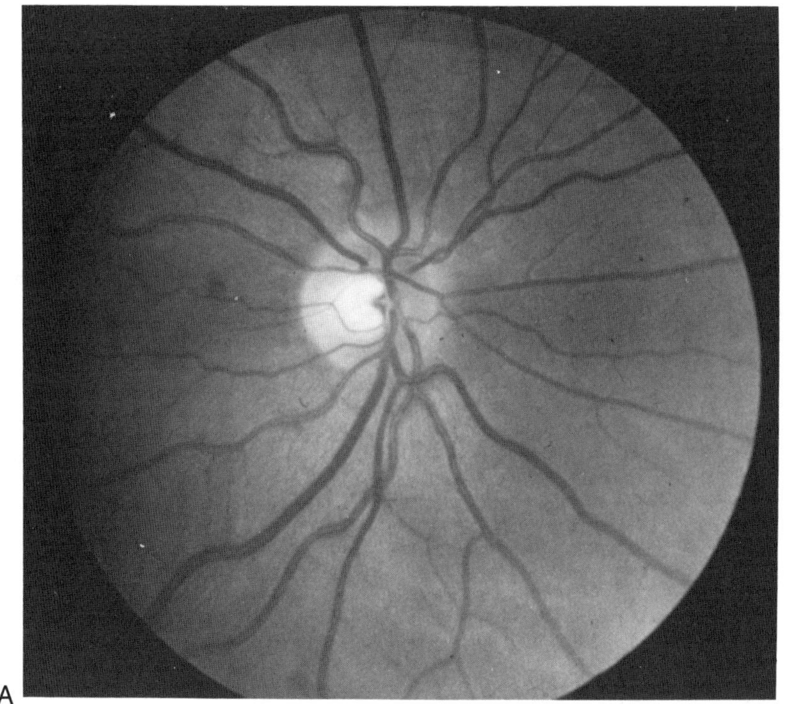


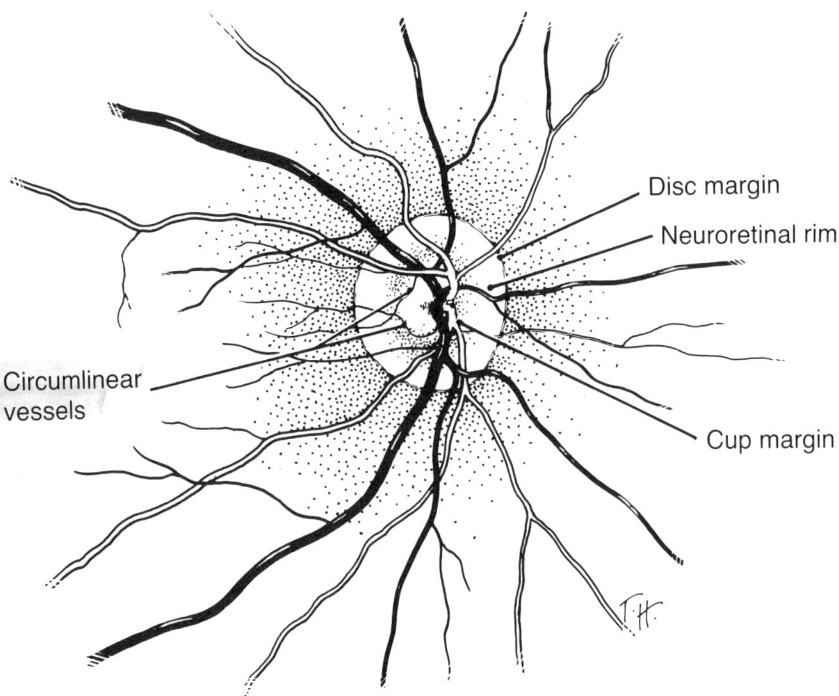


**Fig. 5-1 (A, B)** The normal optic nerve head as seen with the ophthalmoscope. The normal central cup is marked by the area of pallor. Surrounding the cup is the disc rim made up of axons, glial cells, and capillaries. The edge of the cup is marked by circumlinear vessels.

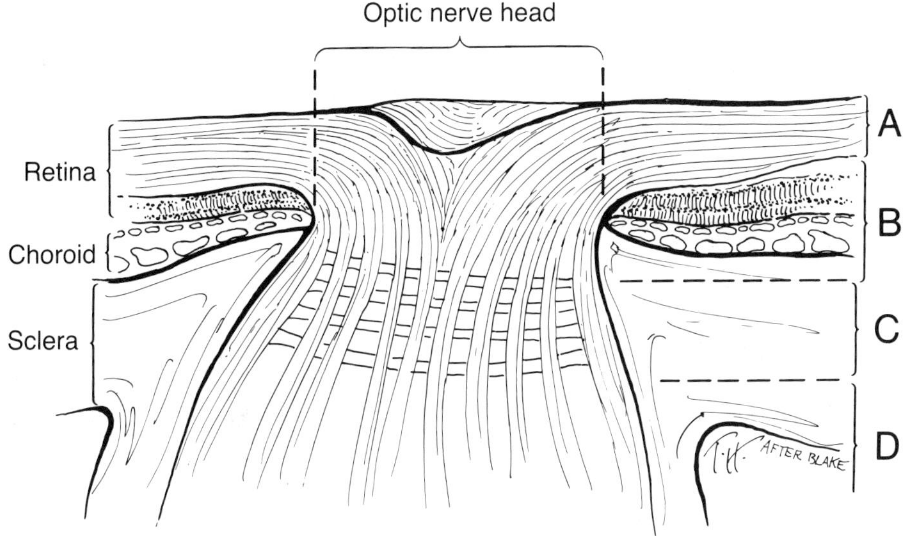


**Fig. 5-2** Histologic anatomy of the optic nerve head showing **(A)** the surface layer, **(B)** the prelaminar portion, **(C)** the region of the lamina cribrosa, and **(D)** the retrolaminar portion. (From Shields, 1987, with permission.)

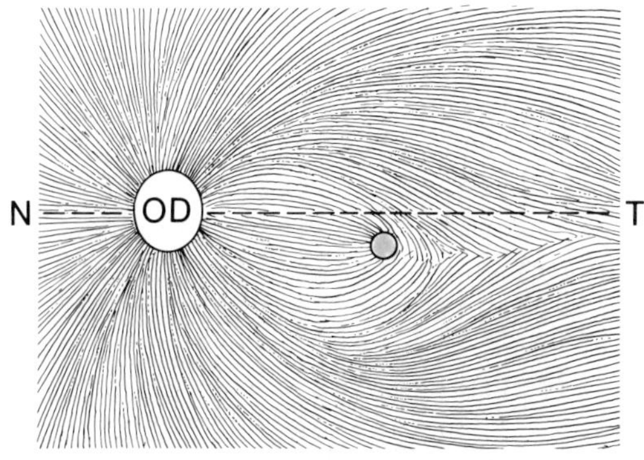


**Fig. 5-3** Drawing of the normal anatomy of the nerve fiber layer of the retina (left eye). Ganglion cell axons converge on the optic nerve head. Fibers from the temporal retina are above and below the macula and are divided into superior and inferior halves by the horizontal raphe. The center of the macula is located slightly below the horizontal, and fibers from the macula (papillomacular bundle) enter the disc slightly below the midportion of the temporal side of the disc. N, nasal; T, temporal; OD, optic disc; open circle, fovea. (From Quigley, 1986, with permission.)

the retina and optic nerve determines the characteristic appearance of the nerve fiber bundle visual field defects seen in glaucoma.

### Glial

Astrocytes are the predominant glial element in the surface layer and prelaminar and laminar portions of the optic nerve. Oligodendroglia predominate in the retrolaminar portion.

### Vascular (Fig. 5-4)

The blood vessels of the optic nerve head consist of capillaries and small arterioles and venules. The only larger vessels normally present are the central retinal artery and vein and, occasionally, a cilioretinal artery.

I. The capillaries of the optic nerve head resemble retinal capillaries and do not normally leak fluorescein.
II. The surface layer portion of the optic

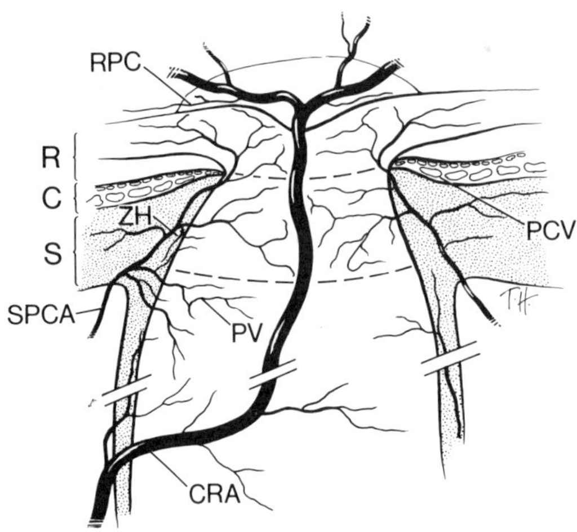


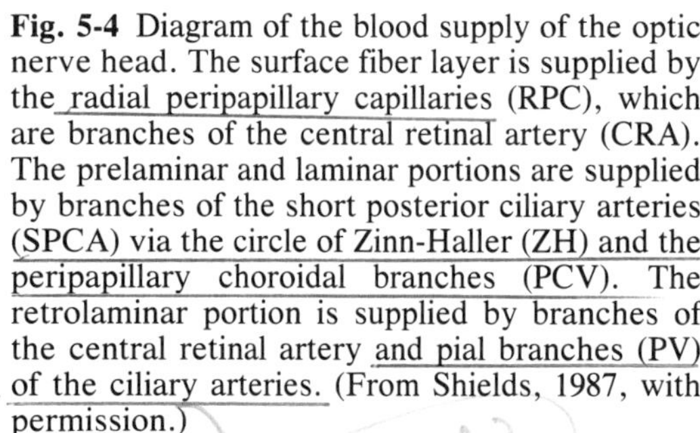

**Fig. 5-4** Diagram of the blood supply of the optic nerve head. The surface fiber layer is supplied by the radial peripapillary capillaries (RPC), which are branches of the central retinal artery (CRA). The prelaminar and laminar portions are supplied by branches of the short posterior ciliary arteries (SPCA) via the circle of Zinn-Haller (ZH) and the peripapillary choroidal branches (PCV). The retrolaminar portion is supplied by branches of the central retinal artery and pial branches (PV) of the ciliary arteries. (From Shields, 1987, with permission.)

nerve head receives its blood supply from branches of the central retinal artery.

III. The prelaminar and laminar portions receive their blood supply mainly from branches of the short posterior ciliary arteries. There may be some contribution from the peripapillary choroid, but this is not certain.

IV. The retrolaminar portion receives blood from both the short posterior ciliary arteries and the central retinal artery.

### Connective Tissue

Collagenous tissue similar to sclera makes up the scleral canal and lamina cribrosa through which the optic nerve axons pass as they leave the eye. The lamina cribrosa has two large openings for the central retinal vessels and multiple small openings for the optic nerve fiber bundles. These small openings are larger and have thinner walls in the superior and inferior portions of the lamina (Fig. 5-5).

## CLINICAL APPEARANCE OF THE OPTIC NERVE IN GLAUCOMA

### Optic Nerve Damage

The optic nerve damage of glaucoma is distinguished from other types of optic neuropathy by the loss of glial and vascular tissue as well as axons and the backward bowing of the lamina cribrosa. This produces the characteristic appearance called "cupping."

The earliest changes of glaucoma are due to the gradual loss of nerve fiber bundles at the optic nerve head. The result is thinning of the visible rim of neuroretinal tissue at the optic disc. The loss of disc rim may be either localized or generalized. As the disc rim becomes thinner, the optic cup enlarges.

### Clinical Features of Glaucomatous Optic Nerve Disease

#### Enlargement of the Optic Cup (Fig. 5-6)

The optic cup size is usually expressed as a cup/disc ratio, that is, the ratio of the diameter of the cup to the diameter of the entire disc. The cup/disc ratio is determined for both horizontal and vertical meridians separately. Estimates of cup/disc ratio, even by experienced observers, are highly variable. Also, the cup/disc ratio is mainly dependent on the size of the optic disc itself, which shows great variability in the population. For these reasons, the cup/disc ratio by itself is of limited value. In the normal population, the average cup/disc ratio is about 0.25. Only 6% of the normal population can be expected to have a cup disc ratio greater than 0.5. A large cup, therefore, should raise the suspicion of glaucoma.

A documented increase in the size of the optic cup over time is generally a sign of progressive glaucomatous damage.

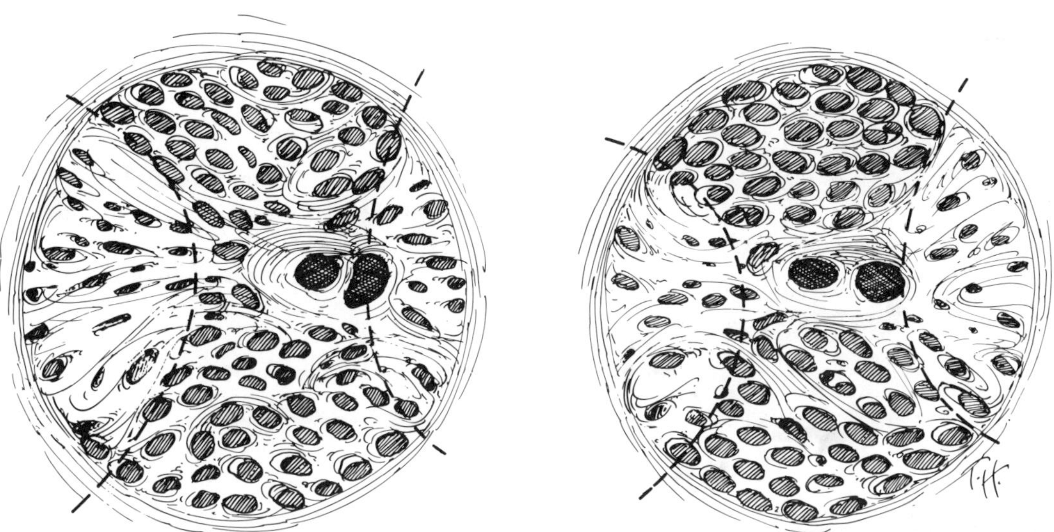

**Fig. 5-5** Drawing of the lamina cribrosa. The two large openings near the center transmit the central retinal vessels. The nerve fiber bundles pass through multiple smaller openings. These openings are larger and have thinner walls superiorly and inferiorly, in the areas of the optic nerve where early glaucomatous damage is usually found. (Courtesy of Harry Quigley, M.D.)

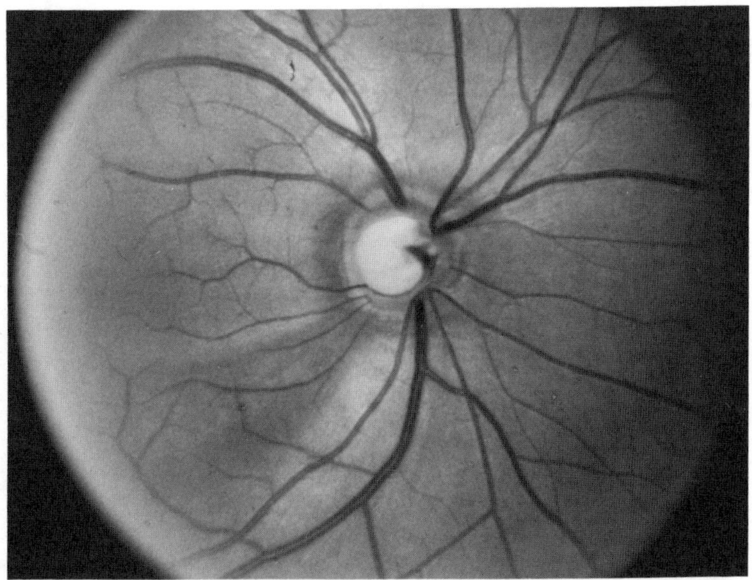

**Fig. 5-6** Glaucomatous optic nerve head showing enlargement of the cup. The vertical cup/disc ratio is approximately 0.8. This disc also shows a defect in the retinal nerve fiber layer extending in an arcuate fashion from the disc margin at the 7 o'clock position.

* large disc < expect larger cup. cup is "spotlight" will show defects early

* small disc expect smaller cup – will show changes very late
– a small Δ is v. significant
– expect to see field Δ's first.

### Loss of Disc Rim Area

Loss of disc rim area appears to be a much better indicator of glaucomatous damage than cup/disc ratio. Of the normal population, 95% has a disc rim area greater than 1.09 $mm^2$, whereas about 75% of glaucoma patients have disc rim areas less than this.

### Asymmetry of Cupping (Fig. 5-7)

About 60% of the normal population has no detectable difference in cup/disc ratio between the two eyes. Only about 6.5% of the normal population has a difference in cup/disc ratio of more than 0.1 between the two eyes, and only 1% of the normal population has a difference greater than 0.2. Significant asymmetry of cupping, therefore, is highly indicative of glaucoma.

### Vertical Elongation of the Cup (Fig. 5-8)

The optic cup is normally concentric with the disc margin. A cup that shows a significant degree of vertical elongation indicates loss of nerve fibers at the superior and inferior poles of the disc. This finding is characteristic of glaucoma.

### Localized Thinning or Notching of the Disc Rim (Fig. 5-9)

If the loss of disc rim is very localized, a small notch is produced. Even more generalized loss of disc rim, however, will produce local areas where the rim is thinner than elsewhere.

### Disc Hemorrhages (Fig. 5-10)

Splinter hemorrhages in the superficial nerve fiber layer of the optic disc occur frequently in glaucoma. They are an ominous sign: they usually indicate continuing damage and are frequently associated with progressive visual field loss.

### Sharply Angled Vessels Crossing the Disc Margin (Fig. 5-11)

As the disc rim is lost in glaucoma, the blood vessels come to lie directly against the

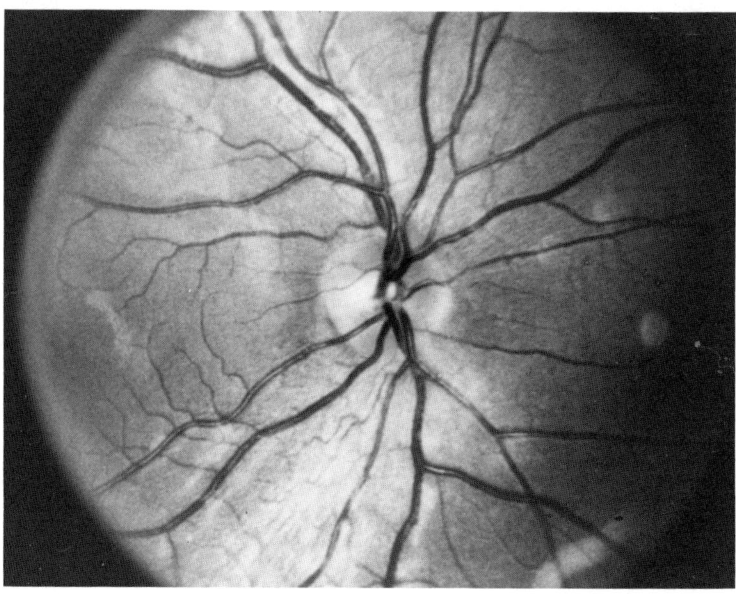

A

**Fig. 5-7** Asymmetry of cupping in a 16-year-old boy with secondary glaucoma due to trauma in the left eye. **(A)** The right vertical cup/disc ratio is approximately 0.3. (*Figure continues.*)

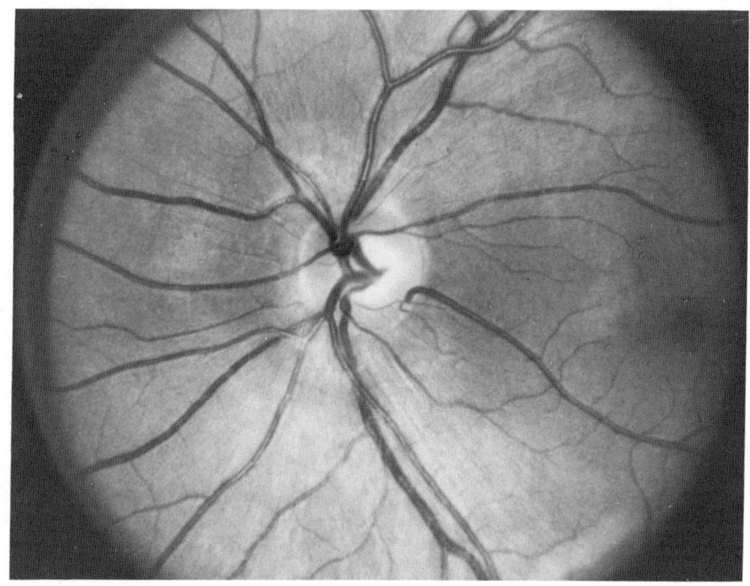


**Fig. 5-7** (*Continued*). (**B**) The vertical cup/disc ratio in the left eye is 0.6.

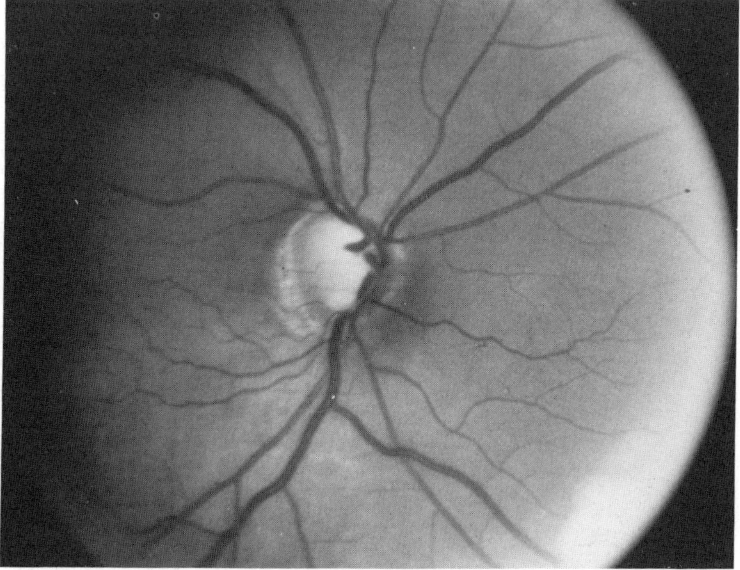

**Fig. 5-8** Optic disc showing vertical enlargement of the cup in glaucoma. The disc rim is thinner at the top and bottom of the nerve head than at the sides, resulting in a vertically oval cup.

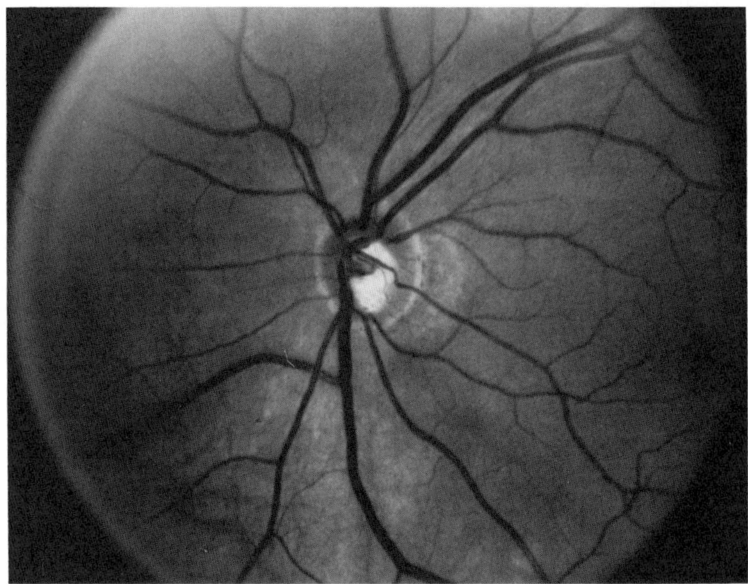

**Fig. 5-9** Optic disc showing localized notching of the disc rim inferiorly. The loss of the tissue overlying the lamina cribrosa exposes the laminar holes in the region of the notch, the so-called laminar dot sign.

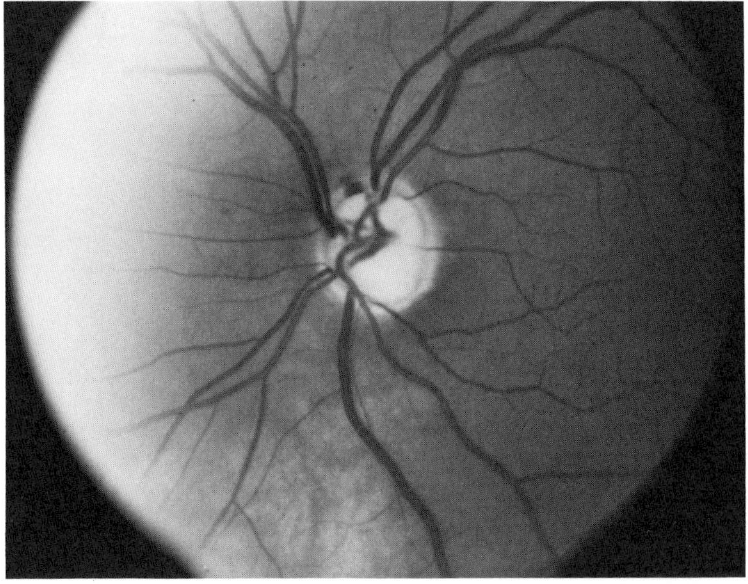

**Fig. 5-10** Optic disc showing a hemorrhage on the disc rim at the 11 o'clock position. When seen in glaucoma patients, such hemorrhages may be a sign of progressive disease.

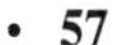

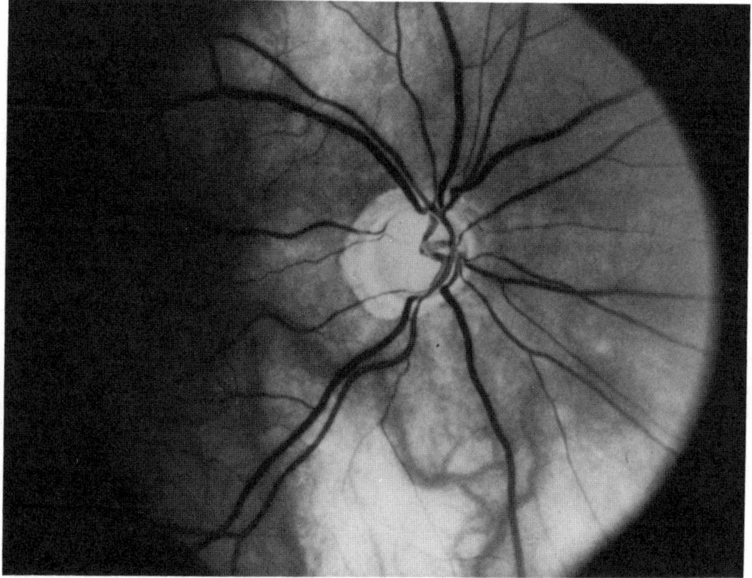

**Fig. 5-11** Optic disc showing sharply angled retinal vessels crossing the disc edge. This is especially well seen in the vein at the 6 o'clock position and the smaller vessel at the 10 o'clock position. This disc also shows the peripapillary atrophy frequently seen in glaucoma.

edge of the scleral canal. They often demonstrate a sharply angled bend as they cross from disc to retina.

#### Peripapillary Atrophy (Fig. 5-11)

Atrophy of the peripapillary retina is a common finding in glaucomatous eyes.

#### Baring of the Circumlinear Vessel (Fig. 5-12)

Circumlinear vessels are small branches of the central retinal vessels that outline the margin of the cup. They are present in about 50% of eyes. As the glaucomatous cup enlarges, the cup margin recedes from the circumlinear vessel and a small area of pallor appears between the vessel and the margin of the cup. The specificity of this finding for acquired optic nerve changes, however, is limited.

#### Retinal Nerve Fiber Layer Defects (See Fig. 5-6)

Red free photography can be used to highlight the retinal nerve fiber layer. The loss of axons can often be easily seen in the photograph as defects in the nerve fiber layer. Large arcuate defects are characteristically seen in glaucoma.

Nerve fiber layer defects may be either diffuse or localized. Diffuse loss is more difficult to detect clinically but may be seen as a generalized loss of the normal striated appearance of the retinal nerve fiber layer. Localized loss is usually best seen one or two disc diameters above or below the upper and lower poles of the disc. Since the normal nerve fiber layer partially obscures the retinal blood vessels, a very sharp, clear image of a retinal blood vessel in one area compared to other areas of the fundus is often a sign of loss of nerve fibers.

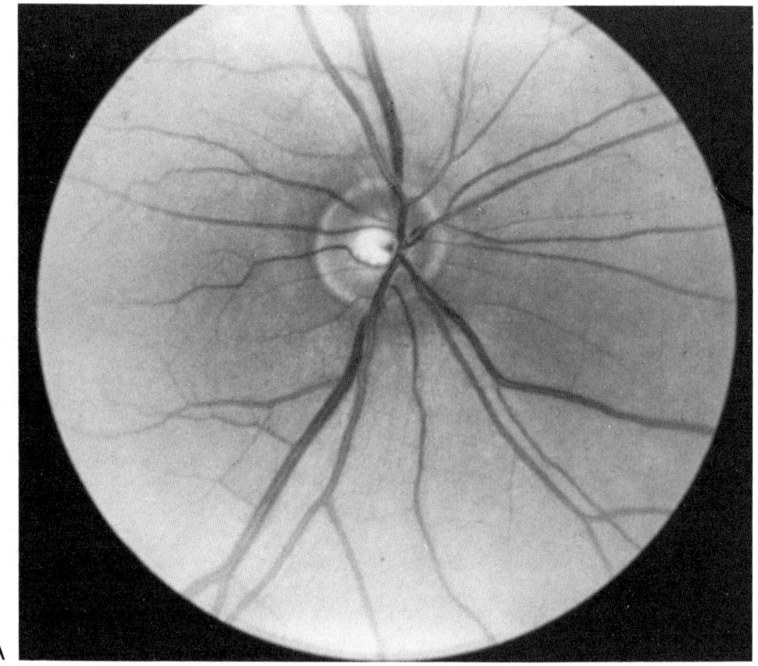


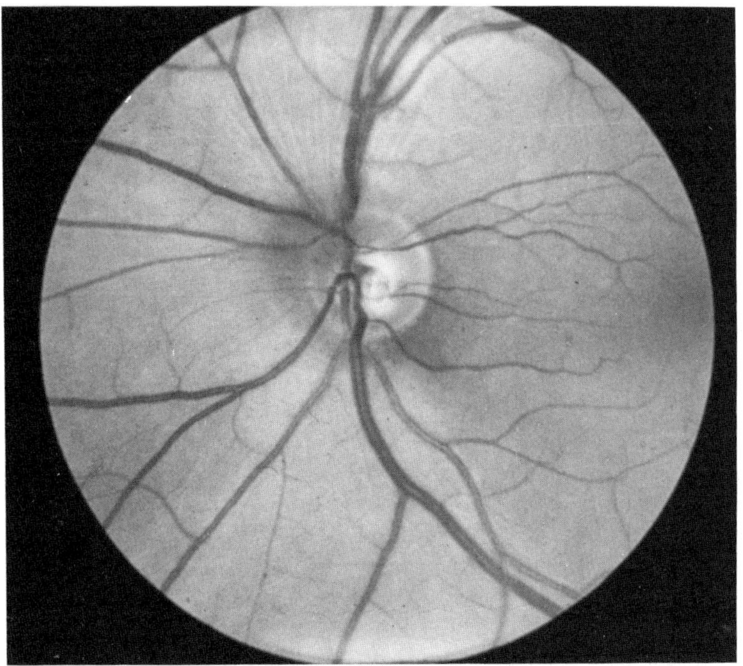


**Fig. 5-12** **(A)** The right eye of a patient with chronic open-angle glaucoma shows an inferior and superior circumlinear vessel in the normal position at the margin of the cup. **(B)** The left eye of the same patient shows baring of the inferior circumlinear vessel due to loss of disc rim in this area.

### Conditions Other Than Glaucoma in Which the Appearance of Optic Nerve Head May Resemble Glaucomatous Cupping

I. Congenital anomalies of the optic disc

A variety of congenital anomalies of the optic nerve may simulate glaucomatous cupping and be associated with nerve-fiber-bundle-type visual field loss. Colobomas, optic pits, large physiologic cups, tilted discs, myopia, and optic nerve drusen are among the lesions said to mimic glaucoma.

II. Compressive lesions of the chiasm and optic nerve

Optic atrophy due to compressive lesions of the optic nerve or chiasm does not generally resemble glaucomatous cupping. Glaucomatous and nonglaucomatous optic atrophy can usually be differentiated by clinical examination. Occasionally, however, the optic nerve in a patient with nonglaucomatous optic atrophy may appear to be cupped to a degree that glaucoma is suspected. In glaucoma, the degree of cupping is usually greater than or equal to the area of pallor. When the area of pallor is greater than the area of cupping, a nonglaucomatous disease process must be considered.

III. Ischemic optic neuropathy

Cupping resembling that seen in glaucoma sometimes follows acute ischemic insults to the optic nerve.

## EXAMINATION TECHNIQUES

### Direct Ophthalmoscopy

I. Advantages are ease of use, high magnification, and ability to use with a small pupil.
II. Disadvantages are the small field of view and lack of stereopsis.

### Slit-Lamp with Goldmann-Style Contact Lens

I. Advantages are stereopsis and use of slit-lamp optics.
II. Disadvantages are patient discomfort and necessity of placing the lens and a contact solution on the cornea.

### Slit-Lamp with High-Power Concave (Hruby) Lens

I. Advantages are stereopsis, use of slit-lamp optics, and lack of direct corneal contact.
II. Disadvantages are small field of view and difficulties with maintaining patient fixation.

### Slit-Lamp with High-Power Convex Lens (Fig. 5-13)

These lenses convert the slit-lamp to an indirect ophthalmoscope and produce an inverted image of the fundus.

I. Advantages are ease of use, stereopsis, use of slit-lamp optics, wide field of view, and lack of direct corneal contact.
II. Disadvantages are the inverted image and need for a well-dilated pupil.

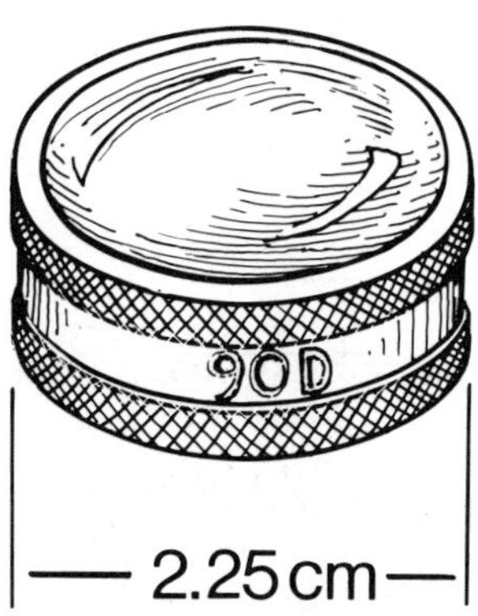


**Fig. 5-13** The 90 diopter lens can be used with the slit-lamp to obtain a high quality, stereoscopic view of the posterior pole. The image is inverted, as with an indirect ophthalmoscope.

Patient: 266TK    right eye

OPTIC DISK PARAMETERS

| SECTION: | TOP | RIGHT | BOTTOM | LEFT | TOTAL | UNITS |
|---|---|---|---|---|---|---|
| CUP/DISK: | 0.490 | 0.539 | 0.530 | 0.584 | 0.535 | - |
| RIM AREA: | 0.280 | 0.229 | 0.264 | 0.213 | 0.986 | square mm |
| DISK AREA: | 0.371 | 0.325 | 0.371 | 0.325 | 1.39 | square mm |
| VOLUME: | 0.022 | 0.016 | 0.018 | 0.092 | 0.148 | cubic mm |
| ELEVATION: | 0.015 | 0.011 | 0.022 | 0.000 | 0.048 | cubic mm |
| DISK DIAMETER: | 1.40 | 1.26 | | | | mm |

**Fig. 5-14** The printout from the Rodenstock Optic Disc Analyzer. This and similar devices use computerized image analysis to map the optic nerve and quantitate the shape, size, and configuration of the nerve head.

## Photographic Techniques

Optic disc photography is extremely useful in glaucoma patients. It allows one to compare the appearance of a patient's optic disc at different times. It also allows one to study the disc at length without causing the patient undue discomfort. Whenever possible, stereo disc photographs should be taken of all glaucoma patients as part of their routine management.

When photography is unavailable or not practical, drawings of the disc may be substituted. This technique is considerably less reliable or reproducible than photography.

Red-free photography using green or blue filters and high-contrast black and white film allows one to see the retinal nerve fiber layer easily. This may prove to be a very useful technique for detecting and evaluating nerve fiber loss in glaucoma.

## Computerized Image Analysis (Fig. 5-14)

Devices are now coming onto the market that perform computerized image analysis of the optic disc. These devices provide quantitative information about the topography of the optic disc. At present, they are very expensive and still experimental; however, in the future some type of objective, quantitative optic disc image analysis may prove to be the standard technique for evaluating the optic nerve head in glaucoma.

## SUGGESTED READINGS

Anderson DR: What happens to the optic disc and retina in glaucoma? Ophthalmology 90:766, 1983

Airaksinen PJ, Drance SM, Schulzer M: Neuroretinal rim area in early glaucoma. Am J Ophthalmol 99:1, 1985

Drance SM: Hemorrhage on the disc: another risk factor in glaucoma. p. 153. In Symposium on Glaucoma, Transactions of the New Orleans Academy of Ophthalmology. CV Mosby, St. Louis, 1981

Drance SM, Airaksinen PJ: Signs of early damage in open-angle glaucoma. p. 17. In Weinstein GW (ed): Open-Angle Glaucoma. Churchill Livingstone, New York, 1986

Kirsch DR, Anderson RE: Clinical recognition of glaucomatous cupping. Am J Ophthalmol 75:442, 1973

Minckler DS, Spaeth GL: Optic nerve damage in glaucoma. Surv Ophthalmol 26:128, 1981

Quigley H: Pathophysiology of the optic nerve in glaucoma. p. 30. In McAllister JA, Wilson PR (eds): Glaucoma. Butterworths, London, 1986

Shields MB: Textbook of Glaucoma. 2nd Ed. Williams & Wilkins, Baltimore, 1987

Spaeth GL: Appearances of the optic disc in glaucoma: a pathogenetic classification. p. 114. In Symposium on Glaucoma, Transactions of the New Orleans Academy of Ophthalmology. CV Mosby, St. Louis, 1981

# 6

# Perimetry in Glaucoma

For over 100 years loss of the visual field has been recognized as the major clinical manifestation of glaucomatous optic nerve damage. As optic nerve fibers are lost in the course of the disease, the ganglion cells of the retina from which those fibers arose die. If enough ganglion cells in a particular area of the retina disappear, visual perception from that area is also lost. These localized areas of loss of vision appear as defects in the visual field and can be measured and mapped by a device called a perimeter.

The visual field as plotted by a perimeter is a representation of retinal sensitivity at various locations. In a three dimensional graph, the x and y axes define location in terms of degrees from fixation while the z axis defines retinal sensitivity. The resulting plot has a characteristic shape and has been termed the hill of vision (Fig. 6-1).

The visual field abnormalities seen in glaucoma patients have a characteristic appearance and are very useful in establishing the diagnosis. Frequent measurement of the visual field over time often allows the detection of progressive glaucomatous visual loss and is important in making therapeutic decisions. An understanding of the principles of perimetry and the manifestations of glaucomatous visual field loss are essential in the management of patients with glaucoma.

## PERIMETRY MEASURES

### Differential Light Threshold

I. The differential light threshold (DLT) refers to the ability of the visual system to detect a difference in contrast between two areas of different luminance. In the case of perimetry, the contrast is between the background luminance of the perimeter bowl and the test target (Fig. 6-2).

II. The DLT is measured in units of brightness per unit area called apostilbs (asb).

III. The dynamic range of a perimeter refers to the range of brightness of the available test targets. On the Octopus and Goldmann perimeters, the brightest target is 1000 asb. On the Humphrey perimeter, the brightest target is 10,000 asb. Most perimeters can produce targets as dim as 1 asb or less.

IV. Because of the large dynamic range of most perimeters, and the tremendous range of adaptation of the retina, many automated perimeters express the apostilb brightness of the targets using a logarithmic scale. The usual unit is the decibel (dB). Apostilbs are converted to decibels by a formula. Different perimeters use different conversion formulas.

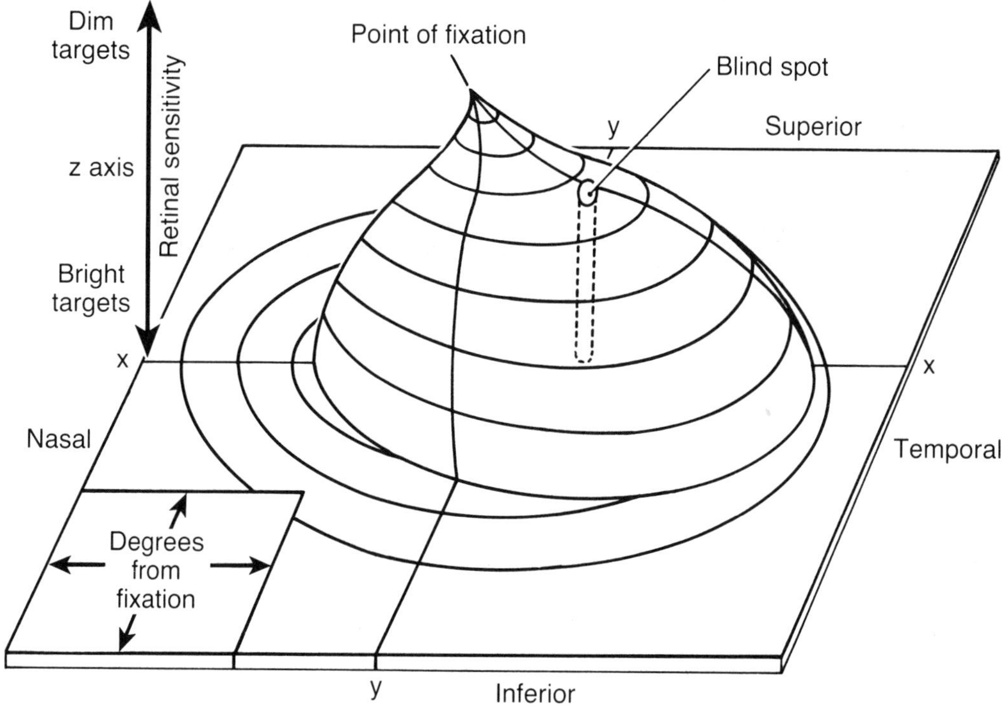


**Fig. 6-1** The hill of vision as represented on a three-dimensional plot of retinal sensitivity (z axis) and location in the visual field (x and y axes) in terms of degrees from fixation. (From Anderson, 1987, with permission.)

For example, the Octopus uses the following formula:

$$dB = 10 \times \log(1000/asb)$$

The Humphrey perimeter uses a different formula:

$$dB = 10 \times \log(10{,}000/asb)$$

V. In addition to varying target brightness, most perimeters can also produce targets of different size. Goldmann perimetry uses a code involving Roman numerals, Arabic numerals, and letters to describe the size and brightness of the targets. This nomenclature has become the standard method for describing perimetric targets. The Goldman equivalents are as follows:

A. Target size

$$I = 0.25\ mm^2$$
$$II = 1.00\ mm^2$$
$$III = 4.00\ mm^2$$
$$IV = 16.00\ mm^2$$
$$V = 64.00\ mm^2$$

B. Target brightness (luminance)

| | |
|---|---|
| 4e = 1000 asb = 0 dB | 2e = 100 asb = 10 dB |
| 4d = 800 asb = 1 dB | 2d = 80 asb = 11 dB |
| 4c = 630 asb = 2 dB | 2c = 63 asb = 12 dB |
| 4b = 500 asb = 3 dB | 2b = 50 asb = 13 dB |
| 4a = 400 asb = 4 dB | 2a = 40 asb = 14 dB |
| 3e = 315 asb | 1e = 32 asb |

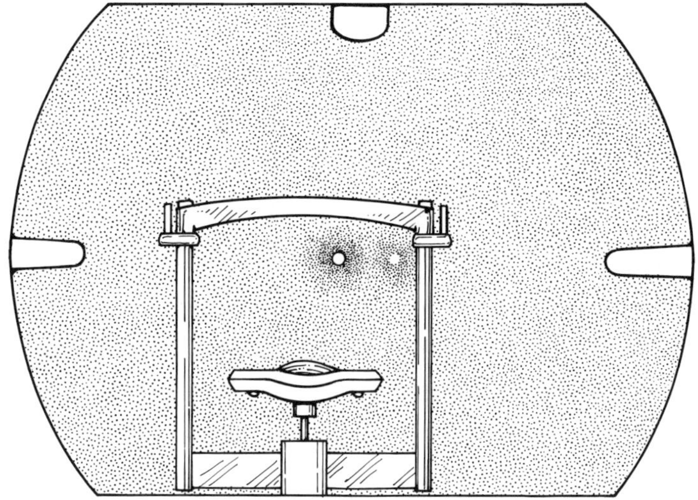

**Fig. 6-2** The bowl of a Goldmann perimeter showing the contrast between the luminance of the test target and the background. The bright light near the center is the fixation target. The dimmer light to the right is the test target. The difference between the luminance of the test target and the background is expressed in apostilbs and the value is often converted to decibels. By varying the contrast between target and background, a patient's threshold can be determined at multiple locations in the visual field.

3e = 5 dB
3d = 252 asb
= 6 dB
3c = 198 asb
= 7 dB
3b = 158 asb
= 8 dB
3a = 126 asb
= 9 dB

= 15 dB
1d = 25 asb
= 16 dB
1c = 20 asb
= 17 dB
1b = 16 asb
= 18 dB
1a = 13 asb
= 19 dB

Decibel equivalents are not generally used with manual perimetry. They are given here only for comparison with automated perimeters.

### Difference between Threshold and Sensitivity

I. Threshold is a property of the target. High-threshold targets are very bright. A threshold target is just bright enough to be seen 50% of the time it is presented in a particular location.
   A. Suprathreshold targets are brighter than threshold and in theory should always be seen.
   B. Infrathreshold targets are dimmer than threshold and in theory should never be seen.

II. Sensitivity is a property of the retina and is measured by determining the threshold in different areas.

III. There is an inverse relationship between threshold and sensitivity. If the threshold is very high in a particular area (i.e., only very bright targets can be seen), sensitivity in that area is very low.

## GLAUCOMATOUS FIELD DEFECTS

I. Localized defects are almost all of the nerve fiber bundle variety.
   A. The appearance and location of the visual field defects seen in glaucoma

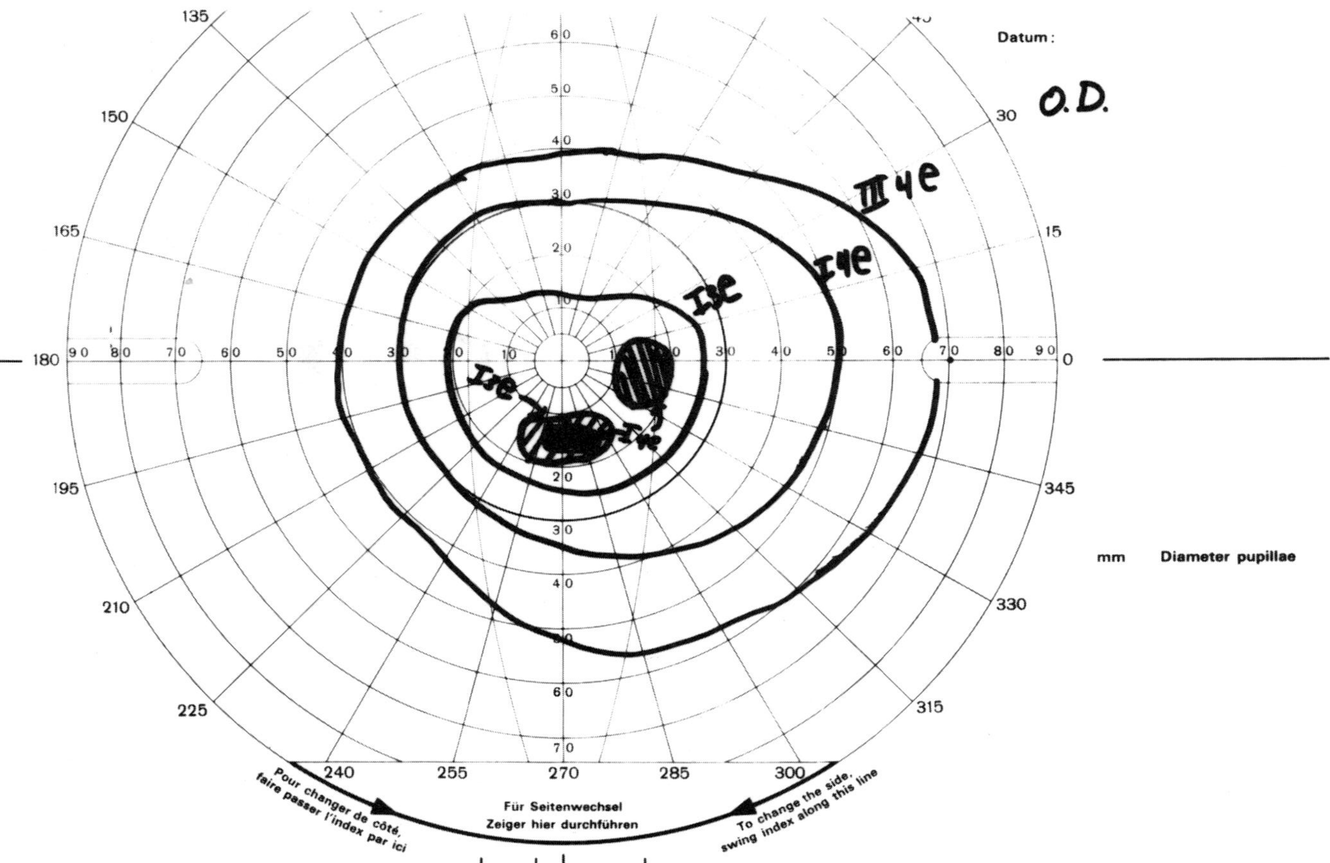


**Fig. 6-3** Example of a paracentral scotoma with a dense nucleus below fixation found using manual kinetic perimetry in a patient with glaucoma.

are determined by the anatomy of the retinal nerve fiber layer and the optic nerve head (see Fig. 5-3).

B. Arcuate and paracentral defects (Figs. 6-3 to 6-6) occur within 20° of fixation. These defects can be quite close to fixation, especially on the temporal side and may involve fixation with loss of central vision, although this is unusual until late in the disease.

C. Nasal steps (Figs. 6-7, 6-8) may occur centrally or peripherally and are often associated with scotomas near the nasal horizontal in the midperiphery.

D. Temporal sector defects (Figs. 6-9, 6-10) are unusual as isolated findings, but often occur in association with other defects.

E. Blind spot enlargement (Figs. 6-11, 6-12) is often found in glaucoma patients.

II. Diffuse defects are much less specific

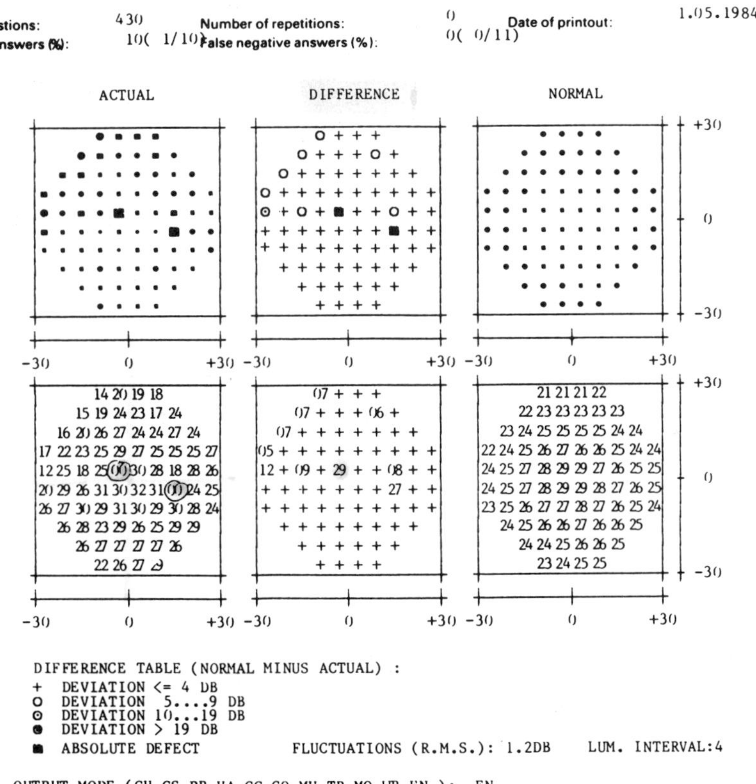


| Symb. | | | | | | | | | |
|---|---|---|---|---|---|---|---|---|---|
| dB | 51–36 | 35–31 | 30–26 | 25–21 | 20–16 | 15–11 | 10–6 | 5–1 | 0 |
| asb | 0,008–0,25 | 0,31–0,8 | 1–2,5 | 3,1–8 | 10–25 | 31–80 | 100–250 | 315–800 | 1000 |

A 1 asb = 0,318 cd/m²

**Fig. 6-4** Example of a paracentral scotoma just above and nasal to fixation found in the right eye of a patient with glaucoma using automated static perimetry. The box on the lower left of the comparison printout (**A**) represents the actual threshold values in decibels at the 76 test locations tested in this program. The double zero on the right in this box is the blind spot. The double zero to the upper left of the center is the scotoma. The central box shows the difference between the measured thresholds and the age corrected normal values (shown in the right box). The scotoma is represented by the number 29. (*Figure continues.*)

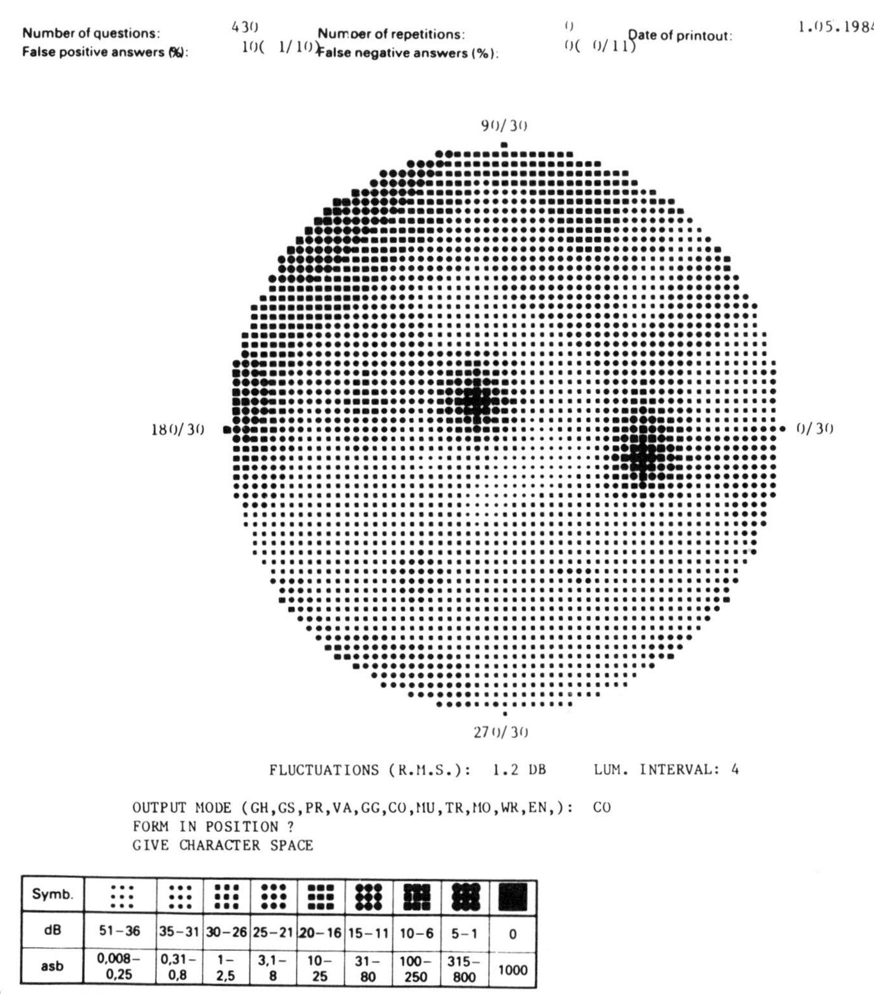


| Symb. | | | | | | | | | |
|---|---|---|---|---|---|---|---|---|---|
| dB | 51–36 | 35–31 | 30–26 | 25–21 | 20–16 | 15–11 | 10–6 | 5–1 | 0 |
| asb | 0,008–0,25 | 0,31–0,8 | 1–2,5 | 3,1–8 | 10–25 | 31–80 | 100–250 | 315–800 | 1000 |

B 1 asb = 0,318 cd/m²

**Fig. 6-4** (*Continued*). (**B**) The gray-scale interpolation provides a visual representation of the threshold values as a gray-scale code. The blind spot is the dark area to the right, while the scotoma is the dark area to the left.

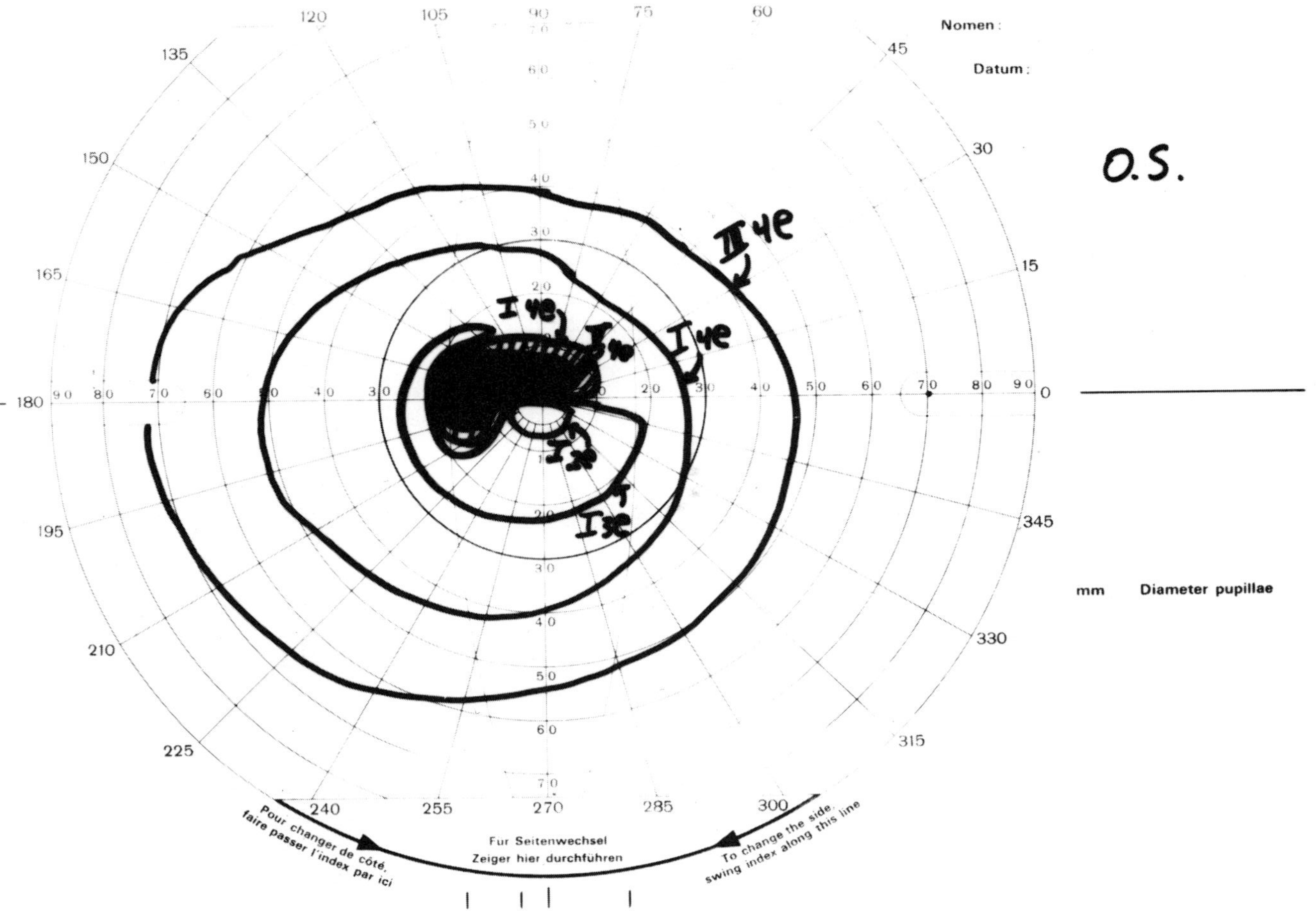


**Fig. 6-5** Manual kinetic perimetry shows a dense arcuate or Bjerrum-type scotoma arising from the superior portion of the blind spot in the left eye of a glaucoma patient.

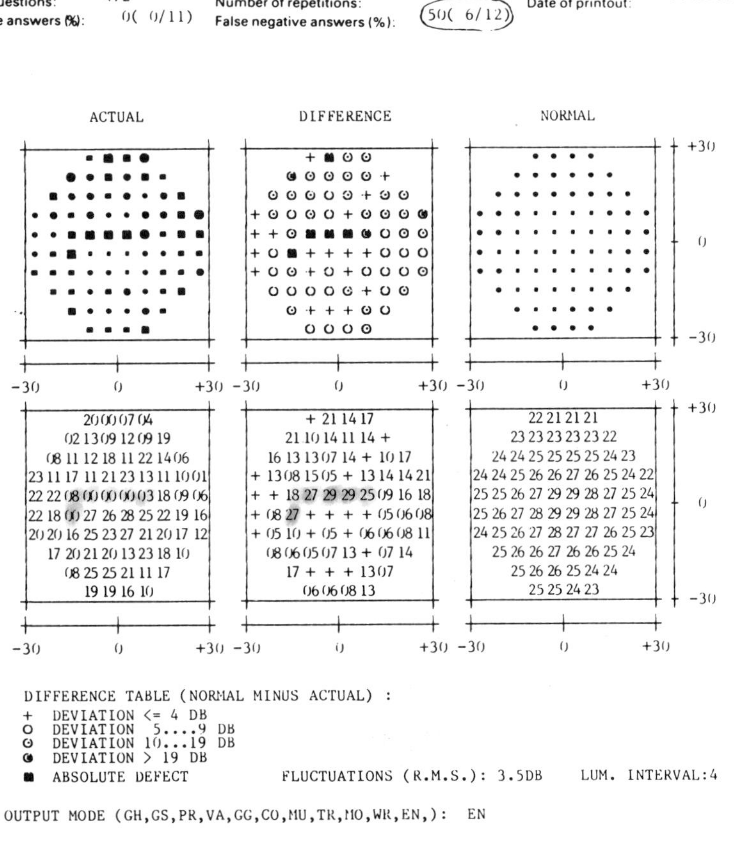


| Symb. | | | | | | | | | |
|---|---|---|---|---|---|---|---|---|---|
| dB | 51–36 | 35–31 | 30–26 | 25–21 | 20–16 | 15–11 | 10–6 | 5–1 | 0 |
| asb | 0,008–0,25 | 0,31–0,8 | 1–2,5 | 3,1–8 | 10–25 | 31–80 | 100–250 | 315–800 | 1000 |

A 1 asb = 0,318 cd/m²

**Fig. 6-6** (**A**) Automated static perimetry of the same patient in Figure 6-5 shows a dense superior arcuate scotoma. (*Figure continues.*)

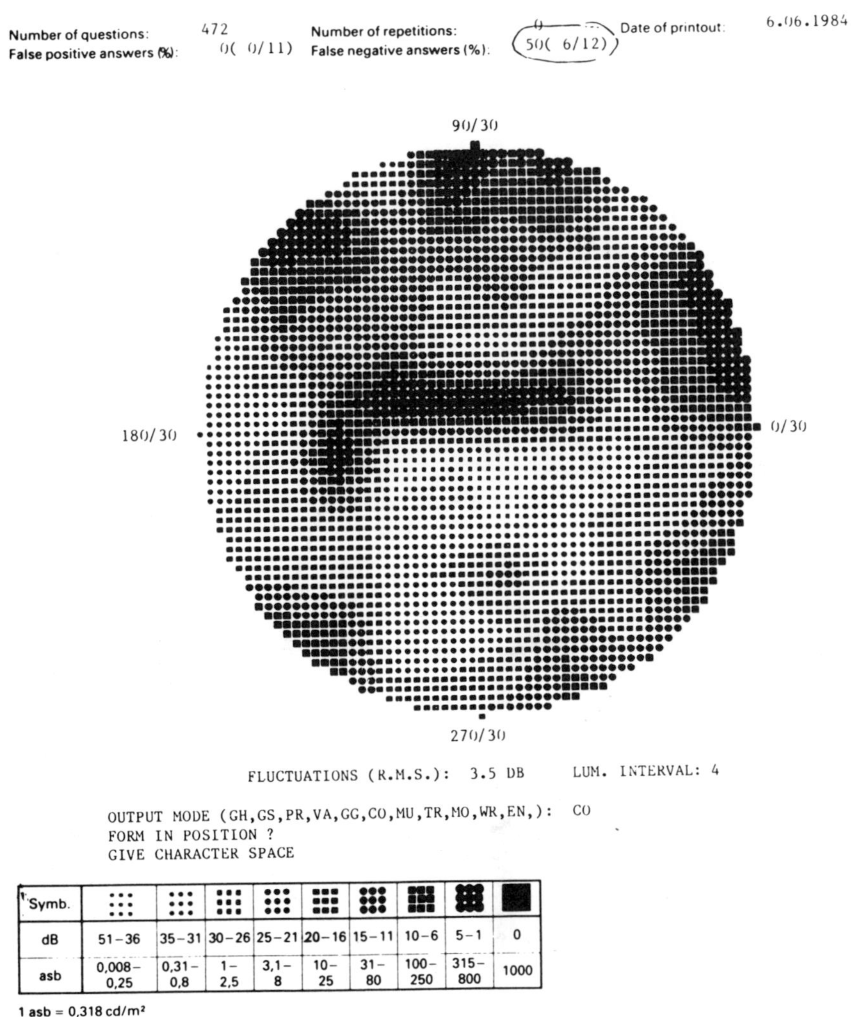


| Symb. | | | | | | | | | |
|---|---|---|---|---|---|---|---|---|---|
| dB | 51–36 | 35–31 | 30–26 | 25–21 | 20–16 | 15–11 | 10–6 | 5–1 | 0 |
| asb | 0,008–0,25 | 0,31–0,8 | 1–2,5 | 3,1–8 | 10–25 | 31–80 | 100–250 | 315–800 | 1000 |

B 1 asb = 0,318 cd/m²

**Fig. 6-6** (*Continued*). (**B**) Gray-scale interpolation of decibel values shown in Figure A.

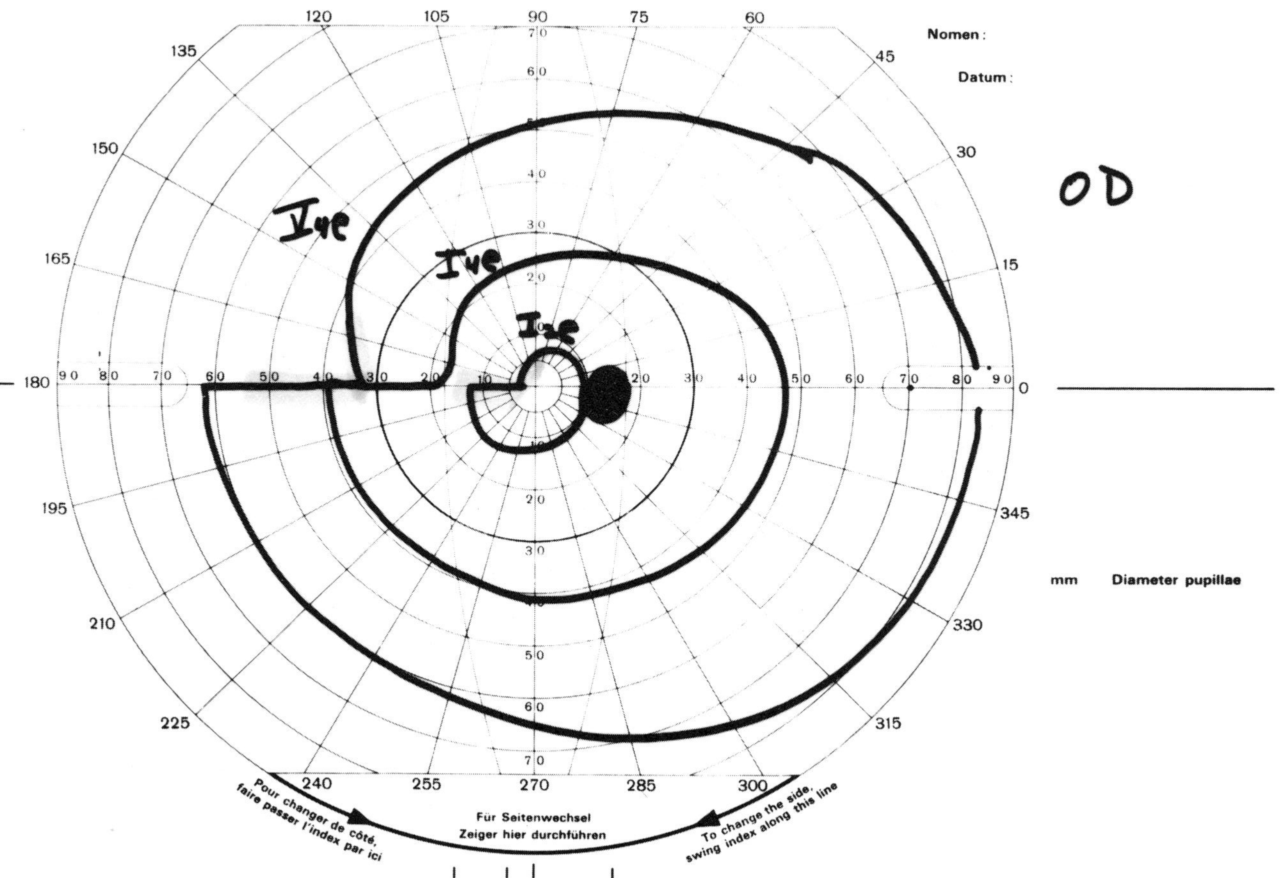


**Fig. 6-7** Superior nasal step seen in the right eye on manual kinetic perimetry.

Number of questions: 463 Number of repetitions: 30 Date of printout: 11.18.1983
False positive answers (%): 0( 0/12) False negative answers (%): 10( 1/10)

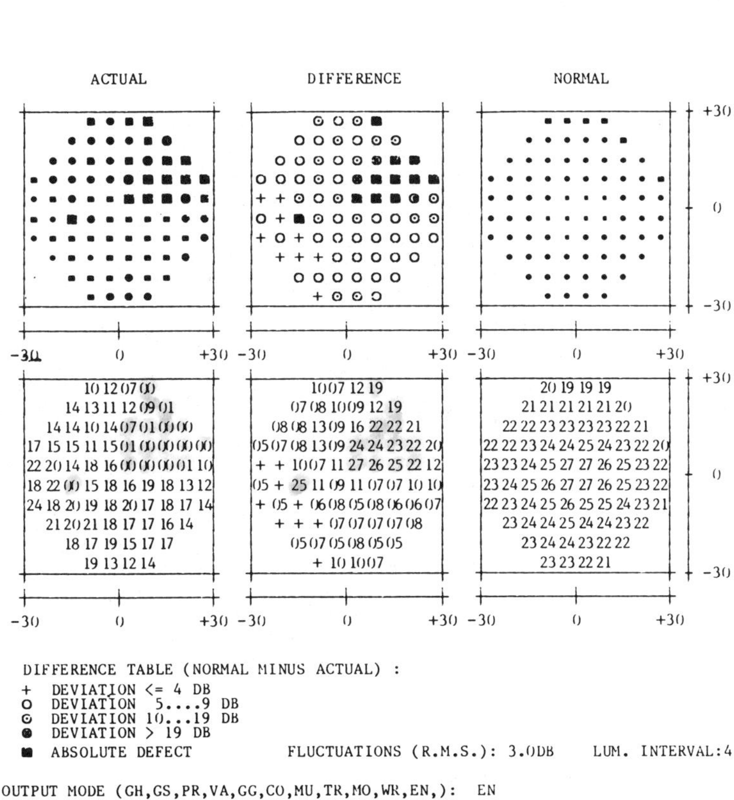


| Symb. | | | | | | | | | |
|---|---|---|---|---|---|---|---|---|---|
| dB | 51–36 | 35–31 | 30–26 | 25–21 | 20–16 | 15–11 | 10–6 | 5–1 | 0 |
| asb | 0,008–0,25 | 0,31–0,8 | 1–2,5 | 3,1–8 | 10–25 | 31–80 | 100–250 | 315–800 | 1000 |

A 1 asb = 0,318 cd/m²

**Fig. 6-8** **(A)** Automated static perimetry shows a dense superior nasal step in the left eye of a glaucoma patient. Nasal steps generally show a sharp edge at the horizontal meridian. (*Figure continues.*)

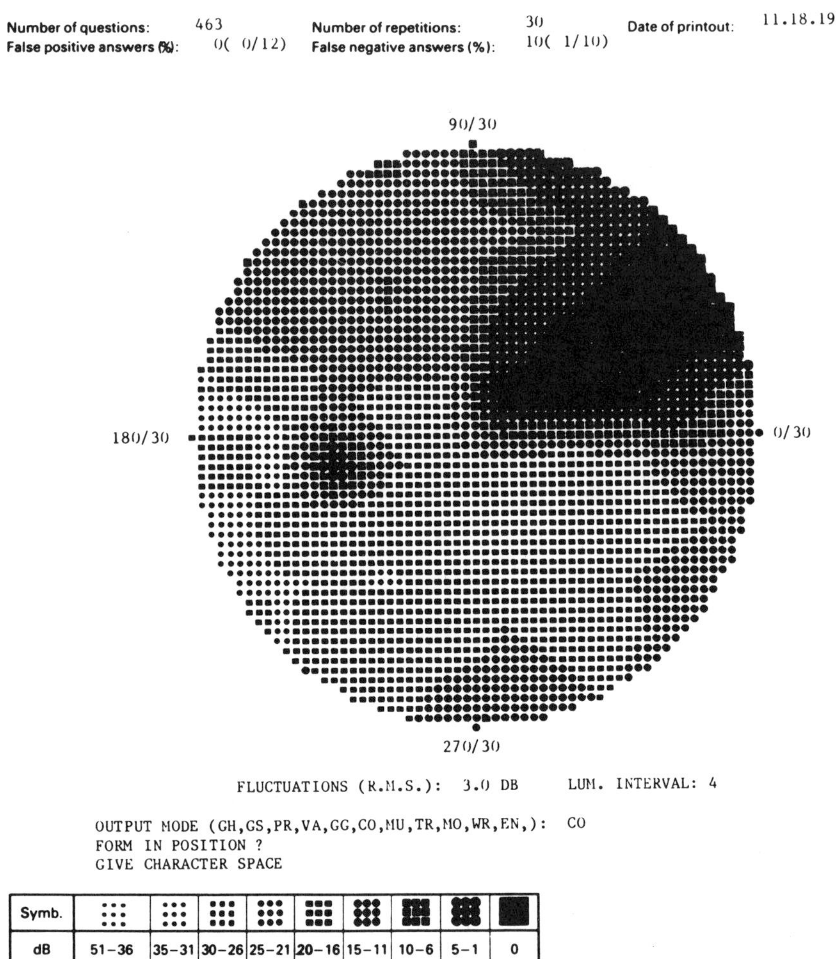


| Symb. | | | | | | | | | |
|---|---|---|---|---|---|---|---|---|---|
| dB | 51–36 | 35–31 | 30–26 | 25–21 | 20–16 | 15–11 | 10–6 | 5–1 | 0 |
| asb | 0,008–0,25 | 0,31–0,8 | 1–2,5 | 3,1–8 | 10–25 | 31–80 | 100–250 | 315–800 | 1000 |

B 1 asb = 0,318 cd/m²

**Fig. 6-8** (*Continued*). (**B**) Gray-scale interpolation of decibel values shown in Figure A.

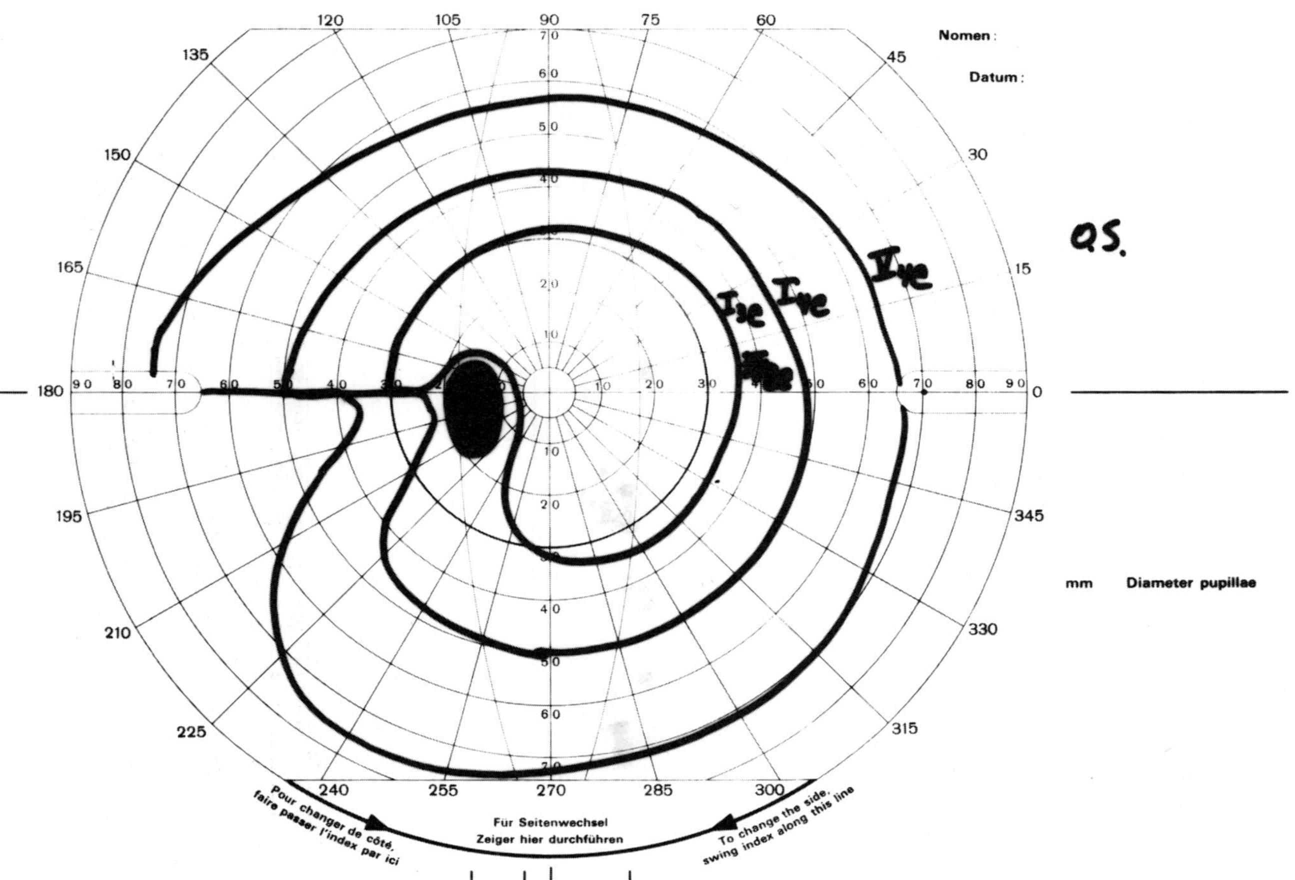


**Fig. 6-9** Unusual isolated temporal sector seen in the left eye of a glaucoma patient with manual kinetic perimetry.

Number of questions: 494 Number of repetitions: 0 Date of printout: 1.26.1987
False positive answers (%): 25( 3/12) False negative answers (%): 25( 3/12)

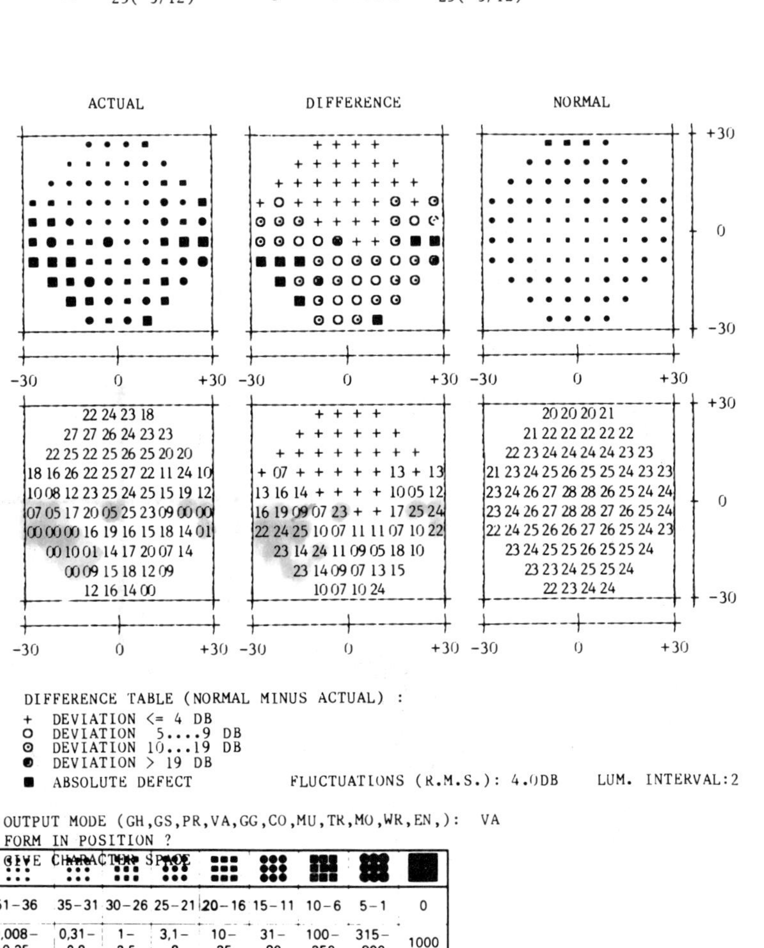


| Symb. | | | | | | | | | |
|---|---|---|---|---|---|---|---|---|---|
| dB | 51–36 | 35–31 | 30–26 | 25–21 | 20–16 | 15–11 | 10–6 | 5–1 | 0 |
| asb | 0,008–0,25 | 0,31–0,8 | 1–2,5 | 3,1–8 | 10–25 | 31–80 | 100–250 | 315–800 | 1000 |

A 1 asb = 0,318 cd/m²

**Fig. 6-10** (**A**) Automated static visual field of the right eye of a glaucoma patient shows a temporal sector defect at the lower right periphery of the field. There is also an inferior paracentral scotoma and nasal step in this figure. (*Figure continues.*)

Number of questions: 494 Number of repetitions: 0 Date of printout: 1.26.1987
False positive answers (%): 25( 3/12) False negative answers (%): 25( 3/12)

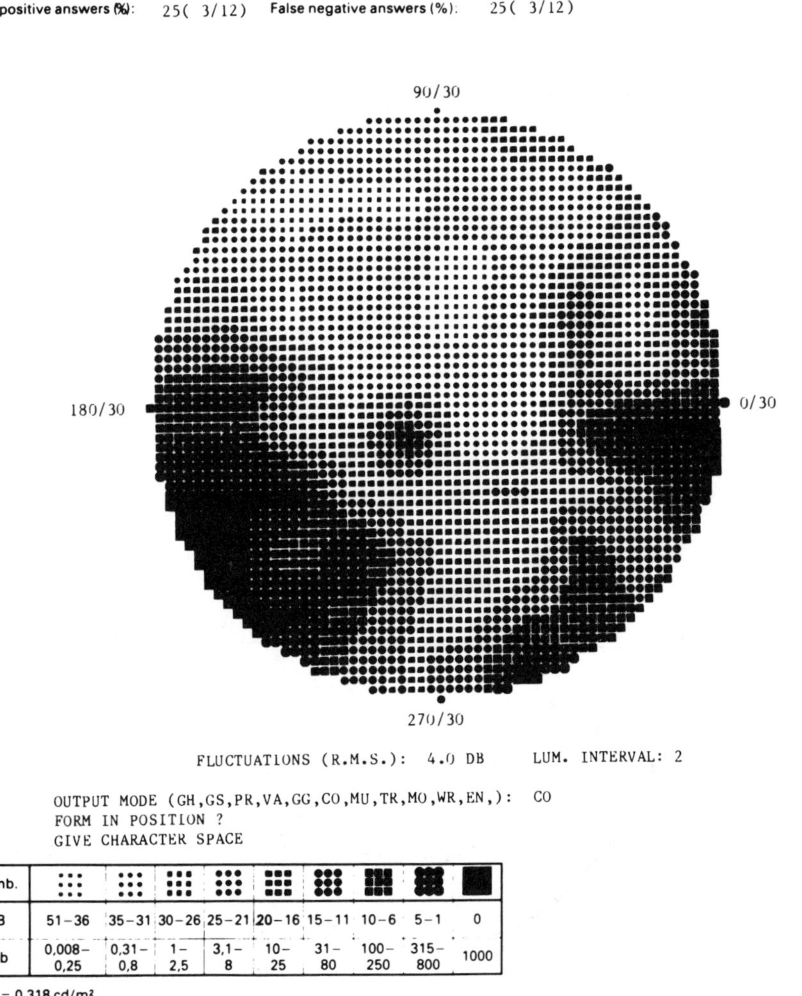


FLUCTUATIONS (R.M.S.): 4.0 DB LUM. INTERVAL: 2

OUTPUT MODE (GH,GS,PR,VA,GG,CO,MU,TR,MO,WR,EN,): CO
FORM IN POSITION ?
GIVE CHARACTER SPACE

| Symb. | | | | | | | | | |
|---|---|---|---|---|---|---|---|---|---|
| dB | 51–36 | 35–31 | 30–26 | 25–21 | 20–16 | 15–11 | 10–6 | 5–1 | 0 |
| asb | 0,008–0,25 | 0,31–0,8 | 1–2,5 | 3,1–8 | 10–25 | 31–80 | 100–250 | 315–800 | 1000 |

B 1 asb = 0,318 cd/m²

**Fig. 6-10** (*Continued*). (**B**) Gray-scale interpolation of decibel values shown in Figure A.

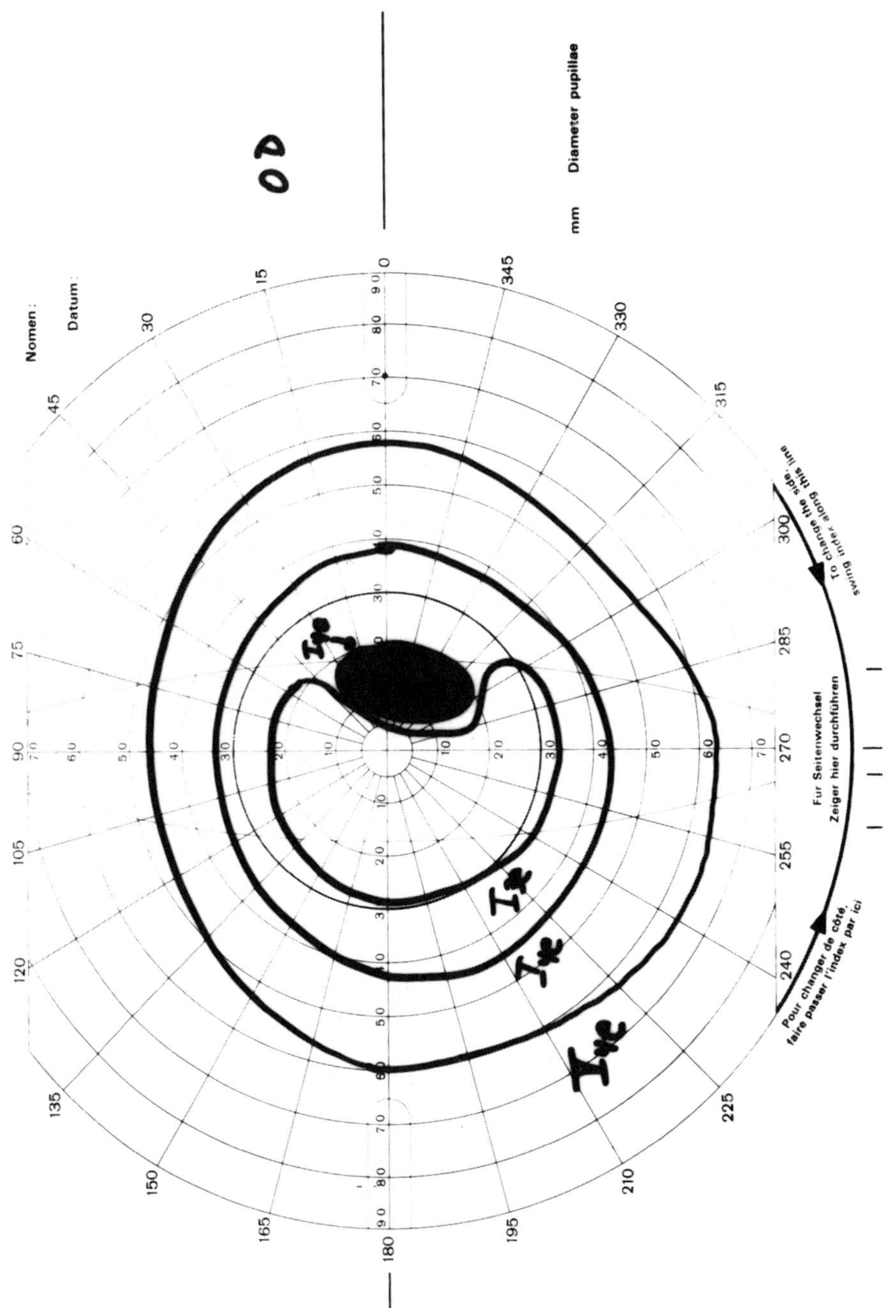


Fig. 6-11 Marked enlargement of the blind spot seen on manual perimetry.

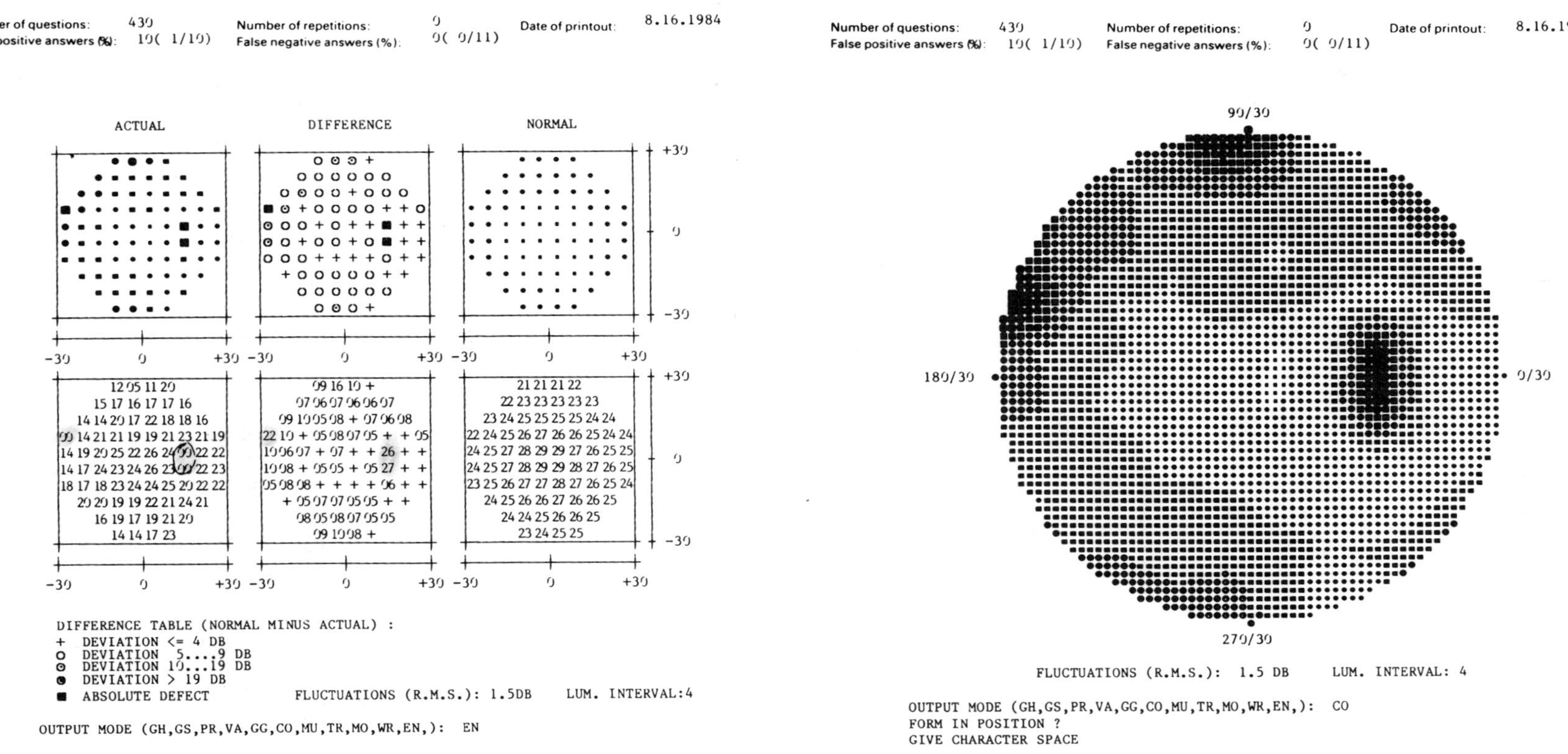


**Fig. 6-12 (A, B)** Enlargement of the blind spot seen on automated perimetry (right eye). This visual field also shows some generalized depression of sensitivity as well as a superior nasal defect.

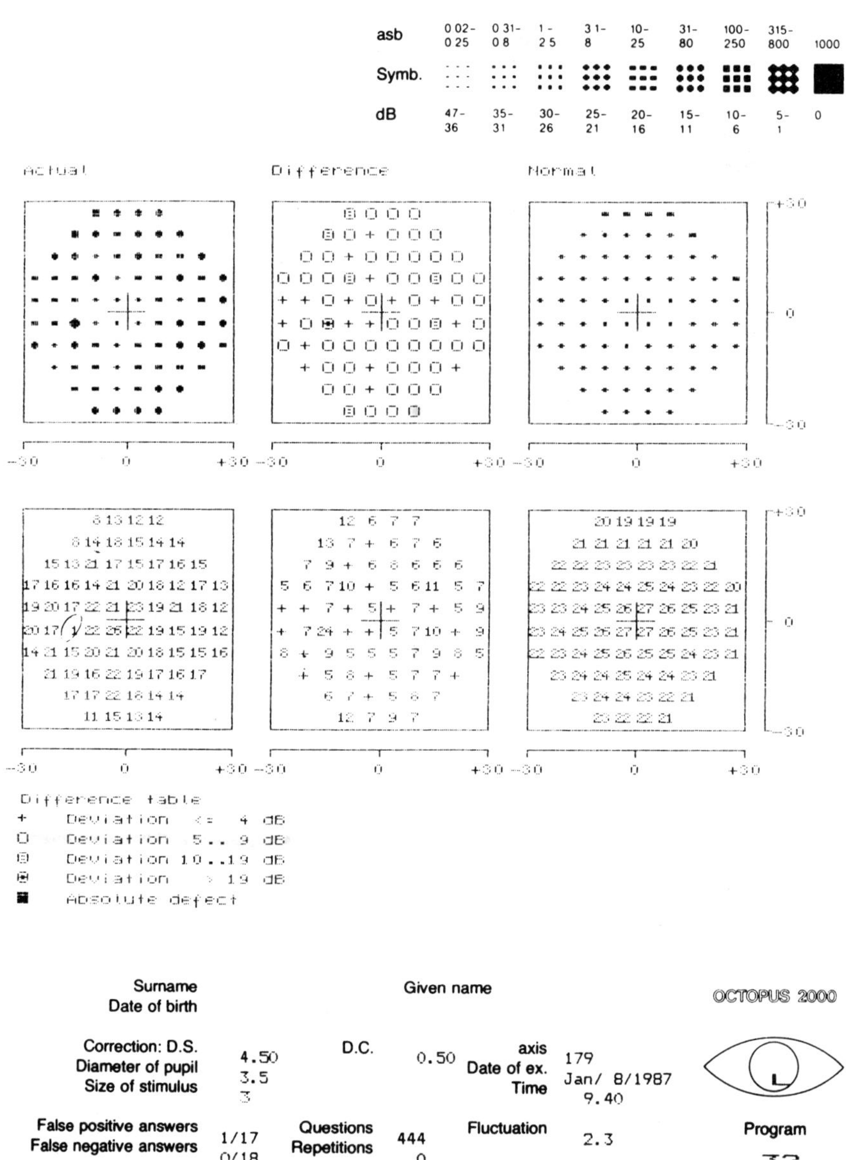


**Fig. 6-13** (**A**) Automated visual field shows a mild, generalized loss of sensitivity. This is best seen in the middle box of the comparison print-out where most test locations are depressed between 5 and 10 dB compared to the age-corrected normal values. (*Figure continues.*)

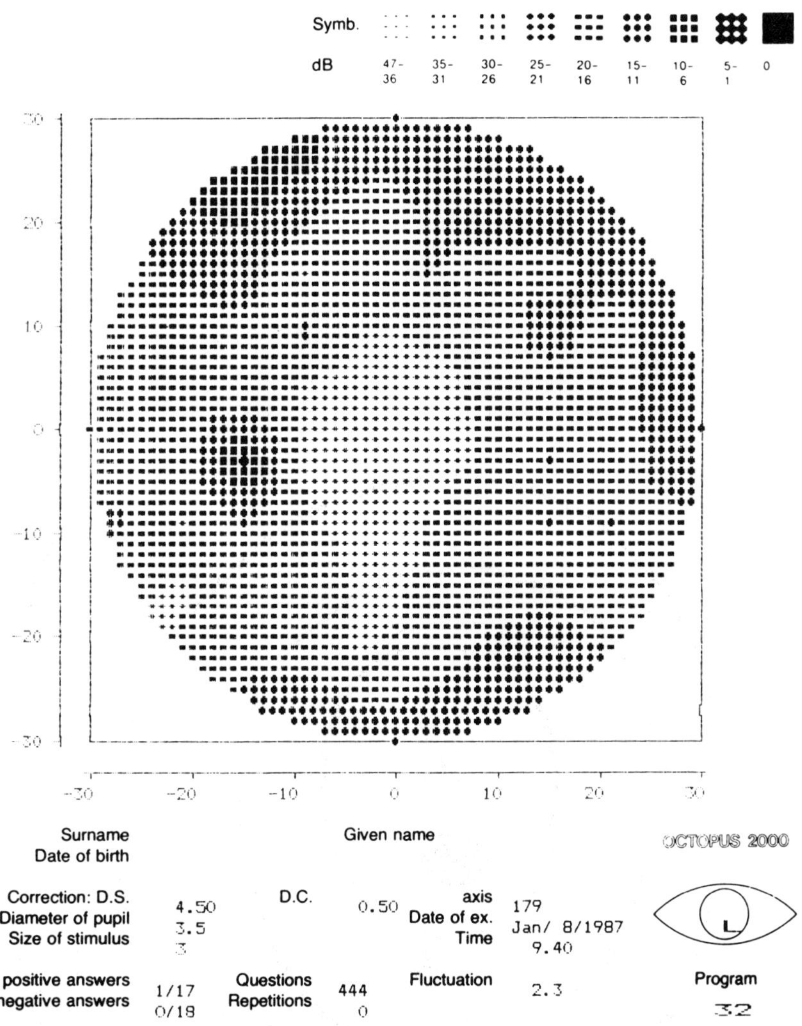


**Fig. 6-13** (*Continued*). (**B**) Gray-scale interpolation of decibel values shown in Figure A.

but are often also found.

A. Generalized loss of sensitivity (Fig. 6-13, 6-14) has many causes, of which glaucoma is only one.

B. Nasal contraction (Fig. 6-15) appears to be somewhat more specific for glaucoma.

III. Advanced or end-stage defects (Figs. 6-16 to 6-18) can appear quite irregular. There may be two or more islands of vision that are not connected. If a central island of vision is retained, visual acuity may be good.

IV. Differential diagnosis of visual field defects resembling those of glaucoma

A. Nonglaucomatous nerve-fiber-bundle-like defects

1. Lesions of the retina

a) Juxtapapillary choroiditis

b) Myopia with peripapillary atrophy

c) Branch retinal artery or vein occlusions

d) Focal retinal lesions such as

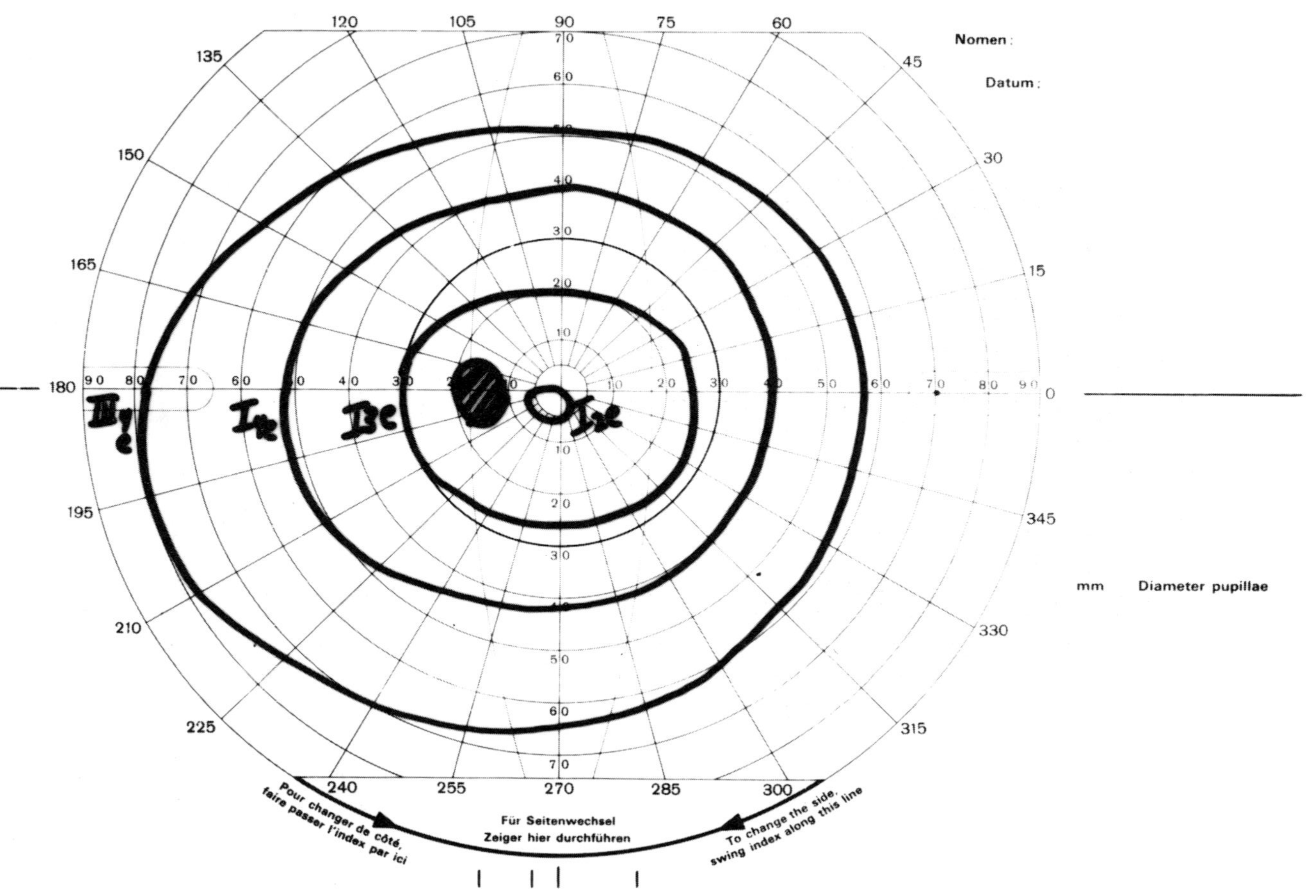


**Fig. 6-14** Generalized depression of the visual field (**A**) on manual perimetry. All of the isopters are smaller than one would expect when compared with a completely normal visual field (**B**). (*Figure continues.*)

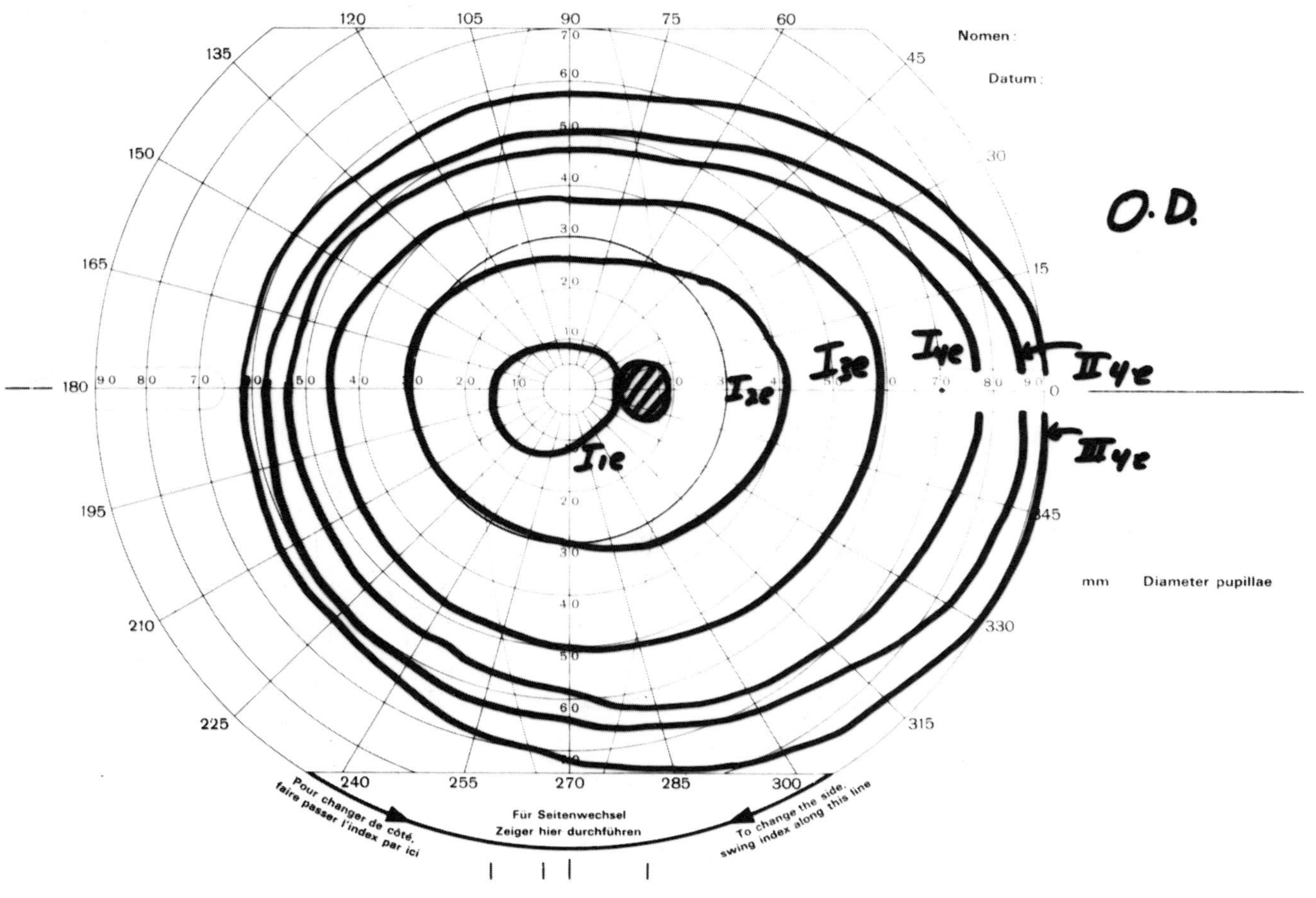


Fig. 6-14 (*Continued*). (B)

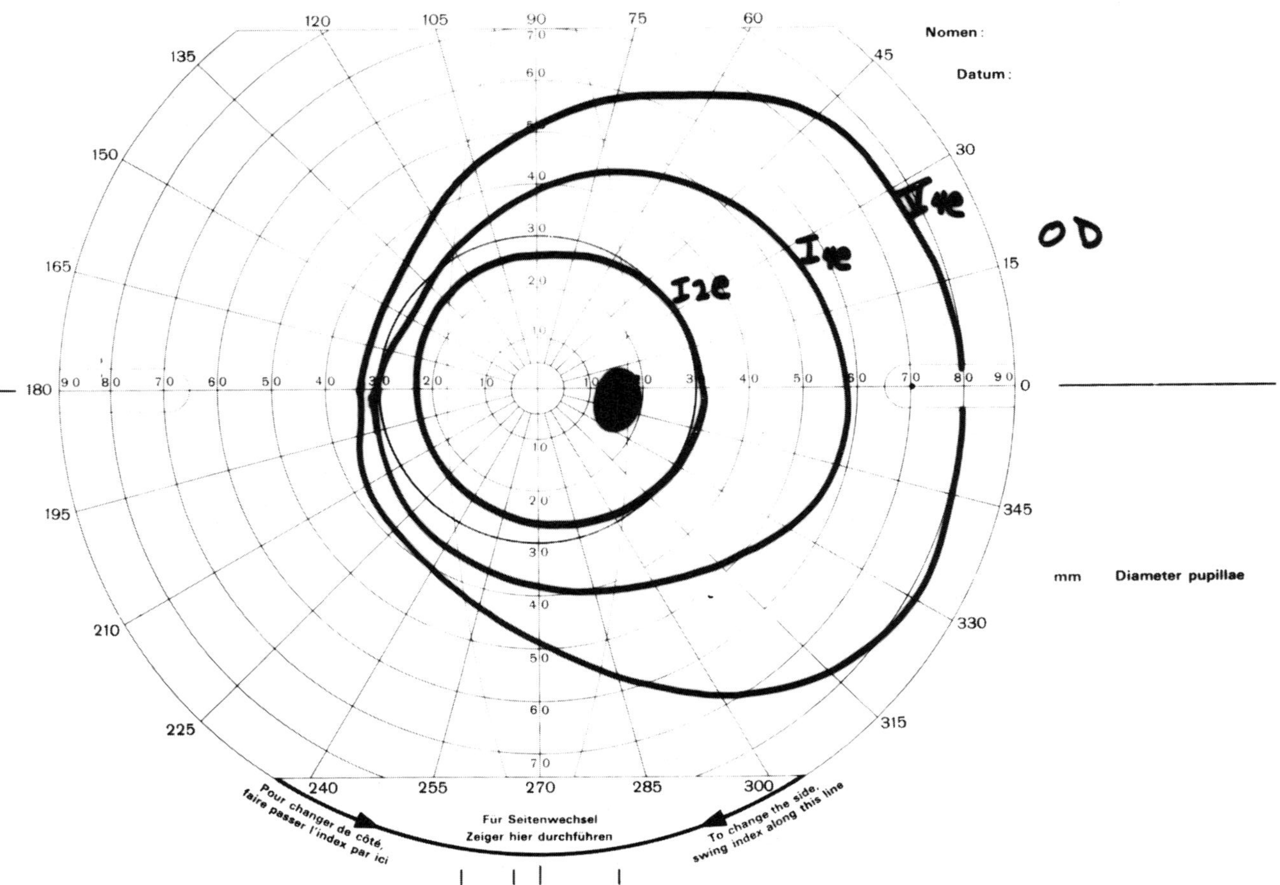


**Fig. 6-15** Contraction of the nasal isopters seen on manual perimetry in the right eye of a glaucoma patient. There is a loss of sensitivity in the nasal half of the field without an actual nasal step being present.

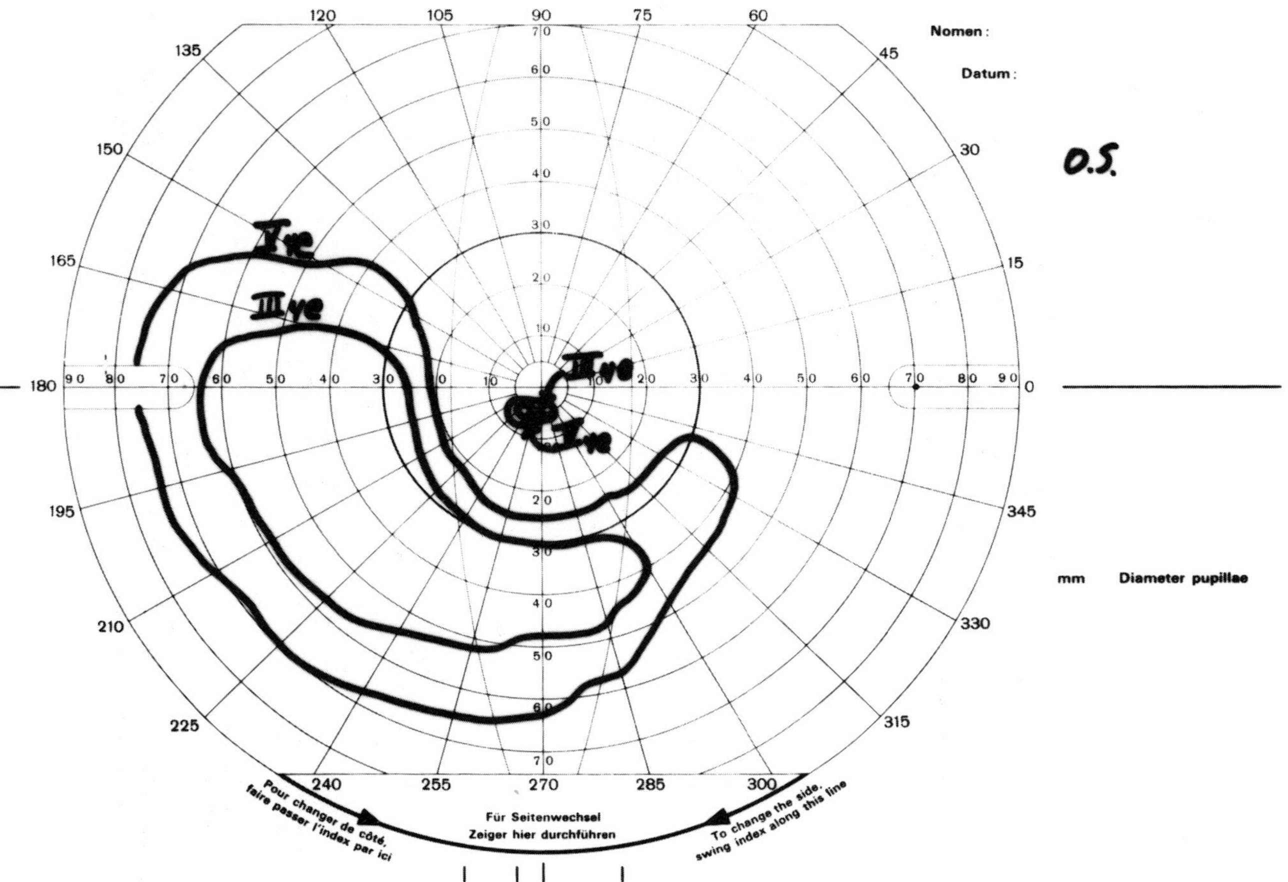


**Fig. 6-16** The left eye of a patient shows advanced glaucomatous field loss. Two arcuate scotomas arise superiorly and inferiorly from the blind spot. These have joined to break the field into central and temporal islands.

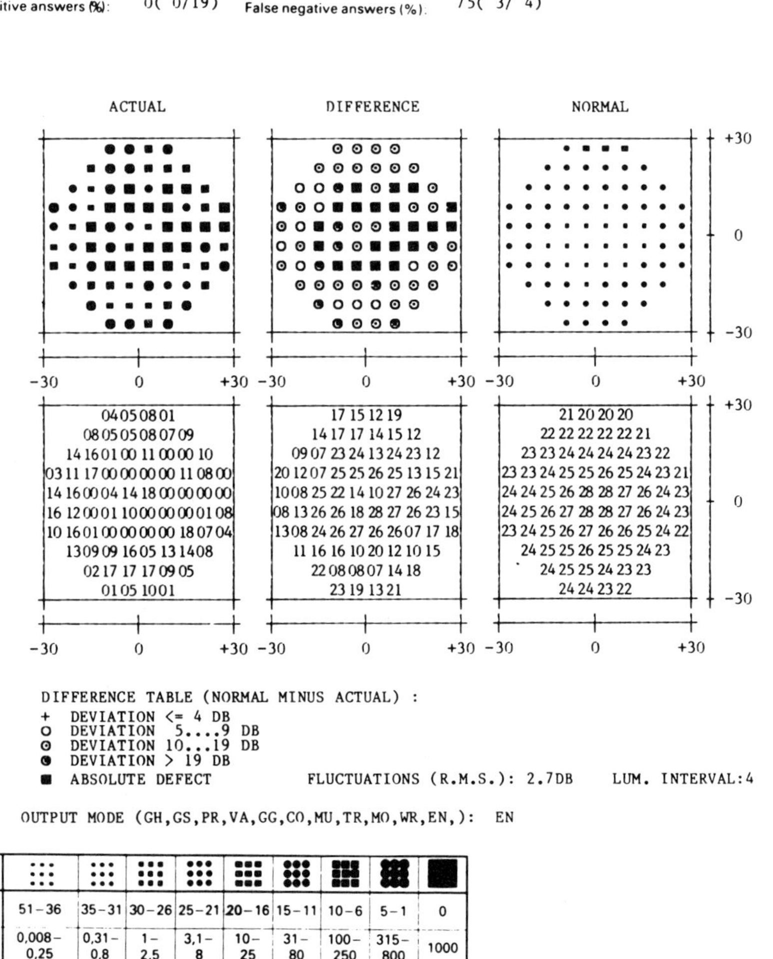


**Fig. 6-17** **(A)** Automated visual field of the left eye of a patient similar to that in Figure 6-16. A double arcuate scotoma produces disconnected central and peripheral islands of vision. (*Figure continues.*)

Number of questions: 477 Number of repetitions: 0 Date of printout: 2.15.1985
False positive answers (%): 0( 0/19) False negative answers (%): 75( 3/ 4)

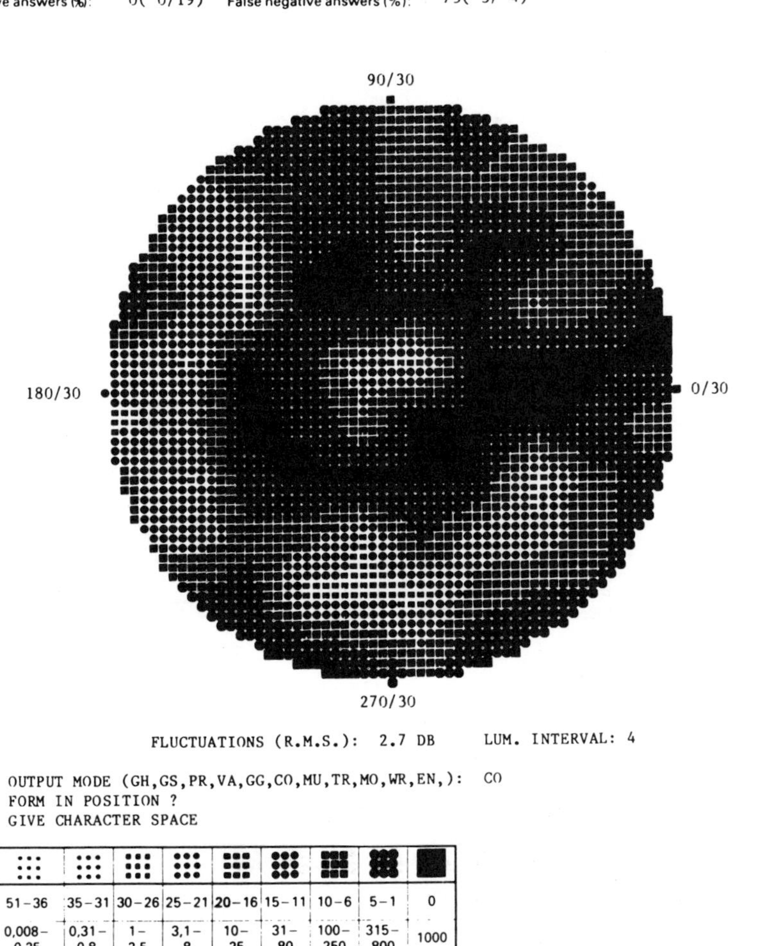


| Symb. | | | | | | | | | |
|---|---|---|---|---|---|---|---|---|---|
| dB | 51–36 | 35–31 | 30–26 | 25–21 | 20–16 | 15–11 | 10–6 | 5–1 | 0 |
| asb | 0,008–0,25 | 0,31–0,8 | 1–2,5 | 3,1–8 | 10–25 | 31–80 | 100–250 | 315–800 | 1000 |

B 1 asb = 0,318 cd/m²

**Fig. 6-17** (*Continued*). (**B**) Gray-scale interpolation of decibel values shown in Figure A.

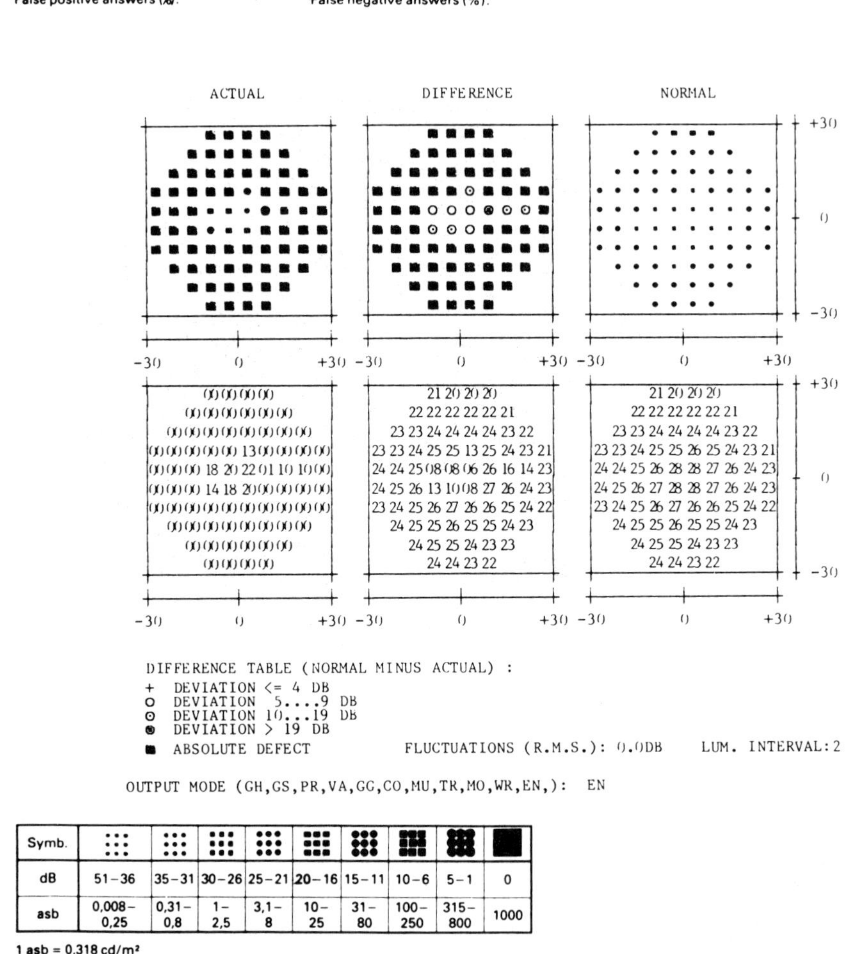


**Fig. 6-18** (**A**) Automated visual field of the left eye of a patient shows complete loss of the peripheral field with only a small central island of vision remaining.

Number of questions: 233 Number of repetitions: 0 Date of printout: 1.09.1984
False positive answers (%): 0( 0/ 11) False negative answers (%): 0( 0/ 0)

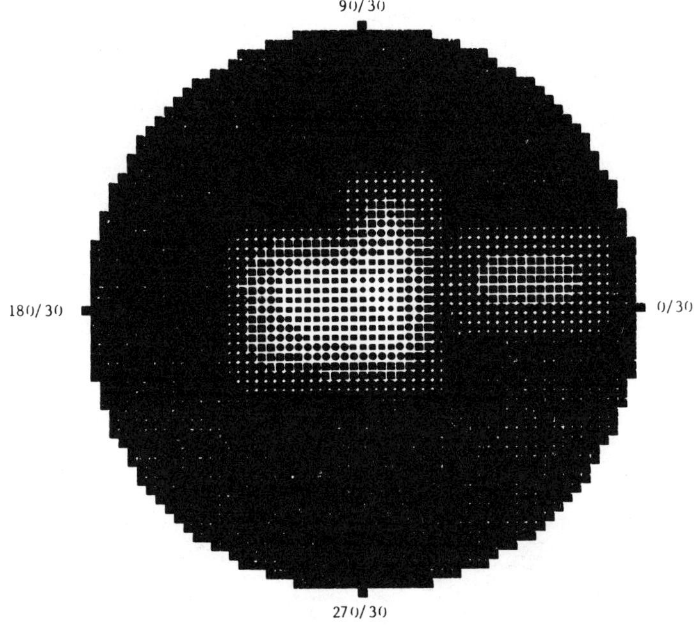


FLUCTUATIONS (R.M.S.): 0.0 DB LUM. INTERVAL: 2

OUTPUT MODE (GH,GS,PR,VA,GG,CO,MU,TR,MO,WR,EN,): CO
FORM IN POSITION ?
GIVE CHARACTER SPACE

| Symb. | | | | | | | | | |
|---|---|---|---|---|---|---|---|---|---|
| dB | 51–36 | 35–31 | 30–26 | 25–21 | 20–16 | 15–11 | 10–6 | 5–1 | 0 |
| asb | 0,008–0,25 | 0,31–0,8 | 1–2,5 | 3,1–8 | 10–25 | 31–80 | 100–250 | 315–800 | 1000 |

B 1 asb = 0,318 cd/m²

**Fig. 6-18** (*Continued*). (**B**) Gray-scale interpolation of decibel values shown in Figure A.

toxoplasmosis, infarcts, tumors, etc.
   e) Retinoschisis
   f) Retinitis pigmentosa
2. Lesions of the optic nerve head
   a) Optic disc coloboma
   b) Optic pit
   c) Papilledema with optic atrophy
   d) Optic nerve drusen
   e) Ischemic optic neuropathy and optic nerve infarct
   f) Papillitis
3. Compressive lesions of optic nerve and chiasm

B. Generalized loss of retinal sensitivity
   1. Age is associated with a gradual loss of retinal sensitivity. Otherwise normal elderly patients may have constricted visual fields.
   2. Miosis is associated with an apparent decrease in retinal sensitivity when the pupil size is less

than 3 mm. This effect may be especially pronounced in patients with lens opacities. For this reason, the pupil size should be recorded whenever perimetry is performed.

3. Media opacities
   a) Corneal opacities or edema
   b) Cataract
4. Functional problems
   a) Incorrect refractive correction in the perimeter during the visual field test
   b) Psychiatric illness
   c) Patient inexperience with perimetry
   d) Fatigue
   e) Lack of interest or understanding by patient
   f) Improper room lighting or perimeter calibration
5. Diffuse retinal disease such as diabetic retinopathy or prior panretinal photocoagulation

## DETERMINING IF THE VISUAL FIELD IS NORMAL

I. Clinical correlation with the patient's other findings is essential, especially optic disc appearance. If a visual field defect is present in the absence of optic disc cupping, a diagnosis other than glaucoma should be considered.

II. Comparison with age-corrected normal values

A. Since retinal sensitivity diminishes with age, the visual field must be interpreted in light of the expected findings for the patient's age. Age-corrected normal values are available for manual perimetry in the literature, but are not usually readily at hand in the normal clinical setting. Proper evaluation of manual visual fields depends on the experience of the clinician in having an accurate concept of the normal field (see Fig. 6-14B).

B. Some automated perimeters provide normal values and compare the patient to normal in the printout of the results (Fig. 6-19). The clinician, however, must recognize the considerable variation present in the normal population, especially in older persons. Depressed sensitivity is not necessarily abnormal, even if the perimeter says the sensitivity in a particular portion of the visual field is below the age-corrected norm.

C. Probability maps are available with the Humphrey Visual Field Analyzer, which tell the examiner the probability that any test location is abnormal given its location in the visual field and the age of the patient (Fig. 6-20).

III. Automated perimeters produce a large amount of numeric data when the visual field is measured. In addition the visual field measurements are subject to considerable variability. To facilitate interpretation of the visual field results, a variety of statistical techniques have been applied to visual field data. These are called visual field indices and a knowledge of them may help identify abnormal visual fields. Some automated perimeters will provide printouts of visual field indices. (For more detail see papers by Flammer, Enger and Sommer, and Statpac User's Guide.)

A. Mean sensitivity (MS) is the average threshold value of all the test locations in a single visual field. It can be useful in detecting diffuse changes.

B. Total loss (TL) is the sum of the differences between the age-corrected normal value for each test location and the measured threshold for each test location. In calculating total loss, test locations with differences of less than 4 dB are ignored as are test locations where the threshold measurement is greater than the age

| | | | |
|---|---|---|---|
| Surname, given names: | PUBLIC JOHN Q | | |
| Date of birth: | 12.28.1938 | | |
| Patient number/eye: | K004.83R | | |
| Examination number, date, time: | 1 | 10.14.1983 | 1.20 |
| Correction, (sph., cyl., + axis): | + 3.50 | + 0.00 | + 0 |
| Diameter of pupil, headposition: | 4.00 | 10 | |
| Size of stimulus: | 3 | | |
| Fixationring: | | | |
| Program number: | 32 | | |

| | | | | | |
|---|---|---|---|---|---|
| Number of questions: | 567 | Number of repetitions: | 0 | Date of printout: | 1.19.1987 |
| False positive answers (%): | 0( 0/14) | False negative answers (%): | 0( 0/14) | | |

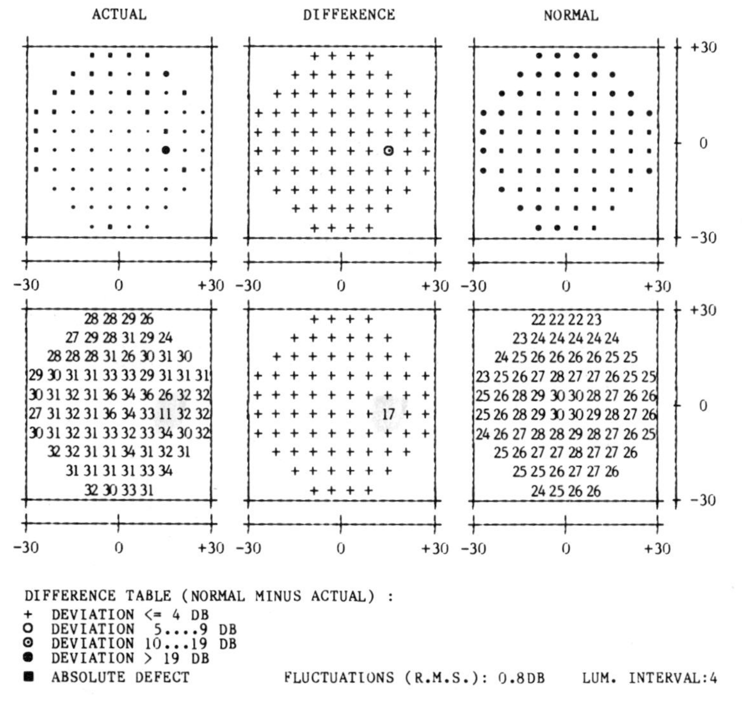


OUTPUT MODE (GH,GS,PR,VA,GG,CO,MU,TR,MO,WR,EN,): VA
FORM IN POSITION ?
GIVE CHARACTER SPACE

| Symb. | | | | | | | | | |
|---|---|---|---|---|---|---|---|---|---|
| dB | 51–36 | 35–31 | 30–26 | 25–21 | 20–16 | 15–11 | 10–6 | 5–1 | 0 |
| asb | 0,008–0,25 | 0,31–0,8 | 1–2,5 | 3,1–8 | 10–25 | 31–80 | 100–250 | 315–800 | 1000 |

A 1 asb = 0,318 cd/m²

**Fig. 6-19** Normal visual field on automated static testing showing (**A**) the comparison, (**B**) gray-scale, and (**C**) threshold value printouts of the Octopus perimeter. Other automated perimeters usually produce similar printouts. The box on the lower left of the comparison printout marked "actual" shows the threshold values in decibels as measured during the test. The box on the lower right marked "normal" shows the expected age-corrected normal values. The box marked difference in the center is the difference between the expected threshold value and the value actually measured. The "17" in the difference box is the location of the blind spot. (*Figure continues.*)

Surname, given names: PUBLIC JOHN Q
Date of birth: 12.28.1938
Patient number/eye: K004.83R
Examination number, date, time: 1 10.14.1983 1.20
Correction, (sph., cyl., + axis): + 3.50 + 0.00 + 0
Diameter of pupil, headposition: 4.00 10
Size of stimulus: 3
Fixationring:
Program number: 32

Number of questions: 567 Number of repetitions: 0 Date of printout: 1.19.1987
False positive answers (%): 0( 0/14) False negative answers (%): 0( 0/14)

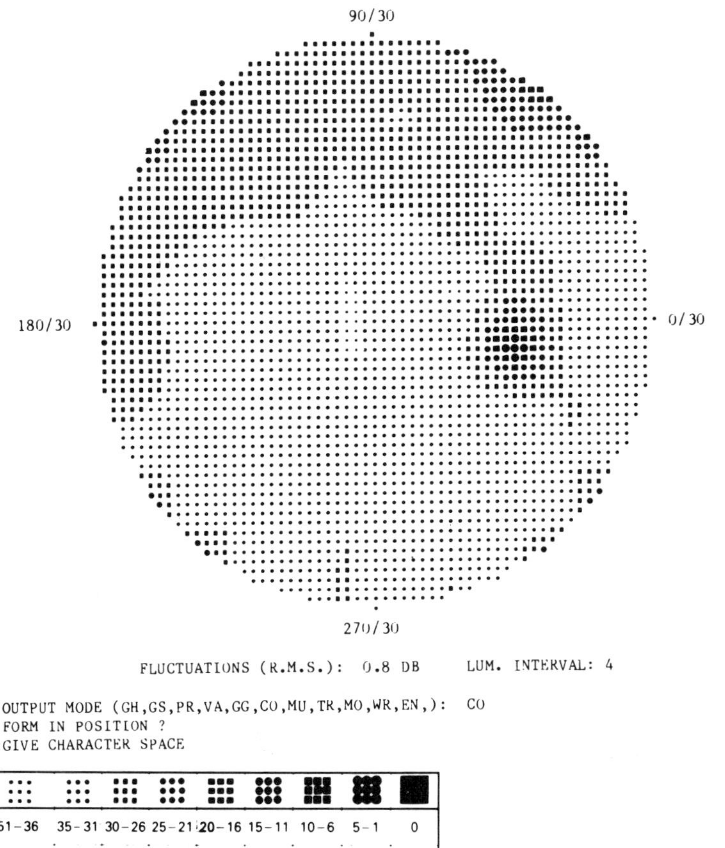


| Symb. | ⁝⁝ | ⁝⁝ | ⁝⁝ | ⁝⁝ | ▪▪ | ●● | ■■ | ●● | ■ |
|---|---|---|---|---|---|---|---|---|---|
| dB | 51–36 | 35–31 | 30–26 | 25–21 | 20–16 | 15–11 | 10–6 | 5–1 | 0 |
| asb | 0,008–0,25 | 0,31–0,8 | 1–2,5 | 3,1–8 | 10–25 | 31–80 | 100–250 | 315–800 | 1000 |

B 1 asb = 0,318 cd/m²

**Fig. 6-19** (*Continued*). The gray-scale printout (**B**) is a graphic representation of the measured threshold values. Each threshold value is assigned a different shade of gray. Areas of low sensitivity (the blind spot or other scotomata) show up as dark areas. Areas of normal sensitivity are lighter. (*Figure continues.*)

Surname, given names: PUBLIC JOHN Q
Date of birth: 12.28.1938
Patient number/eye: K004.83R
Examination number, date, time: 1 10.14.1983 1.20
Correction, (sph., cyl., + axis): + 3.50 + 0.00 + 0
Diameter of pupil, headposition: 4.00 10
Size of stimulus: 3
Fixationring:
Program number: 32

Number of questions: 567 Number of repetitions: 0 Date of printout: 1.19.1987
False positive answers (%): 0( 0/14) False negative answers (%): 0( 0/14)

Y

| | | | | | | | | | | | |
|---|---|---|---|---|---|---|---|---|---|---|---|
| | | | | 28 | 27<br>29 | 29<br>29 | 26 | | | | |
| | | | 27 | 29 | 28 | 31 | 29 | 24 | | | |
| | | 28 | 28 | 28 | 31 | 26 | 30 | 31<br>31 | 30 | | |
| | 29 | 30 | 31 | 31<br>31 | 33 | 33 | 29 | 31 | 31 | 31 | |
| | 30 | 31 | 32 | 31 | 36 | 34 | 36 | 26 | 32 | 32 | |
| X | 26<br>28 | 31 | 32 | 31 | 36 | 34 | 33 | 11 | 32 | 32<br>32 | X |
| | 30 | 31 | 32 | 31 | 33<br>33 | 32<br>32 | 33 | 34 | 30 | 32 | |
| | | 32 | 32 | 31 | 31 | 34 | 31 | 32<br>32 | 31 | | |
| | | | 32<br>30 | 31 | 31 | 31 | 33 | 34 | | | |
| | | | | 32 | 30 | 33 | 31 | | | | |

Y

FLUCTUATIONS (R.M.S.): 0.8 DB LUM. INTERVAL: 4

OUTPUT MODE (GH,GS,PR,VA,GG,CO,MU,TR,MO,WR,EN,): EN

| Symb. | | | | | | | | | |
|---|---|---|---|---|---|---|---|---|---|
| dB | 51–36 | 35–31 | 30–26 | 25–21 | 20–16 | 15–11 | 10–6 | 5–1 | 0 |
| asb | 0,008–<br>0,25 | 0,31–<br>0,8 | 1–<br>2,5 | 3,1–<br>8 | 10–<br>25 | 31–<br>80 | 100–<br>250 | 315–<br>800 | 1000 |

C 1 asb = 0,318 cd/m²

**Fig. 6-19** (*Continued*). The threshold value printout (**C**) shows the actual measured thresholds including the 10 test locations where threshold is determined twice. The root mean square (RMS) is an index of short-term fluctuation and is calculated from the ten doubly determined test locations.

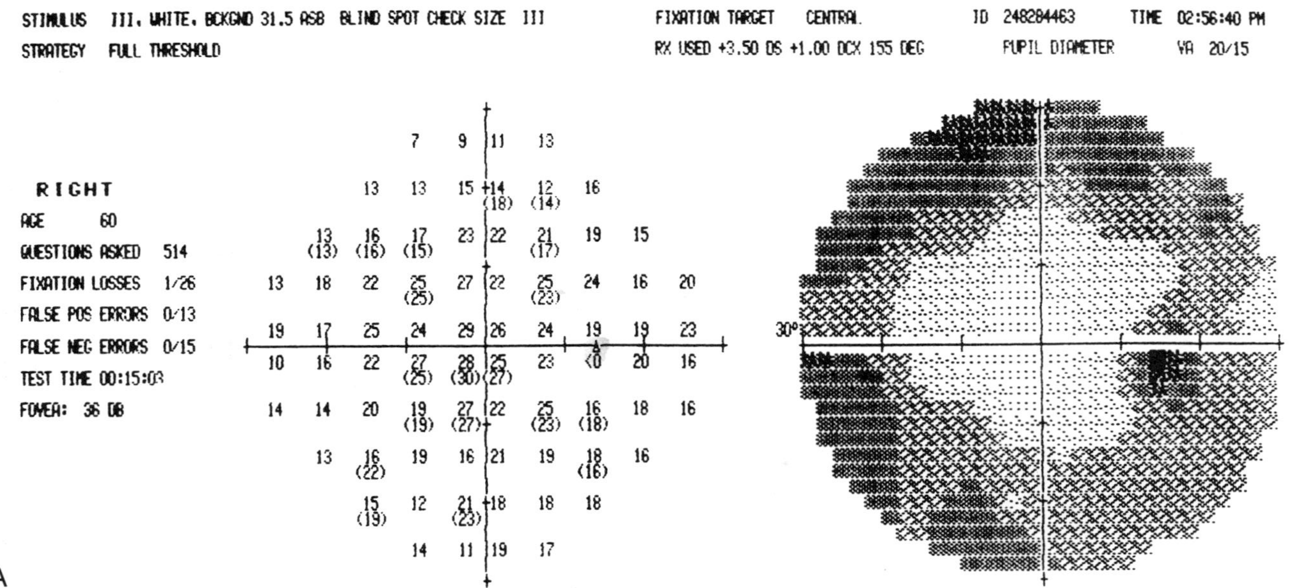


**Fig. 6-20** (**A**) The gray-scale and threshold value printout and (**B**) total and pattern-deviation probability plots of the Humphrey Visual Field Analyzer. The gray-scale and value table show a diffuse depression of retinal sensitivity most pronounced in the periphery of the field. (*Figure continues.*)

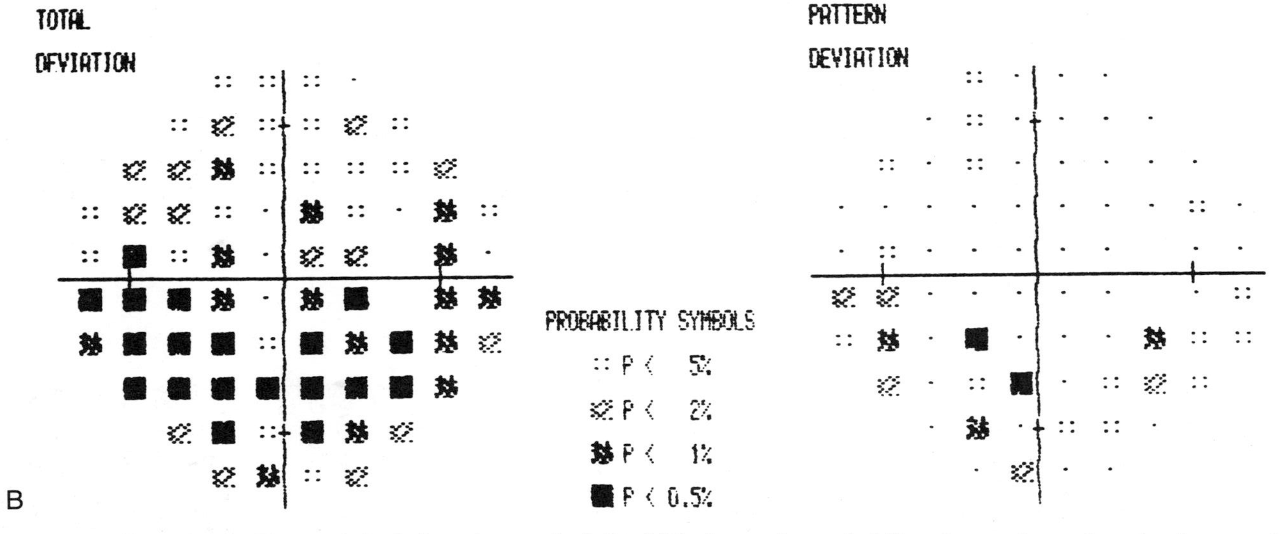


**Fig. 6-20** (*Continued*). The total deviation plot on the left of (**B**) shows the probability that each test location is normal compared to the normal, age-matched population. The darker symbols represent points more likely to be abnormal. The pattern deviation on the right subtracts the effect of any generalized depression and shows the probability of each test location being normal relative to the patient's own hill of vision. In this particular patient, most of the abnormality seen in the total deviation is due to generalized depression. The pattern deviation shows, however, that there is a small, localized nerve-fiber-bundle-type defect in the inferior portion of the visual field that is not seen on simple inspection of the gray-scale and threshold value printout.

corrected normal. Total loss reflects both local and diffuse loss of sensitivity, but does not distinguish between them.

C. Mean defect (MD) is the average difference between the threshold value and the age-corrected normal value for each test location. It is sensitive to generalized depression of the visual field.

D. Short-term fluctuation (SF) is a measure of the variability of the patient's responses during a single visual field examination. Many perimeters provide an estimate of SF as the root mean square (RMS). Calculation of the SF or RMS requires that the threshold at some test locations be determined more than once. (Fig. 6-19C) Caution is necessary in interpreting visual fields with large SF.

E. Corrected loss variance (CLV) measures the local nonuniformity of the visual field corrected for the SF. It is sensitive to the presence of localized defects and tends to ignore diffuse loss.

F. Skewness (Q) measures the distribution of the deviations of measured from expected values. It is sensitive to small changes in a few test locations.

G. Spatial correlation (SC) is similar to the CLV but considers the location of defects. It is sensitive to defects clustered in one area of the visual field.

H. Pattern standard deviation (PSD) is a measure of the uniformity of the visual field and is determined by comparing the shape of the patient's measured field to an age-corrected reference field. A low PSD indicates a smooth hill of vision. A high PSD indicates an irregular hill and may be due to variability in the patient's responses or to actual localized visual field defects.

I. Corrected pattern standard deviation (CPSD) is a measure of the uniformity of the shape of the hill of vision after the effect of short-term fluctuation has been removed. It is similar to the CLV. A high CPSD usually indicates the presence of true localized visual field defects even in the presence of a high SF or generalized loss of sensitivity. The PSD and CPSD are related by

$$CPSD^2 = PSD^2 - SF^2$$

IV. Indices of patient reliability

A. False-positive responses occur when the patient responds to a target that is not there. Detection of false-positive responses requires that the patient be given an auditory clue prior to presentation of the test target.

B. False-negative responses occur when the patient fails to respond to a maximally suprathreshold target that should be seen. Detection of false-negative responses does not require an auditory clue.

C. In order to obtain a reliable visual field, the patient must maintain fixation of the central fixation target during the test. If a patient does not fixate, the visual field results may not be reliable. Fixation loss refers to the patient responding to a target placed in the blind spot. Not all perimeters record this, but all perimeters provide some mechanism for monitoring fixation.

The Octopus perimeter uses an optical detector of eye movements to monitor fixation. The Humphrey perimeter uses suprathreshold targets presented in the blind spot to check fixation losses, and records any patient response to a blind spot target as a fixation loss. The best fixation monitor is probably direct observation of a patient's eye by the perimetrist during the test.

Visual field results must be interpreted in light of the patient's reliability.

## DETECTING PROGRESSIVE CHANGE IN THE VISUAL FIELD

I. At the present time there is no satisfactory technique for detecting progressive visual field loss with great certainty unless the change is quite large.

II. Detection of progressive visual field loss in glaucoma patients is confounded by the existence of long-term fluctuation. Long-term fluctuation (LTF) refers to variability of a patient's visual field response to several examinations performed on different days, usually over a period of weeks or months.
   A. LTF is larger in glaucoma patients than in normals.
   B. LTF is larger in more extensively damaged visual fields.
   C. LTF may be large enough to look like progression when only a few fields are available. As a general rule, in order to detect progression at least four visual fields should be performed over a reasonable period of time.
   D. In patients with large amounts of short and long-term fluctuation, great caution must be used when deciding if a change represents true progression of visual field defects.
   E. Some patients will show an apparent improvement in their visual field after two or three examinations. This has been termed the learning effect and may require more than one baseline examination in some patients.

III. Simple visual inspection of visual field results is the traditional technique for detecting progression (Fig. 6-21).
   A. One looks for an easily detectable and reproducible change in the size and/or depth of a defect or the appearance of new defects.
   B. Simple inspection is very unreliable for automated perimetry unless the changes are quite large.

IV. Arbitrary criteria
   A. One can define a set of quantitative criteria as significant and apply them to any field. For example, one might decide that a change in a single point of 10 dB or more, or a change in two adjacent points of 6 dB or more represents true progression.
   B. Such criteria are arbitrary and not usually based on any scientific data.

V. Statistical analysis of visual field data applies a statistical test and looks for statistical significance.
   A. The Delta program on the Octopus system, for example, is a paired t-test that compares the mean sensitivities of two fields or two groups of fields (Fig. 6-22).
   B. Analysis of variance is a technique that compares the mean sensitivities of multiple fields and can detect significant changes over time.
   C. Regression analysis and correlation coefficients on various visual field indices can be performed to see if there is significant correlation of a change with time (Fig. 6-23). The statistical package available with the Humphrey Visual Field Analyzer utilizes regression analysis.
   D. Statistically significant change as detected by a statistical test does not always, however, reflect clinically meaningful change. The judgment of the clinician is still required.
   E. Statistical tests are all heavily dependent on sample size. The number of test locations evaluated and the number of available examinations will have important effects on the outcome of any statistical test.
   F. Patients with large amounts of fluctuation can appear to be progressing even if, in fact, they are not. Tests of statistical significance can be skewed by large amounts of long-term fluctuation.

VI. Population studies are now being done to define prospectively the expected behavior of the glaucomatous visual field

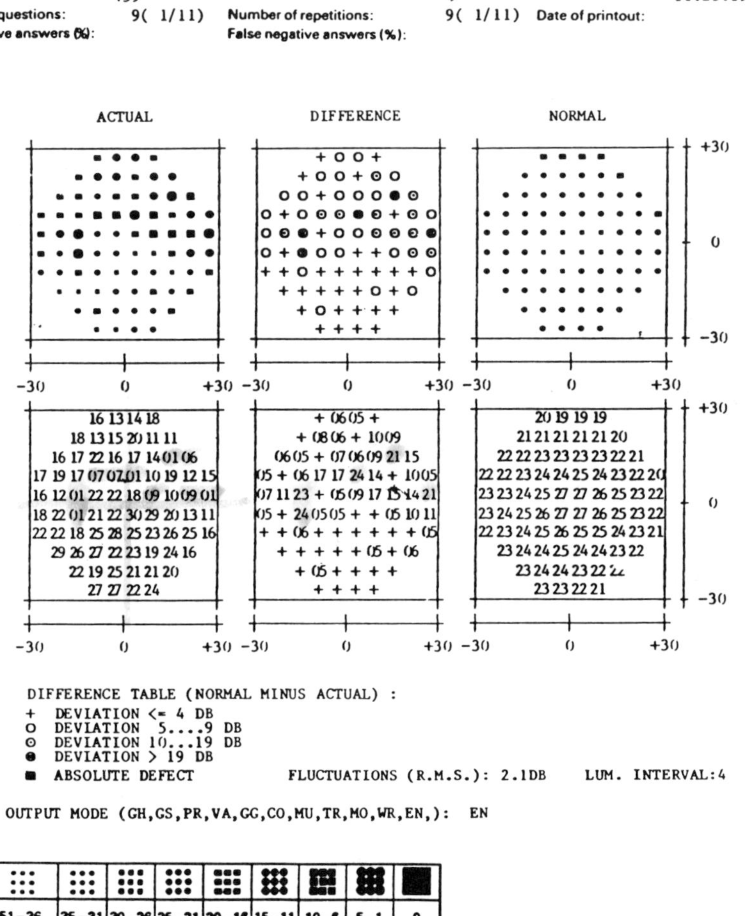


| Symb. | | | | | | | | | |
|---|---|---|---|---|---|---|---|---|---|
| dB | 51–36 | 35–31 | 30–26 | 25–21 | 20–16 | 15–11 | 10–6 | 5–1 | 0 |
| asb | 0,008–0,25 | 0,31–0,8 | 1–2,5 | 3,1–8 | 10–25 | 31–80 | 100–250 | 315–800 | 1000 |

A 1 asb = 0,318 cd/m²

**Fig. 6-21** Visual fields obtained on a patient over a period of nearly 3 years show progressive glaucomatous loss in the left eye. The superior arcuate scotoma has become denser and larger over time. The dates of the examinations were **(A, B)** 11/23/83, **(C, D)** 9/26/84, **(E, F)** 7/18/85, **(G, H)** 1/10/86, **(I, J)** 5/22/86, **(K, L)** 9/25/86. (*Figure continues.*)

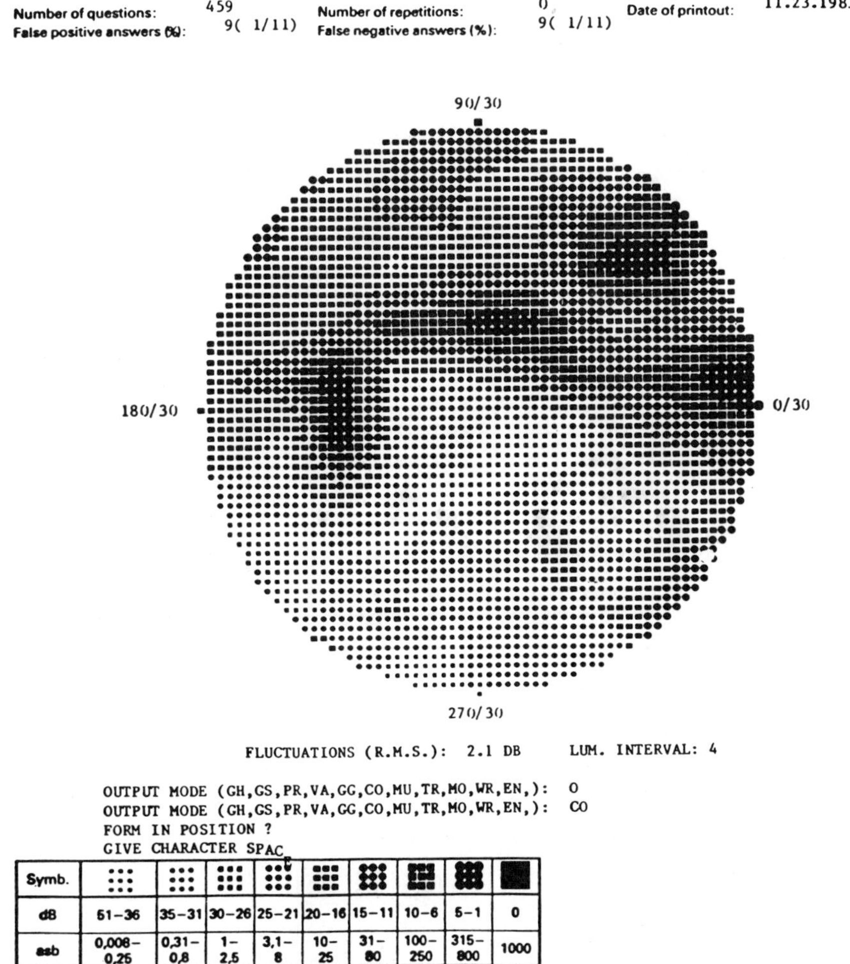


| Symb. | | | | | | | | | |
|---|---|---|---|---|---|---|---|---|---|
| dB | 51–36 | 35–31 | 30–26 | 25–21 | 20–16 | 15–11 | 10–6 | 5–1 | 0 |
| asb | 0,008–0,25 | 0,31–0,8 | 1–2,5 | 3,1–8 | 10–25 | 31–80 | 100–250 | 315–800 | 1000 |

B 1 asb = 0,318 cd/m²

**Fig. 6-21** (*Continued*). (**B**)

Number of questions: 444 Number of repetitions: 0 Date of printout: 9.26.1984
False positive answers (%): 10( 1/10) False negative answers (%): 0( 0/11)

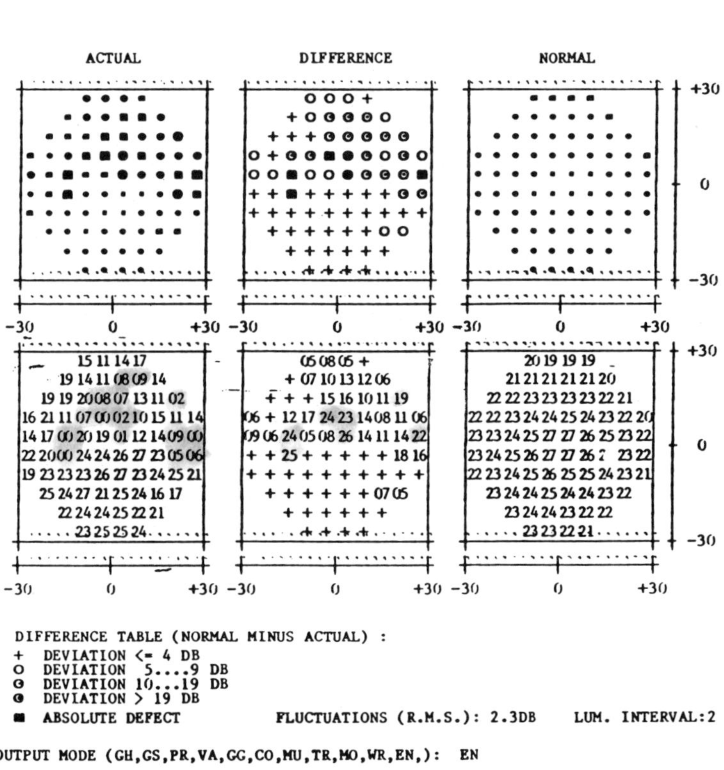


DIFFERENCE TABLE (NORMAL MINUS ACTUAL) :
+ DEVIATION <= 4 DB
O DEVIATION 5....9 DB
⊖ DEVIATION 10...19 DB
◐ DEVIATION > 19 DB
■ ABSOLUTE DEFECT FLUCTUATIONS (R.M.S.): 2.3DB LUM. INTERVAL:2

OUTPUT MODE (GH,GS,PR,VA,GG,CO,MU,TR,MO,WR,EN,): EN

| Symb. | ⁙ | ⁙ | ⁙ | ⁙ | ⁙ | ⁙ | ⁙ | ⁙ | ■ |
|---|---|---|---|---|---|---|---|---|---|
| dB | 51–36 | 35–31 | 30–26 | 25–21 | 20–16 | 15–11 | 10–6 | 5–1 | 0 |
| asb | 0,008–0,25 | 0,31–0,8 | 1–2,5 | 3,1–8 | 10–25 | 31–80 | 100–250 | 315–800 | 1000 |

C 1 asb = 0,318 cd/m²

Fig. 6-21 (*Continued*). (C)

Number of questions: 444 Number of repetitions: 0 Date of printout: 9.26.1984
False positive answers (%): 10( 1/10) False negative answers (%): 0( 0/11)

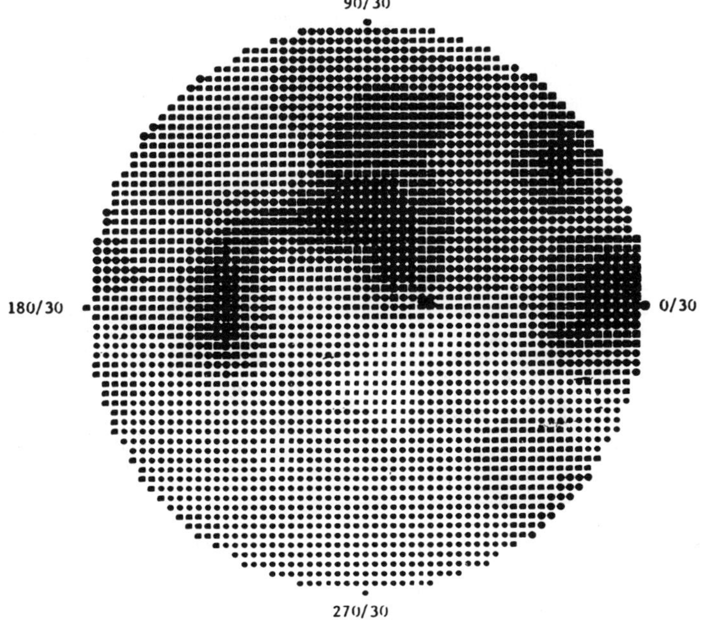


FLUCTUATIONS (R.M.S.): 2.3 DB LUM. INTERVAL: 2

OUTPUT MODE (GH,GS,PR,VA,GG,CO,MU,TR,MO,WR,EN,): CO
FORM IN POSITION ?
GIVE CHARACTER SPACE

| Symb. | | | | | | | | | |
|---|---|---|---|---|---|---|---|---|---|
| dB | 51–36 | 35–31 | 30–26 | 25–21 | 20–16 | 15–11 | 10–6 | 5–1 | 0 |
| asb | 0,008–0,25 | 0,31–0,8 | 1–2,5 | 3,1–8 | 10–25 | 31–80 | 100–250 | 315–800 | 1000 |

D 1 asb = 0,318 cd/m²

**Fig. 6-21** (*Continued*). **(D)**

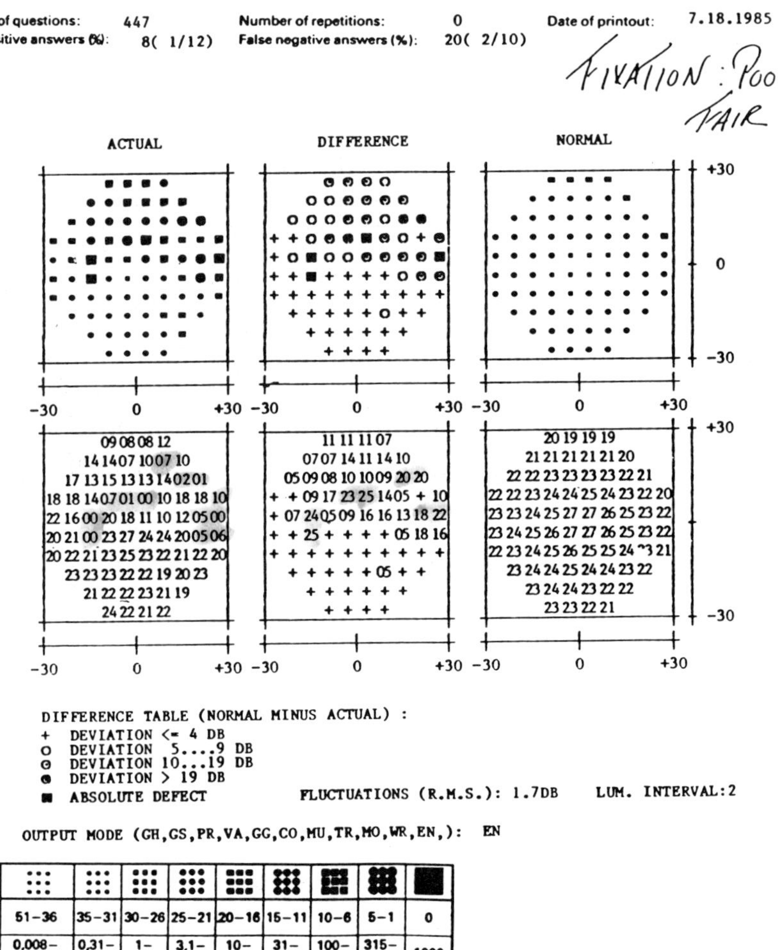


| Symb. | | | | | | | | | |
|---|---|---|---|---|---|---|---|---|---|
| dB | 51–36 | 35–31 | 30–26 | 25–21 | 20–16 | 15–11 | 10–6 | 5–1 | 0 |
| asb | 0,008–0,25 | 0,31–0,8 | 1–2,5 | 3,1–8 | 10–25 | 31–80 | 100–250 | 315–800 | 1000 |

E 1 asb = 0,318 cd/m²

**Fig. 6-21** (*Continued*). **(E)**

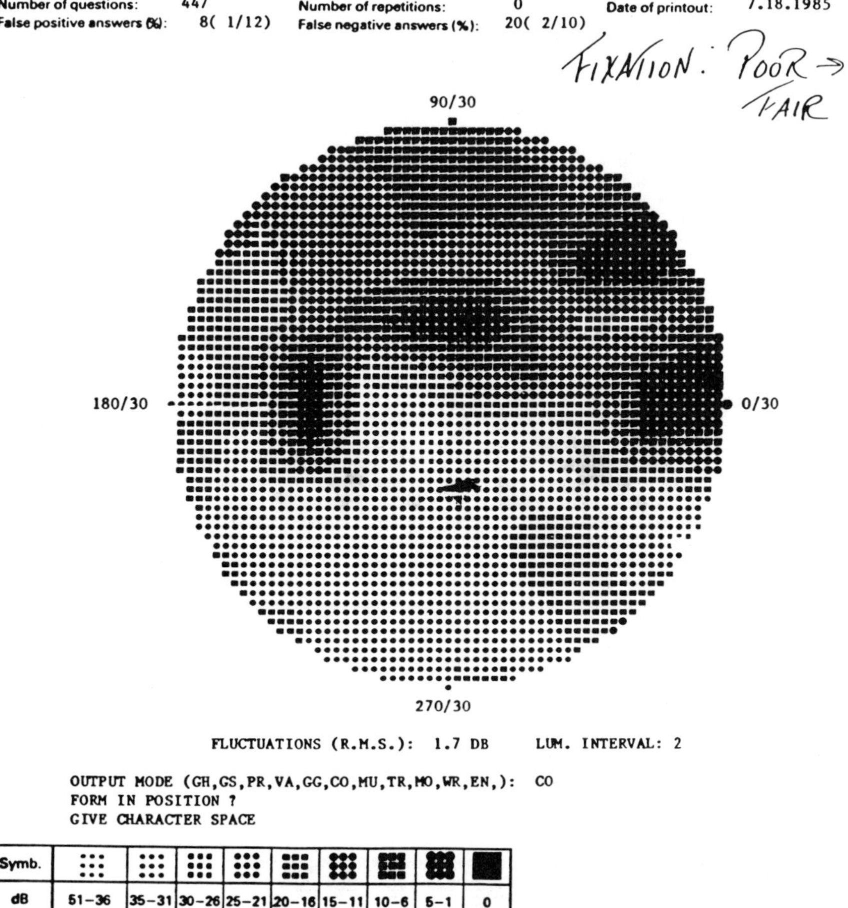


| Symb. | | | | | | | | | |
|---|---|---|---|---|---|---|---|---|---|
| dB | 51–36 | 35–31 | 30–26 | 25–21 | 20–16 | 15–11 | 10–6 | 5–1 | 0 |
| asb | 0,008–0,25 | 0,31–0,8 | 1–2,5 | 3,1–8 | 10–25 | 31–80 | 100–250 | 315–800 | 1000 |

F 1 asb = 0,318 cd/m²

**Fig. 6-21** (*Continued*). **(F)**

Number of questions: 511 Number of repetitions: 0 Date of printout: 1.10.1986
False positive answers (%): 0( 0/13) False negative answers (%): 8( 1/12)

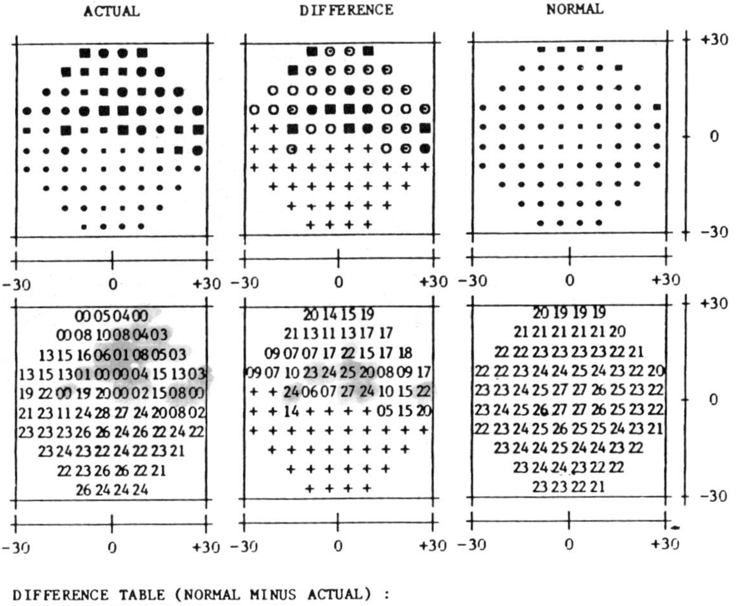


DIFFERENCE TABLE (NORMAL MINUS ACTUAL) :
+ DEVIATION <= 4 DB
O DEVIATION 5....9 DB
Θ DEVIATION 10...19 DB
◕ DEVIATION > 19 DB
■ ABSOLUTE DEFECT FLUCTUATIONS (R.M.S.): 3.8DB LUM. INTERVAL:2

OUTPUT MODE (CH,CS,PR,VA,GG,CO,MU,TR,MO,AR,EN):

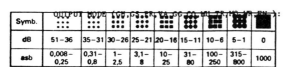

| Symb. | | | | | | | | | |
|---|---|---|---|---|---|---|---|---|---|
| dB | 51–36 | 35–31 | 30–26 | 25–21 | 20–16 | 15–11 | 10–6 | 5–1 | 0 |
| asb | 0,008–0,25 | 0,31–0,8 | 1–2,5 | 3,1–8 | 10–25 | 31–80 | 100–250 | 315–800 | 1000 |

G 1 asb = 0,318 cd/m²

Fig. 6-21 (*Continued*). (G)

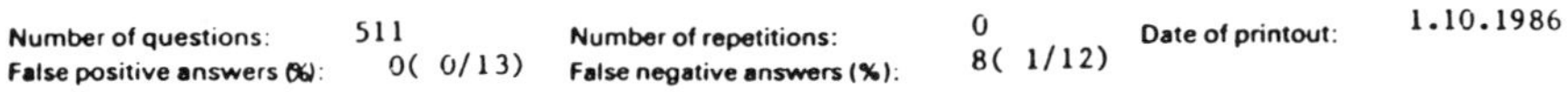


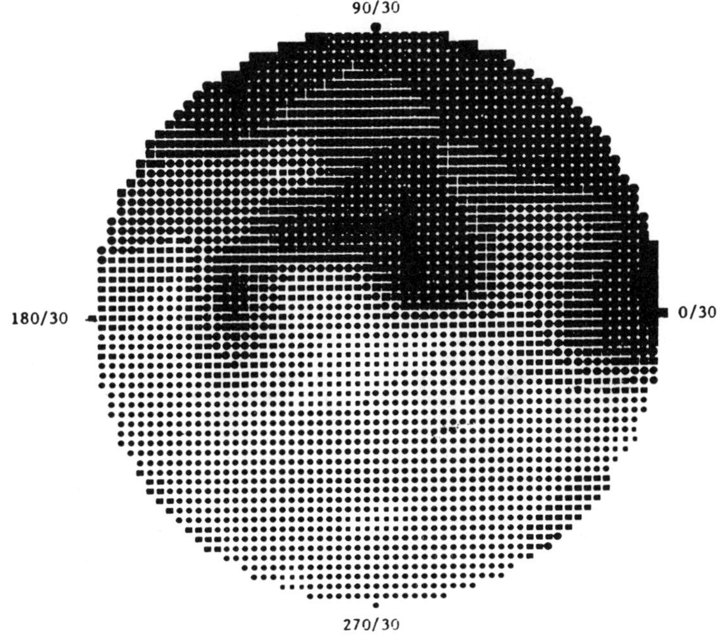


FLUCTUATIONS (R.M.S.): 3.8 DB LUM. INTERVAL: 2

OUTPUT MODE (GH,GS,PR,VA,GG,CO,MU,TR,MO,WR,EN,): CO
FORM IN POSITION ?
GIVE CHARACTER SPACE

| Symb. | | | | | | | | | |
|---|---|---|---|---|---|---|---|---|---|
| dB | 51–36 | 35–31 | 30–26 | 25–21 | 20–16 | 15–11 | 10–6 | 5–1 | 0 |
| asb | 0,008–0,25 | 0,31–0,8 | 1–2,5 | 3,1–8 | 10–25 | 31–80 | 100–250 | 315–800 | 1000 |

H 1 asb = 0,318 cd/m²

**Fig. 6-21** (*Continued*). **(H)**

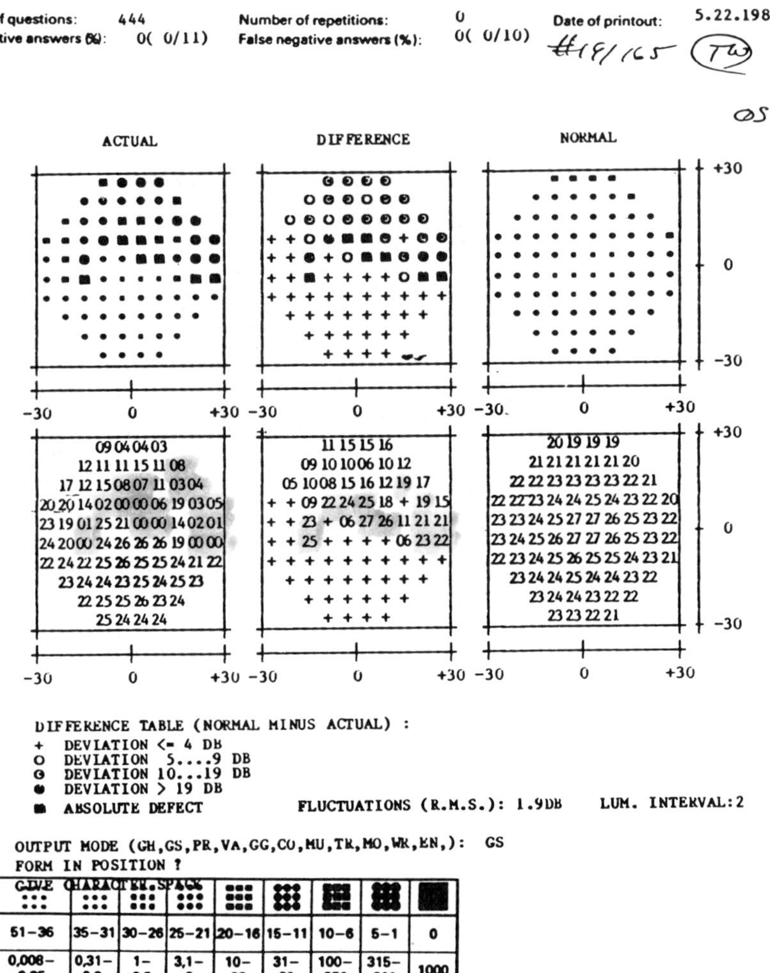
Number of questions: 444
Number of repetitions: 0
Date of printout: 5.22.1986
False positive answers (%): 0( 0/11)
False negative answers (%): 0( 0/10)
OS
ACTUAL
DIFFERENCE
NORMAL
+30
0
-30
DIFFERENCE TABLE (NORMAL MINUS ACTUAL) :
+ DEVIATION <= 4 DB
O DEVIATION 5....9 DB
DEVIATION 10...19 DB
DEVIATION > 19 DB
ABSOLUTE DEFECT
FLUCTUATIONS (R.M.S.): 1.9DB
LUM. INTERVAL:2
OUTPUT MODE (GH,GS,PR,VA,GG,CO,MU,TR,MO,WR,EN,): GS
FORM IN POSITION ?
GIVE CHARACTER SPACE
Symb.
dB 51–36 35–31 30–26 25–21 20–16 15–11 10–6 5–1 0
asb 0,008–0,25 0,31–0,8 1–2,5 3,1–8 10–25 31–80 100–250 315–800 1000
1 asb = 0,318 cd/m²

Fig. 6-21 (*Continued*). (I)

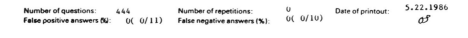

Number of questions: 444    Number of repetitions: 0    Date of printout: 5.22.1986
False positive answers (%): 0( 0/11)    False negative answers (%): 0( 0/10)

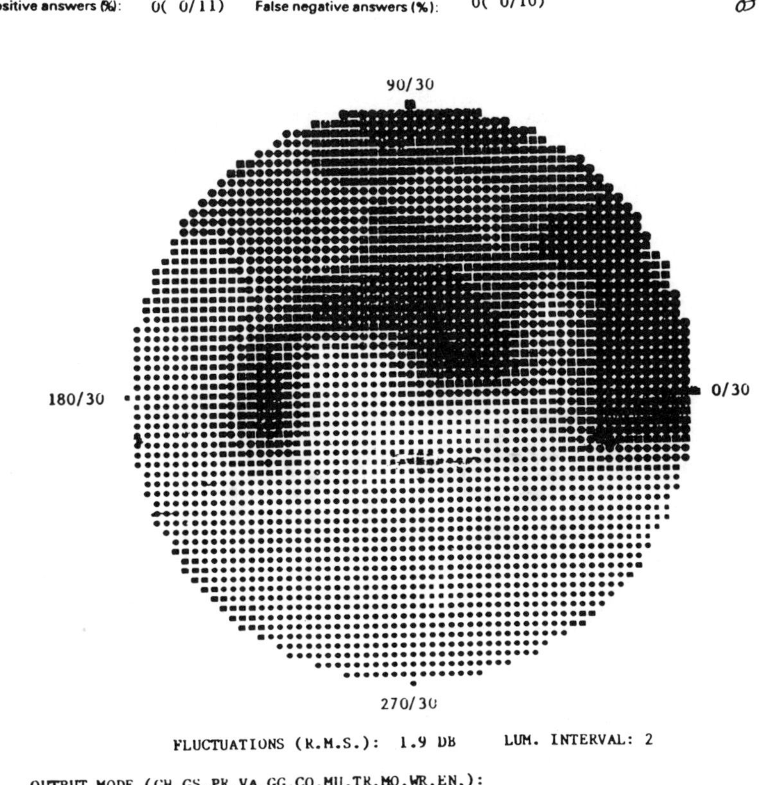


| Symb. | | | | | | | | | |
|---|---|---|---|---|---|---|---|---|---|
| dB | 51–36 | 35–31 | 30–26 | 25–21 | 20–16 | 15–11 | 10–6 | 5–1 | 0 |
| asb | 0,008–0,25 | 0,31–0,8 | 1–2,5 | 3,1–8 | 10–25 | 31–80 | 100–250 | 315–800 | 1000 |

J    1 asb = 0,318 cd/m²

Fig. 6-21 (*Continued*). (J)

| Number of questions: | 396 | Number of repetitions: | 0 | Date of printout: | 9.25.1986 |
|---|---|---|---|---|---|
| False positive answers (%): | 0( 0/ 9) | False negative answers (%): | 20( 2/10) | | |

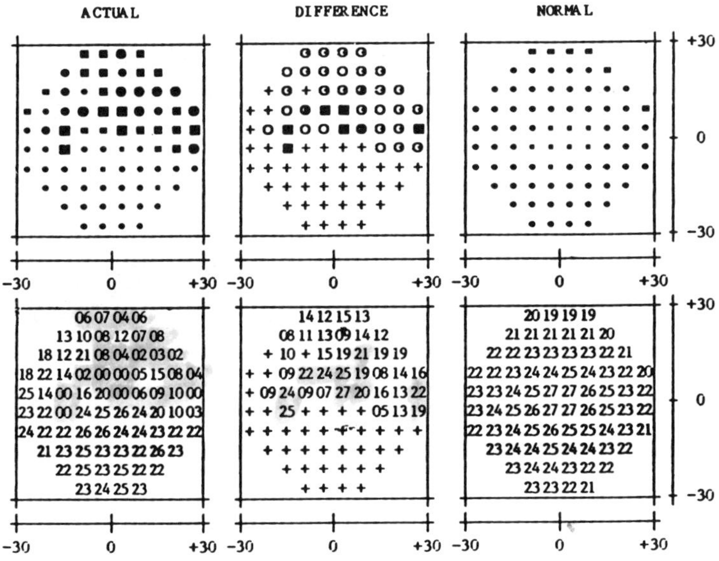


DIFFERENCE TABLE (NORMAL MINUS ACTUAL) :
+ DEVIATION <= 4 DB
O DEVIATION 5....9 DB
Ø DEVIATION 10...19 DB
● DEVIATION > 19 DB
■ ABSOLUTE DEFECT

FLUCTUATIONS (R.M.S.): 1.5DB LUM. INTERVAL:2

OUTPUT MODE (GH,GS,PR,VA,GG,CO,MU,TR,MO,WR,EN,): EN

| Symb. | | | | | | | | | |
|---|---|---|---|---|---|---|---|---|---|
| dB | 51–36 | 35–31 | 30–26 | 25–21 | 20–16 | 15–11 | 10–6 | 5–1 | 0 |
| asb | 0,008–0,25 | 0,31–0,8 | 1–2,5 | 3,1–8 | 10–25 | 31–80 | 100–250 | 315–800 | 1000 |

K 1 asb = 0,318 cd/m²

Fig. 6-21 (*Continued*). (**K**)

Number of questions: 396   Number of repetitions: 0   Date of printout: 9.25.1986
False positive answers (%): 0( 0/ 9)   False negative answers (%): 20( 2/10)

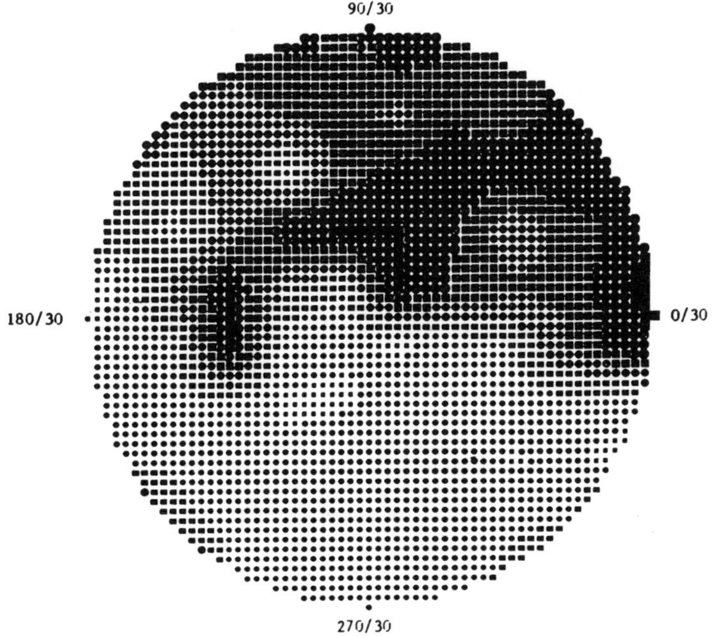


FLUCTUATIONS (R.M.S.): 1.5 DB   LUM. INTERVAL: 2

OUTPUT MODE (GH,GS,PR,VA,GG,CO,MU,TR,MO,WR,EN,): CO
FORM IN POSITION ?
GIVE CHARACTER SPACE

| Symb. | | | | | | | | | |
|---|---|---|---|---|---|---|---|---|---|
| dB | 51–36 | 35–31 | 30–26 | 25–21 | 20–16 | 15–11 | 10–6 | 5–1 | 0 |
| asb | 0,008–0,25 | 0,31–0,8 | 1–2,5 | 3,1–8 | 10–25 | 31–80 | 100–250 | 315–800 | 1000 |

L   1 asb = 0,318 cd/m²

**Fig. 6-21** (*Continued*). **(L)**

Number of questions: Number of repetitions: Date of printout:
False positive answers (%): False negative answers (%):

| | EX1 | EX2 | EX3 | EX4 | EX5 | EX6 | SUMMARY |
|---|---|---|---|---|---|---|---|
| DATE OF EXAM : DAY | 11.23 | 09.26 | 07.18 | 01.10 | 05.22 | 09.25 | |
| YEAR | 1983 | 1984 | 1985 | 1986 | 1986 | 1986 | |
| PROGRAM / EXAMINATION | 32/01 | 32/02 | 32/03 | 32/04 | 32/05 | 32/06 | |
| TOTAL LOSS (WHOLE FIELD) | 378 | 419 | 447 | 575 | 511 | 521 | 475 ± 29 |
| MEAN LOSS (PER TEST LOC) | | | | | | | |
| WHOLE FIELD | 5.1 | 5.7 | 6.0 | 7.8 | 6.9 | 7.0 | 6.4 ± 0.4 |
| QUADRANT UPPER NASAL | 10.7 | 12.7 | 13.2 | 17.4 | 16.1 | 16.9 | 14.5 ± 1.1 |
| LOWER NASAL | 2.2 | 2.4 | 2.3 | 2.1 | 2.7 | 1.9 | 2.3 ± 0.1 |
| UPPER TEMP. | 5.9 | 7.3 | 8.4 | 11.4 | 8.6 | 9.1 | 8.4 ± 0.7 |
| LOWER TEMP. | 1.4 | 0.0 | 0.0 | 0.0 | 0.0 | 0.0 | 0.2 ± 0.2 |
| ECCENTRICITY 0 - 10 | 6.8 | 8.3 | 7.8 | 9.4 | 9.0 | 9.3 | 8.5 ± 0.4 |
| 10 - 20 | 5.0 | 5.7 | 5.8 | 7.6 | 6.5 | 7.4 | 6.3 ± 0.4 |
| 20 - 30 | 4.7 | 4.9 | 5.6 | 7.4 | 6.5 | 6.3 | 5.9 ± 0.4 |
| MEAN SENSITIVITY | | | | | | | |
| WHOLE FIELD (N: 23.1) | 18.0 | 17.1 | 16.2 | 15.2 | 16.1 | 15.8 | 16.4 ± 0.4 |
| QUAD.UPP.NAS.(N: 22.4) | 11.4 | 9.6 | 9.0 | 5.1 | 6.1 | 5.5 | 7.8 ± 1.1 |
| LOW.NAS.(N: 23.4) | 21.5 | 21.4 | 19.8 | 21.4 | 21.4 | 21.5 | 21.2 ± 0.3 |
| UPP.TMP.(N: 22.5) | 15.8 | 14.5 | 13.6 | 10.8 | 13.5 | 13.0 | 13.5 ± 0.7 |
| LOW.TMP.(N: 24.1) | 23.4 | 23.3 | 22.4 | 23.9 | 23.8 | 23.5 | 23.4 ± 0.2 |
| ECC. 0 - 10 (N: 25.9) | 19.5 | 17.3 | 17.2 | 16.2 | 16.6 | 15.9 | 17.1 ± 0.5 |
| 10 - 20 (N: 23.9) | 18.6 | 17.7 | 17.2 | 15.9 | 17.1 | 16.0 | 17.1 ± 0.4 |
| 20 - 30 (N: 22.0) | 17.3 | 16.9 | 15.5 | 14.7 | 15.6 | 15.7 | 16.0 ± 0.4 |
| NO. OF DISTURBED POINTS | 40 | 35 | 37 | 38 | 34 | 35 | 37 ± 1 |
| R.M.S. FLUCTUATION | 2.1 | 2.3 | 1.7 | 3.8 | 1.9 | 1.5 | 2.2 |
| TOTAL FLUCTUATION | | | | | | | 2.9 |

| Symb. | | | | | | | | | |
|---|---|---|---|---|---|---|---|---|---|
| dB | 51–36 | 35–31 | 30–26 | 25–21 | 20–16 | 15–11 | 10–6 | 5–1 | 0 |
| asb | 0,008–0,25 | 0,31–0,8 | 1–2,5 | 3,1–8 | 10–25 | 31–80 | 100–250 | 315–800 | 1000 |

A 1 asb = 0,318 cd/m²

**Fig. 6-22** Delta Program printout of the patient in Figure 6-21. (**A**) The series printout summarizes each visual field in chronologic order. One can see a gradual increase in total loss over time, indicating progressive loss. Reviewing the mean sensitivity shows that the greatest decrease in sensitivity has been in the upper nasal quadrant. (*Figure continues.*)

Number of questions: Number of repetitions: Date of printout:
False positive answers (%): False negative answers (%):

| | | | | | | | | | |
|---|---|---|---|---|---|---|---|---|---|
| | | | -8. | -7 | -10 | -13. | | | |
| | | -6. | -3 | -4 | -1. | -1 | -5 | | |
| | 0. | -6. | -3. | -4 | -7 | -7 | -3 | -1 | |
| 3. | 1: | 0 | -5 | -4 | -2 | -5 | 0. | -6 | -10 |
| 9. | 2. | | -1. | 0 | -10 | -8 | -1 | -3 | 0 |
| 4. | 0: | | 2. | 3. | -2: | -3: | -2. | -4 | -7 |
| 3: | 1: | 2. | 2: | -1: | -2: | 2: | -2: | -4: | 4. |
| | -5: | -2: | -3: | 2: | 0: | 2. | 6. | 7. | |
| | | 0: | 4. | -1: | 3: | 1: | 3: | | |
| | | | -1: | -2: | 1: | -1: | | | |

DIFFERENCE TABLE : MEAN B MINUS MEAN A (NEGATIVE VALUES: DECREASED SENSITIVITY)
0-0 ALL RESULTS ZERO <> LOW NORMAL VALUES
DOTS INDICATE THAT SOME (.) OR ALL (:) RESULTS ARE IN NORMAL RANGE (FULLY VALID)

CONFIDENCE INTERVAL FOR MEAN DIFFERENCE / T-TEST
(1) PATHOL. AREA (UNDOTTED) - 4.5 ± 1.3 (T-TEST: ALTERATION IS INDICATED)
(2) WHOLE FIELD - 1.6 ± 1.0 (T-TEST: ALTERATION IS INDICATED)

| Symb. | | | | | | | | | |
|---|---|---|---|---|---|---|---|---|---|
| dB | 51–36 | 35–31 | 30–26 | 25–21 | 20–16 | 15–11 | 10–6 | 5–1 | 0 |
| asb | 0,008–0,25 | 0,31–0,8 | 1–2,5 | 3,1–8 | 10–25 | 31–80 | 100–250 | 315–800 | 1000 |

B 1 asb = 0,318 cd/m²

**Fig. 6-22** (*Continued*). (**B**) A paired t test comparing the sensitivities of the first two fields with the last two fields shows a statistically significant change in the visual field over time.

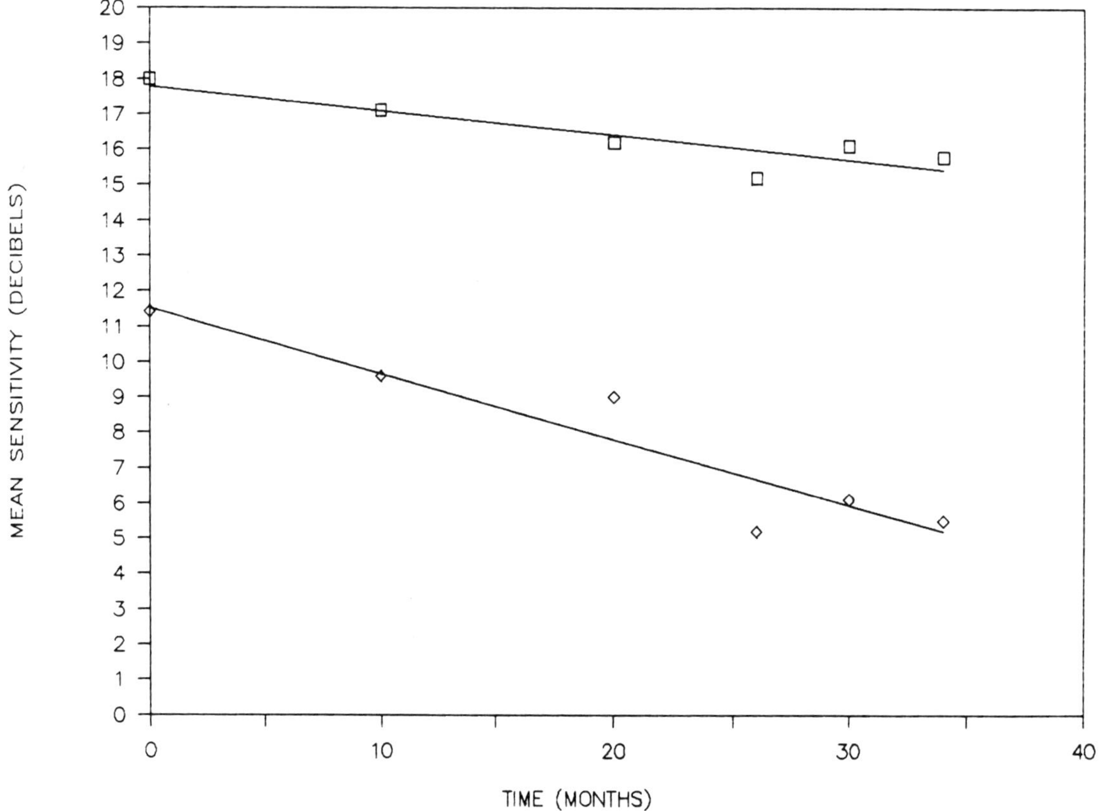


**Fig. 6-23** Regression analysis performed on the visual fields of the patient in Figure 6-21. There has been a significant deterioration of the overall mean sensitivity of the whole visual field (open squares), while the deterioration of the upper nasal area (diamonds) has been even more pronounced.

and apply what is learned to the development of clinically relevant criteria for visual field change.

## SUGGESTED READINGS

Anderson DR: Perimetry With and Without Automation. 2nd Ed. CV Mosby, St. Louis, 1987

Drance SM, Anderson D: Automatic Perimetry in Glaucoma: A Practical Guide. Grune & Stratton, Orlando, 1985

Ellenberger C: Perimetry: Principles, Technique and Interpretation. Raven Press, New York, 1980

Enger C, Sommer A: Recognizing glaucomatous field loss with the Humphrey Statpac. Arch Ophthalmol 105:1355, 1987

Flammer J: The concept of visual field indices. Graefes Arch Clin Exp Ophthalmol 224:389, 1986

Heijl A, Lindgren G, Olsson J, et al: Statpac User's Guide. Allergen Humphrey, San Leandro, CA, 1986

Keltner JL, Johnson CA: Comparative material on automated and semiautomated perimeters—1986. Ophthalmology Suppl:1–25, 1986

Keltner JL, Johnson CA: Current status of automatic perimetry. Arch Ophthalmol 104:347, 1986

Lieberman MF, Drake MV: A Simplified Guide to Computerized Perimetry. Slack, Thorofare, NJ, 1987

Silverstone DE, Hirsch J: Automated Visual Field Testing: Techniques of Examination and Interpretation. Appleton-Century-Crofts, East Norwalk, CT, 1986

Tate GW, Lynn JR: Principles of Quantitative Perimetry: Testing and Interpreting the Visual Field. Grune & Stratton, Orlando, 1977

Whalen WR, Spaeth GL: Computerized Visual Fields: What They Are and How to Use Them. Slack, Thorofare, NJ, 1985

# 7

# Pharmacology

# Therapeutic Drugs

## CHOLINERGIC (PARASYMPATHETIC) AGENTS

I. These agents are often referred to as "miotics" because of their effect on the iris sphincter muscle.
II. Acetylcholine is the main neurotransmitter released at parasympathetic nerve terminals.
III. Acetylcholine is inactivated by the enzyme cholinesterase.
IV. Specific acetylcholinesterase is found in neurons, red blood cells, and neuromuscular junctions and is the main cholinesterase found in the iris/ciliary body and lens.
V. Pseudocholinesterase is found in plasma and some tissues and inactivates long-chain choline esters in addition to acetylcholine.
VI. Postganglionic parasympathetic nerves innervate the sphincter pupillae and the ciliary muscle and induce miosis and increased accommodation.
VII. Cholinergic blockade causes mydriasis and cycloplegia.
VIII. Miotic agents include the following.
  A. Direct-acting medications (e.g., pilocarpine).
  B. Dual-acting medications that have both a direct cholinergic effect and an indirect effect by inhibition of cholinesterase (e.g., carbachol).
  C. Indirect-acting medications that function by inactivation of the enzyme cholinesterase (e.g., phospholine iodide). A decrease in cholinesterase activity prevents the normal inactivation of acetylcholine and therefore an accumulation of acetylcholine and cholinergic effects.

### Pilocarpine (Direct-Acting Parasympathomimetic)

#### Ocular Effects

I. Decreases intraocular pressure by increasing aqueous humor outflow facility. Contraction of the ciliary muscle results in traction on the scleral spur, which alters the configuration of the trabecular meshwork.
II. Induces miosis by stimulation of the iris sphincter muscle.
III. Decreases uveoscleral outflow, which can result in a paradoxical rise in intraocular pressure in eyes with markedly reduced trabecular outflow.
IV. Induces ciliary muscle contraction and forward movement of the lens position resulting in:
  A. an increase in myopic refraction.
  B. an increase in the thickness of the lens.
  C. a decrease in anterior chamber depth.
V. Pilocarpine-induced lowering of intraocular pressure does not involve alterations in the rate of aqueous humor formation or in episcleral venous pressure.

## Pilocarpine Preparations (Table 7-1)

I. Solutions

A. Available in concentrations from ½ to 10%.

B. The intraocular pressure-lowering effect following a single drop administration of pilocarpine is dose-related. In most patients a 4% pilocarpine concentration is at the top of the dose–response curve. However, higher concentrations of pilocarpine (6%, 8%, or 10%) may result in a greater lowering of intraocular pressure in eyes with darkly pigmented irides.

C. Maximum aqueous humor concentration following administration of a single drop of pilocarpine occurs in approximately 30 min. Pilocarpine is no longer detectable in the aqueous humor 4 hr after administration.

D. Maximum intraocular pressure reduction occurs within 2 hr after a single drop administration with a duration of at least 8 hr; however, the onset of action, maximum lowering of pressure, and the duration of action are dose-related within any given patient.

E. Recommended frequency of administration is one drop four times a day; however, in some patients less frequent administration may provide satisfactory pressure lowering.

F. The effect of pilocarpine on intraocular pressure may last up to 7 days after use of the medication is stopped.

II. Membrane-controlled delivery system (Ocusert)

A. The Ocusert disc consists of pilocarpine between two polymeric membranes.

B. Pilocarpine is released at a constant rate (zero order delivery), either at 20 μg/hr (Ocusert P-20) or at 40 μg/hr (Ocusert P-40).

C. Ocusert P-20 is roughly comparable in pressure-lowering effect to 1–2%

**Table 7-1.** Miotics (Cholinergic Stimulators)

| Drug | Preparations | Administration | Trade Name |
|---|---|---|---|
| **Direct acting** | | | |
| Pilocarpine Hydrochloride | drops 0.25–10% | every 6 hr | Adsorbocarpine (Al)<br>Akarpine (Ak)<br>Almocarpine (Ay)<br>Isopto Carpine (Al)<br>Ocu-Carpine (Oc)<br>Pilocar (Co)<br>Pilokair (Ph) |
| | ointment | bedtime | Pilopine (Al) |
| Nitrate | drops 1, 2, and 4% | every 6 hr | P.V. Carpine (Al) |
| Membrane release | P 20, P 40 | every 5–7 days | Ocusert (Az) |
| **Carbachol** | drops 0.75, 1.5, 2.25, 3.0% | every 8 hr | Isopto Carbachol (Al) |
| **Cholinesterase inhibitors** | | | |
| Echothiophate iodide | drops 0.03, 0.06, 0.125, 0.25% | every 12 hr | Phospholine iodide (Ay) |
| Demecarium bromide | drops 0.125, 0.25% | every 12 hr | Humorsol (MSD) |
| Physostigmine sulfate | drops 0.25% | every 6 hr | Eserine (Ph) |

Al, Alcon; Az, Alza; Ak, Akorn; Ay, Ayerst; Oc, Ocumed; Co, Coopervision; Ph, Pharmafair; MSD, Merck Sharp Dohme.

pilocarpine drops; Ocusert P-40 is comparable to 4% drops.

D. Duration of the pilocarpine release is stated to be 7 days; however, this varies between patients and the duration of release may be as short as 4–5 days.

E. Both the duration of action and the relative effectiveness of Ocuserts must be established for each patient.

F. Advantages of the Ocusert constant rate delivery system
   1. Reduced ocular side effects (see below) in comparison to pulsed topical drug administration
   2. Continuous drug delivery and associated intraocular pressure-lowering effect
   3. Improved patient compliance secondary to reduced side effects

G. Disadvantages of Ocuserts
   1. More expensive than pilocarpine drops
   2. Occasional discomfort and difficulty in retaining the device within the cul-de-sac
   3. May be less effective than pilocarpine drops

III. Pilocarpine gel (Pilopine)

A. A high-viscosity acrylic vehicle containing the equivalent of 4% pilocarpine.

B. Formulation designed for pilocarpine to be used once daily.

C. Duration of once-a-day administration varies from 18 to 24 hr, therefore the gel's effect in an individual patient should be monitored.

D. Advantages of the gel include
   1. improved compliance because of once daily administration.
   2. better patient tolerance of pilocarpine because of bedtime administration of the gel with major ocular side effects occurring during sleep.

E. Disadvantages of the gel include
   1. irritation and superficial punctate corneal changes.
   2. corneal haze in 20% of patients that persists after use of the gel is discontinued and is of unknown cause and visual consequence.
   3. that in some patients the gel may be less effective than pilocarpine drops but with the same side effects as drop therapy.

### Systemic Toxicity

Systemic toxicity can occur with effects similar to muscarine. Toxicity results from excessive topical administration and systemic accumulation of pilocarpine. Toxicity is rare with the usual doses used in the chronic management of glaucoma. The greatest danger exists following excessive pilocarpine administration over a short period of time in the therapy of acute closed-angle glaucoma.

I. Perspiration (diaphoresis)

II. Increased salivary and lacrimal gland stimulation, increased gastric secretion, and increased respiratory tract mucosal secretion

III. Stimulation of smooth muscles of the

A. gastrointestinal tract including the gallbladder, causing nausea, vomiting, and diarrhea.

B. respiratory tract, causing bronchospasm.

C. genitourinary tract including the ureter and bladder, causing urinary retention.

D. capsular muscle of the spleen, causing leukocytosis.

IV. Weakening of myocardial contractility

V. Increased or decreased blood pressure and pulse depending on the level of autonomic stimulation

### Ocular Side Effects

Ocular side effects are very common with pilocarpine therapy. Side effects vary depending on the age of the patient, preexisting ocular conditions, such as the presence of cataracts or retinal pathologic changes, and the method of pilocarpine administration.

I. Miosis secondary to contraction of iris sphincter muscle
   A. Decreased visual acuity, especially if a cataract is present.
   B. Depression of central and peripheral visual field isopters and exaggerated visual field defects.
   C. Miosis is greatest and of longest duration following the use of higher concentrations of pilocarpine.
   D. Miosis is least with the use of pilocarpine Ocuserts, which also result in a less variable miotic state.
   E. Miosis following use of pilocarpine gel is similar to that following use of pilocarpine solutions, with a duration of miosis lasting 12–18 hr.

II. Ciliary muscle contraction
   A. Browache, which usually diminishes with time and is more common in younger patients
   B. Induced myopia, which is more marked in young individuals but can occur in presbyopic patients
      1. Induced myopia begins approximately 30 min after instillation of a pilocarpine drop with the peak effect at 60–90 min and a duration of 2–4 hr.
      2. Magnitude of the induced myopia after pilocarpine drops is not dependent on the concentration of drug used.
      3. Duration of the induced myopia is longer with increased concentrations of pilocarpine solution.
      4. Magnitude of induced myopia may be less and the duration more constant following use of pilocarpine Ocuserts compared to pilocarpine drops.
   C. Shallowing of the anterior chamber secondary to a forward shift of the lens and an increased thickening of the lens
   D. Retinal detachment secondary to ciliary body contraction exerting vitreoretinal traction
      1. Risk relates to the degree of preexisting retinal pathologic changes: retinal hole, vitreoretinal traction, high myopia, history of a retinal detachment, and the presence of aphakia.
      2. Risk may relate to the concentration of pilocarpine used: greater risk with higher concentrations of pilocarpine solutions and reduced risk with Ocusert delivery.
      3. Dilated peripheral retinal examination is mandatory prior to the initiation of pilocarpine therapy and should be repeated independent of symptoms at regular intervals.
   E. Long-term pilocarpine therapy may be cataractogenic.

## Carbachol (Dual-Action Parasympathomimetic)

### Ocular Effects

I. Produces a direct cholinergic motor endplate stimulation as well as an indirect parasympathomimetic action by inhibition of the enzyme acetylcholinesterase.
II. Effects are similar to pilocarpine.
   A. Increased outflow facility
   B. Induced miosis
   C. Decreased uveoscleral outflow
   D. Induced ciliary muscle contraction with increased myopic refraction, increased lens thickness, and decreased anterior chamber depth

### Preparations (Table 7-1)

I. Available in concentrations of 0.75%, 1.5%, and 3.0%.
II. Carbachol has poor corneal penetration and requires an adjuvant such as benzalkonium chloride to achieve effective concentrations within the eye.

III. If there is adequate ocular penetration, carbachol is a more potent miotic then pilocarpine: 1.5% carbachol three times a day has a greater and more prolonged pressure effect than pilocarpine 2%.

IV. An excellent replacement or alternative drug for pilocarpine when resistance or intolerance develops. Patients who show a lessening intraocular pressure response after long-term pilocarpine administration may demonstrate an excellent intraocular pressure-lowering effect upon switching from pilocarpine to carbachol therapy. The reverse effect also occurs: lack of response to carbachol with a return of pressure-lowering by switching from carbachol to pilocarpine.

V. The effect on intraocular pressure after stopping therapy with carbachol may last up to 7 days.

#### Side Effects

I. Systemic side effects similar to pilocarpine (see above).

II. The ocular side effects of accommodative spasm and pain, as well as miosis, may be greater following carbachol administration.

III. The other ocular side effects are similar to pilocarpine (see above).

### Acecline

I. A synthetic ester with direct motor endplate action and weak anticholinesterase activity.

II. Available in Europe under the trade name Glaucostat.

III. Intraocular pressure effect similar to pilocarpine with less accommodative spasm than carbachol.

## INDIRECT CHOLINERGIC (ANTICHOLINESTERASE) DRUGS (Table 7-1)

### Ocular Effects

I. Increased acetylcholine accumulation by irreversible inhibition of cholinesterase activity

II. Similar ocular effects to the direct-acting miotic agents
  A. Reduced intraocular pressure secondary to increased outflow facility
  B. Miosis
  C. Induced ciliary muscle contraction and forward movement of the lens position
    1. Increased myopic refraction
    2. Increased thickness of the lens
    3. Decreased anterior chamber depth
  D. The effect on intraocular pressure after stopping cholinesterase therapy can last up to 14 days. The effect on the blood–aqueous barrier can last up to 3–4 weeks.

### Anticholinesterase Drugs

#### Phospholine Iodide (Echothiophate Iodide)

I. Available in concentrations of 0.03%, 0.06%, 0.12%, 0.25%.

II. A concentration of 0.03% is equivalent to 1–2% pilocarpine and a concentration of 0.06–4% pilocarpine drops.

III. Higher concentrations have more prolonged duration of effect.

IV. Maximum reduction in intraocular pressure is 4–6 hr with a substantial effect after 24 hr. The medication is used twice daily.

#### Humorsol (Demecarium Bromide)

I. Available in solutions of 0.125% and 0.25%.

II. Administered twice daily

#### Physostigmine (Eserine)

I. The first medical therapy used in the treatment of glaucoma.

II. Available in a 0.25% solution and in an ointment.

III. The drug is light- and heat-sensitive and should not be used if the solution turns red.

IV. A weak cholinesterase inhibitor, it produces miosis in 30 min, persisting for 12–36 hr.

V. Long-term use is limited because of ocular irritation and development of follicular conjunctivitis.

### Systemic Side Effects

I. Systemic absorption suppresses both true cholinesterase in red blood cells and pseudocholinesterase in the plasma.

II. Systemic depletion of cholinesterase begins within 2 weeks of therapy and reaches a plateau after 5–8 weeks. Recovery after discontinuing the drug takes several weeks.

III. Pseudocholinesterase hydrolyzes the muscle relaxant succinylcholine; therefore, use of succinylcholine during induction of general anesthesia can result in prolonged respiratory paralysis in patients receiving topical irreversible cholinesterase inhibitors.

IV. Severe systemic reactions including cardiac and central nervous system depression can result following retrobulbar injection of procaine, which also is hydrolyzed by cholinesterase.

V. Parasympathomimetic reactions of nausea, diarrhea, and abdominal cramps can occur.

VI. Pralidoxime chloride (Protopam) is the antidote for phospholine iodide toxicity, administered intravenously for acute toxicity at a dosage of 500 mg/min for a total dose of 2 g.
   A. Frees cholinesterase from the drug complex by reactivating acetylcholinesterase and prevents further enzyme inhibition.
   B. Protopam does not alter the intraocular pressure effect.
   C. An oral dosage of 500 mg, three times a day for 3–5 days, restores cholinesterase activity.

VII. Systemic toxic effects such as nausea and bradycardia can be treated by high dose injections of atropine, 2–20 mg total dose as a 2 mg intravenous injection every 5 min until symptoms are relieved.

### Ocular Side Effects

I. Cataract formation following long-term use for glaucoma therapy
   A. Anterior subcapsular vacuole formation
   B. Related to both the dose and duration of therapy.
   C. Not observed in patients receiving anticholinesterase therapy for accommodative esotropia.
   D. Cataract formation limits the use of these agents mainly to the treatment of aphakic glaucoma.

II. Iris cysts at the pupillary margin
   A. Proliferation of pigment epithelium and nodular excrescences or cysts can occur at the pupil.
   B. Cyst formation may reverse after the medication is stopped.
   C. Concomitant use of topical neosynephrine may reduce the frequency of iris cyst formation.

III. Disruption of the blood–aqueous barrier
   A. Can result in an exacerbated postoperative inflammatory reaction
   B. Anticholinesterase agents should be discontinued for 4–6 weeks prior to intraocular surgery, with a direct-acting cholinergic agent substituted.

IV. Retinal detachment

May be more frequent following the use of topical anticholinesterase agents than with the direct-acting parasympathomimetic agents.

## ADRENERGIC (SYMPATHETIC) DRUGS

I. Norepinephrine is the main sympathetic neurotransmitter and is synthesized from tyrosine with the enzyme tyrosine hydroxylase being the rate-limiting factor: dopa > dopamine > norepinephrine > epinephrine.

II. Norepinephrine released from the presynaptic axon into the synapse is inactivated by:
   A. 90% reuptake by the axon for restorage in the axon granules.
   B. Inactivation in the synaptic cleft by the enzyme catechol-O-methyl transferase.
   C. Monoamine oxidase when systemically absorbed.

III. Adrenergic stimulation causes pupillary dilation whereas adrenergic blockade causes pupillary constriction. The ciliary muscle has minor adrenergic innervation with stimulation decreasing accommodation.

IV. Alpha receptors are present in the iris dilator, Müller's muscle in the eyelid, and the arteriolar vasculature.

V. Norepinephrine stimulates alpha receptors while epinephrine has both alpha- and beta-adrenergic agonist activity.

VI. Beta-2 receptors predominate intraocularly, particularly in the corneal endothelium, iris, ciliary body, and trabecular meshwork.

VII. Adrenergic agents include
   A. epinephrine preparations that have alpha- and beta-adrenergic agonistic activity.
   B. the prodrug dipivalyl epinephrine (Propine).
   C. beta-adrenergic antagonistic agents.

## Epinephrine Agents

### Ocular Effects

I. Increased outflow facility via stimulation of the intracellular second messenger cyclic adenosine monophosphate.

II. Aqueous humor production may actually increase following the initial delivery of epinephrine therapy.

**Table 7-2.** Epinephrine Preparations (Adrenergic Stimulators)

| Drug | Concentrations | Trade Name |
|---|---|---|
| **Epinephrine** | | |
| Borate | 0.5%, 1% | Epinal (Al) |
| | 0.5%, 1%, 2% | Eppy/N (B-H) |
| Hydrochloride | 0.25%, 0.5%, 1%, 2% | Epifrin (Ag) |
| | 1%, 2% | Glaucon (Al) |
| Bitartrate | 1%, 2% (2% = 1.1% epinephrine base) | Epitrate (Ay) |
| **Dipivefrin** | 0.1% | Propine (Ag) |
| **Combined epinephrine-pilocarpine preparations** | | |
| Bitartrate 1% E-Pilo 1%, 2%, 3%, 4%, 6% | | E-Pilo (Co) |

All preparations administered every 12 hr.
Al, Alcon; Ag, Allergan; Ay, Ayerst; B-H, Barnes-Hind; Co, Coopervision.

III. The magnitude of the reduction in intraocular pressure increases after continued administration secondary to either a decreased aqueous humor production or a further increase in outflow facility.

IV. The intraocular pressure effect persists from 7–14 days after stopping therapy with these agents.

V. Pupillary dilation occurs secondary to adrenergic stimulation of the iris dilator.

### Preparations (Table 7-2)

I. Lowering of intraocular pressure is proportional to the concentration of free epinephrine base (active drug).

II. Intraocular pressure may transiently increase within the first 30–60 min after topical administration.

III. Pressure reduction begins approximately 2 hr after administration, with the peak lowering in pressure 7–8 hr after administration. Duration of pressure reduction is at least 12 hr with the recommended frequency of administration twice daily.

IV. Intraocular pressure reduction is dose-dependent in the range of 0.25% to 1% free epinephrine base. In some patients the 2% concentration may be more effective.

V. Formulations are available as either the bitartate, borate, or epinephrine salt.
   A. Epinephrine bitartate
      1. Active concentration of the preparation is less than the stated percentage: the 2% solution contains approximately 1.1% free epinephrine.
      2. Solution has a low pH, which may cause ocular irritation.
      3. Solutions can degrade over time with discoloration.
   B. Epinephrine borate
      1. Available in 0.5% or 1% concentration of the free base.
      2. Solution has a pH of 7.4.
      3. Solutions can degrade over time with discoloration.
   C. Epinephrine hydrochloride
      1. Available in concentrations of 0.5%, 1%, and 2% of the free base.
      2. Solutions are stable.
      3. Solution has a pH of 3.5, which can cause ocular irritation.

VI. Dipivalyl epinephrine (dipivefrin, Propine)
   A. Dipivefrin is an ester formed by the addition of two pivalic acid groups to epinephrine.
   B. Dipivefrin is more lipophilic than epinephrine with increased corneal penetration.
   C. Dipivefrin is a prodrug.
      1. The drug has to undergo biotransformation prior to exhibiting an epinephrine pharmacologic effect.
      2. Hydrolysis occurs in the cornea with the formation of epinephrine that enters the anterior chamber.
   D. Available as a 0.1% concentration with an intraocular pressure-lowering effect equivalent to 1% epinephrine.

## Systemic Side Effects

I. Cardiovascular, including elevated blood pressure, tachycardia, and arrhythmias

II. Nervous system, including tremor, nervousness, and anxiety

III. Headache

IV. Dipivefrin associated with fewer systemic side effects
   A. The drug is not converted into epinephrine until it enters the anterior chamber.
   B. Dipivefrin, which enters the systemic system via conjunctival adsorption, the mucosal linings of the nasolacrimal system, or adsorption through the gastrointestinal tract, does not have epinephrine pharmacologic activity.

## Intraocular Side Effects

I. Pupil enlargement
   A. May reduce vision.
   B. Complaints of photophobia.
   C. Precipitation of acute closed-angle glaucoma in predisposed patients with an anatomically narrow iridocorneal angle. Epinephrine preparations are contraindicated in such patients unless an iridectomy has been performed.

II. Epinephrine maculopathy
   A. It is a form of cystoid macular edema.
   B. Primarily, it occurs in aphakic eyes without an intact posterior capsule; however, the condition may also occur in phakic eyes.
   C. It occurs in up to 20% of aphakic eyes receiving topical epinephrine.

D. The maculopathy and reduced vision are probably dose-related and reversible when use of the topical medication is discontinued.
E. The possible occurrence of the associated maculopathy does not prevent the use of epinephrine in the aphakic eye; however, careful follow-up examinations are required to detect the complication, which requires discontinuation of the medication.

III. Intraocular side effects are similar following the use of any of the epinephrine preparations and can occur with the use of dipivefrin since it becomes the active drug after entering the eye.

### Local Extraocular Side Effects

Most common of the side effects following topical epinephrine therapy.

I. Irritation and discomfort on instillation
   A. Related to low pH of the epinephrine solution.
   B. Minimized with dipivefrin administration.
II. Reactive hyperemia
   A. Occurs with the use of all epinephrine preparations.
   B. Related to initial vasoconstriction by the epinephrine preparation followed by later vasodilation as the epinephrine effect wears off.
III. Topical drug allergy
   A. Occurs in up to 20% of patients following long-term use of the medication.
   B. The major reason why patients do not tolerate epinephrine therapy.
   C. Reduced allergic reactions following the use of dipivefrin; however, patients with an epinephrine allergy can also show an allergic response to dipivefrin.
IV. Adrenochrome pigmentation
   A. An oxidative and polymerized breakdown product of epinephrine that is related to melanin.
   B. Deposition can occur in the conjunctiva, the cornea ("black cornea"), and the lacrimal system (canaliculus, sac, or nasolacrimal duct).
   C. Breakdown products can deposit in a soft contact lens, turning it black.
   D. Reduced occurrence following the use of topical dipivefrin.
V. Loss of the eyelashes (madarosis)

### Other Alpha-Adrenergic Agents

I. Alpha-adrenergic system consists of the following receptors:
   A. Presynaptic alpha-2 receptors
   B. Postsynaptic alpha-1 receptors
II. Other alpha-adrenergic agonists or antagonists have been shown to alter intraocular pressure; however, none of these agents is currently used for glaucoma therapy.
III. Thymoxamine, an an alpha-adrenergic antagonist
   A. Topical administration results in miosis by inhibiting the iris dilator muscle.
   B. The drug does not influence ciliary muscle contraction, does not alter outflow facility, and does not lower intraocular pressure.
   C. The induced miosis without an effect on intraocular pressure allows opening of a narrow or appositionally closed iridocorneal angle.
      1. Termination of the acute attack
      2. Determination if angle crowding is a component of a possible combined-type glaucoma.
   D. The dilator muscle does not appear to be affected by ischemia during an acute attack of glaucoma, therefore, thymoxamine is still effective in producing miosis.

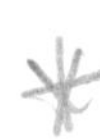

E. Thymoxamine is available in Canada and Europe; however, the drug is not commercially available in the United States.

## Beta-Adrenergic Antagonists

### Ocular Effects

I. Oral, intravenous, or topical administration lowers intraocular pressure by inhibition of aqueous humor formation.
II. Biochemical (or cellular) mechanism of action is unknown. Possible mechanisms include a direct effect on the ciliary epithelium, a reduced blood flow to the ciliary body, or decreased ultrafiltration.
III. Intraocular pressure reduction is greatest after the initial administration ("honeymoon effect") with a slow rise over the next few days to weeks until a maintenance level intraocular pressure is reached.
IV. The effect on intraocular pressure can persist for 14–21 days after stopping therapy with a beta-adrenergic blocker.
V. A late upward drift in the lowering of intraocular pressure occurs in some patients 3 months to a year after initiation of therapy. Some patients may show no effectiveness of therapy with these agents.
VI. There is no effect on pupil size or ciliary muscle tone.
VII. Topical administration of beta-adrenergic antagonists may interact with the topical administration of epinephrine, which has both alpha- and beta-adrenergic agonist activity.
   A. Possible block of epinephrine's beta-adrenergic effect to increase outflow facility; the beta antagonist blocks the epinephrine-induced reduction in intraocular pressure.
   B. Enhanced epinephrine-induced alpha-adrenergic effect on pupil dilation.
   C. The inhibitory interaction, as well as possible additive effects, on the lowering of intraocular pressure, varies between patients. A careful trial with combined therapy of a topical beta blocker and an epinephrine drug is necessary to determine an individual's response.

### Topical Preparations (Table 7-3)

I. Timolol maleate (Timoptic)
   A. Nonspecific beta 1 and 2 antagonist
   B. Commercially available as 0.25% and 0.5% concentrations, although concentrations as low as 0.1% may be effective.
   C. Optimal frequency of administration is one drop twice daily. Some patients respond to once daily administration.
   D. Patients with dark irides may respond better to the 0.5% concentration.
II. Betaxolol hydrochloride (Betoptic)
   A. Beta 1 (cardio) selective antagonist.
   B. Commercially available as a 0.5% solution.
   C. Optimal frequency of administration is one drop twice daily, with some patients responding to once daily administration.
   D. May be less effective in lowering intraocular pressure than nonspecific beta 1 and 2 antagonists.
   E. Major indication is for patients with known asthma or other obstructive pulmonary diseases (see below).
   F. While betoptic has beta 1 cardioselective properties, topical administration has less systemic beta 1 antagonistic effects than the nonselective antagonistic agents for topical administration (see below).
III. Levobunolol hydrochloride (Betagan)
   A. Nonselective beta 1 and 2 antagonist.

**Table 7-3.** Pharmacologic Profile of Topical Ophthalmologic Beta-Adrenergic Antagonists

| Drug | Beta-Blocking Potency (Propanolol = 1) | Plasma Half-Life (hr) | ISA | Cardioselective | Anesthetic Properties |
|---|---|---|---|---|---|
| Befunolol | 2–6 | 1.5 | (+) | – | (+) |
| Betaxolol | 3–10 | 16 | – | ++ | (+) |
| Carteolol | 30 | 5–7 | ++ | – | – |
| Levobunolol | 6 | NA | – | – | – |
| Metipranolol | 2 | 2.5 | – | – | (+) |
| Pindolol | 20 | 3–4 | ++ | – | (+) |
| Timolol | 5–10 | 4–5 | – | – | + |

ISA, intrinsic sympathetic activity.

B. Commercially available as a 0.5% solution.
C. Similar to timoptic in clinical effectiveness.

IV. Other topical agents under investigation or use in countries other than the United States:
A. Metipranolol (nonselective antagonist)
B. Pindolol (nonselective antagonist)

## Ocular Side Effects

I. Irritation
A. Greatest with Betoptic.
B. The other agents rarely produce burning or tearing.
C. Decreased corneal sensation.

II. Ptosis

III. Decreased tear production

IV. Increased epinephrine-induced pupil dilation

V. Visual blurring secondary to possible macular toxicity

VI. Choroidal detachment with hypotony in aphakic eyes

VII. Diffuse, superficial punctate keratitis

## Systemic Side Effects

I. Headache

II. Cardiovascular (beta 1 effect). Can follow use of the topical agents with beta 1 activity. However, there are reduced cardiovascular side effects with Betoptic secondary to low systemic levels of the drug:
A. Bradycardia and arrhythmia
B. Hypotension and syncopy
C. Failure to increase pulse during exercise
D. Congestive heart failure
E. Prolonged atrioventricular conduction time with additive effects to systemic treatment with digitalis and calcium antagonists.

III. Respiratory (beta 2 effect). Can follow use of the topical agents with beta 2 activity. However, beta 1 and 2 selectivity are relative and the use of a topical beta-1-selective agent could result in sufficient blood or tissue drug levels to induce a beta 2 response.
A. Bronchospasm in patients with preexisting disease
B. Decreased forced expiratory volume in 1 sec and vital capacity
C. Respiratory failure and dyspnea

IV. Nervous system
A. Depression
B. Impotence
C. Paresthesias
D. Dizziness
E. Increased signs and symptoms of myasthenia gravis

V. Gastrointestinal system
A. Nausea
B. Diarrhea

VI. Endocrine system
A. Masked symptoms of hypoglycemia

in insulin-dependent diabetes mellitus

B. Possible interference with oral hypoglycemic agents

VII. Timolol is excreted in mothers' milk with potential drug administration to the nursing infant

## CARBONIC ANHYDRASE INHIBITORS (Table 7-4)

### Ocular Effects

I. Systemic administration reduces intraocular pressure due to a decreased (40–60%) rate of aqueous humor formation.
   A. Inhibition of the enzyme carbonic anhydrase in the ciliary epithelium.
   B. Metabolic acidosis occurs following administration of some of the agents, with an associated inhibition of aqueous humor formation.

II. The effect on intraocular pressure can last for 3–5 days after stopping therapy with these agents.

III. Carbonic anhydrase is also present in other structures of the eye including the corneal epithelium and endothelium, the lens, and the retina. Long-term systemic administration of the inhibitors does not affect function of these other structures.

### Preparations

I. Acetazolamide (Diamox)
   A. Available as 125 mg and 250 mg tablets or 500 mg sustained-release capsules.
   B. Lowering of intraocular pressure with the tablet form follows a dose–response curve from 62.5 mg to 250 mg.
      1. Peak lowering of intraocular pressure 2 hr after tablet administration with a duration of up to 6 hr.
      2. Recommended frequency of administration is four times daily; however, many patients respond to less frequent administration and lower doses.
      3. Recommended dosage for children is 5–10 mg/kg prepared as an elixir by the pharmacy.
   C. Lowering of intraocular pressure with the sustained-release capsules peaks in 8 hr and lasts at least 12 hr. Dosage is twice daily administration, with some patients responding to once daily administration.
   D. It is administered parenterally.
      1. Available in powder mixed to 50 mg/ml.
      2. Intravenous administration of 250 mg results in a peak lowering of intraocular pressure at 15–30 min with a duration of 4 hr.
      3. For emergency conditions such as acute closed-angle glaucoma, the recommended parenteral dose is 250 mg intravenously and 250 mg intramuscularly.
      4. Systemic acidosis is greater following parenteral administration.

**Table 7-4.** Carbonic Anhydrase Inhibitors

| Drug | Preparation | Administration | Trade Name |
|---|---|---|---|
| Acetazolamide | Tablet 125, 250 mg | 67.5–250 mg every 6–12 hr | Diamox (Le) |
| | Sequel 500 mg | every 12 hr | Diamox (Le) |
| | Parenteral 50 mg/ml | 250 mg IV/IM | Diamox (Le) |
| Methazolamide | Tablet 50 mg | 25–100 mg every 12 hr | Neptazane (Le) |
| Dichlorphenamide | Tablet 50 mg | 25–50 mg every 6–12 hr | Daranide (MSD) |

Le, Lederle; MSD, Merck Sharp & Dohme.

II. Methazolamide (Neptazane)
   A. Commercially available as a 50 mg tablet.
   B. Lowering of intraocular pressure follows a dose–response. Some patients respond to a dosage of 25 mg twice daily. However, the standard dosage is from 50 mg twice a day up to 100 mg three times a day.
   C. Neptazane has lower plasma protein binding and a longer plasma half life than acetazolamide. The relative drug effectiveness on a per drug weight basis is greater than acetazolamide.

III. Dichlorphenamide (Daranide, Oratrol)
   A. Commercially available as a 50 mg tablet.
   B. Recommended dosage is 25–200 mg up to three times daily.
   C. Action is similar to acetazolamine.

IV. Ethoxzolamide (Cardrase, Ethamide)
   A. Commercially available as a 125 mg tablet.
   B. Recommended dosage is 125 mg four times a day.
   C. Action is similar to acetazolamide.

### Systemic Side Effects

Systemic side effects are very common and frequently limit the clinical acceptance of the carbonic anhydrase inhibitors. Side effects are related to the specific agent and to the total dose administered. Paresthesias of the fingers, toes, and the area around the mouth occur transiently in most patients.

Major side effects that necessitate discontinuation of carbonic anhydrase inhibitor therapy include the following.

I. Renal calculi

The most common serious side effect. Kidney stone formation may relate to an associated alkaline urine, or to reduced urinary excretion of citrate or magnesium by the carbonic anhydrase inhibitor therapy. Stone formation may be less with methazolamide, which does not reduce urinary citrate concentration. However, kidney stones can occur with any of the inhibitors. The prior history of a kidney stone is a contraindication for the long-term administration of any of the carbonic anhydrase inhibitors.

II. Blood dyscrasias

Aplastic anemia, neutropenia, thrombocytopenia, and agranulocytosis have been reported. The incidence of these side effects is extremely low and it is not known if they are idiosyncratic reactions or related to total amount of drug administration. Blood counts prior to and at various times after initiation of therapy have been recommended, especially during the first 6–12 months. It is important to be aware of these side effects, which can be reversed upon stopping the medication.

III. Drug allergy

The carbonic anhydrase inhibitors are sulfonamide drugs and allergic reactions manifested by a skin rash are not uncommon. This requires stopping the drug. These agents should not be used in patients with documented sulfa drug allergy.

IV. Gastrointestinal

Symptoms of abdominal discomfort, nausea, a peculiar metallic taste, a loss of taste for carbonated beverages, and diarrhea are common. Occasionally taking the medication with meals reduces these complaints.

V. Metabolic acidosis

Metabolic acidosis, which occurs with all of the agents, is greatest with acetazolamide and least with methazolamide. Acidosis, which adds to the reduction in intraocular pressure, is related to administration of the higher doses of the drugs. Patients with underlying medical conditions that prevent compensation for alterations in acid–base balance should not receive carbonic anhydrase inhibitors. These medical states include: renal failure, hyperchloremic acidosis, severe pulmonary obstructive disease, hepatic insufficiency, and adrenocortical insufficiency. The degree of metabolic acidosis may trigger the symptom complex of malaise, fatigue, weight loss, anorexia, depression, and decreased libido. Systemic sodium bicarbonate treatment with the carbonic anhydrase inhibitor may reduce the induced acidosis and this symptom complex. Large doses of aspirin combined with carbonic anhydrase inhibitors can result in added acid–base imbalance and salicylate intoxication.

VI. Potassium depletion

Transient reduction of serum potassium levels secondary to increased urinary excretion can occur on initiation of therapy. Long-term potassium depletion can be a significant problem in patients with the following concomitant conditions: treatment with diuretics, especially chlorothiazide derivatives; patients on digitalis or systemic corticosteroid therapy; and in patients with cirrhosis. Potassium levels should be monitored in these patients and supplemental therapy given for significant hypokalemia.

VII. Carbonic anhydrase inhibitors are teratogenic in rats. While documented teratogenicity has not occurred in humans, use of these agents should be avoided during pregnancy, when intraocular pressure tends to be lower due to hormonal alterations.

VIII. Elevation of serum uric acid levels.

IX. Hirsutism has been reported.

X. Severe mental depression and confusion have occasionally been seen with the use of carbonic anhydrase inhibitors. These symptoms are reversible upon stopping the medication.

### Ocular Side Effects

No ocular damage has been reported as a consequence of long-term use of the carbonic anhydrase inhibitors and prolonged inhibition of aqueous humor formation. However, transient and reversible myopia has been reported with the use of these agents. This side effect is also reported with the use of other sulfonamides.

## HYPEROSMOTIC AGENTS

Hyperosmotic agents are effective in the short-term treatment of acutely elevated intraocular pressure. Their most common use, however, remains in the preoperative preparation of the patient for ocular surgery.

### Mechanism of Action

I. Hyperosmotic agents result in a rapid increase in plasma osmolarity, between 20 and 30 mOsmol/L.

II. The smaller the molecular size of the drug, the greater the osmotic qualities.

III. The blood–ocular osmotic gradient draws water from the eye via the retinal and uveal vasculature.

IV. The reduction in intraocular pressure is primarily due to a reduction in vitreous volume.

### Duration of Action

A number of factors determine the degree and duration of the blood–ocular osmotic gradient and therefore the effectiveness of the hyperosmotic drug.

I. Rate of drug metabolism or excretion. This determines the clearing of the agent from the systemic circulation and therefore the duration of the osmotic gradient.

II. Distribution of drug in extracellular or intracellular fluid. Drugs that remain extracellular are more effective osmotic agents.

III. Rate of drug penetration into the eye. Drugs that penetrate the blood–ocular barrier and enter the eye generally are less effective as osmotic agents

## Oral Agents (Table 7-5)

I. Glycerin
   A. This is the most commonly used oral agent.
   B. Administered at a dosage of 1–1.5 g/kg body weight.
   C. Glycerin is denser than water: 1 ml 100% glycerin = 1.24 g (1 g = 0.8 ml glycerine). This must be considered when calculating the total gram dosage of 100% glycerin to be mixed with an equal volume of juice.
   D. Administration of commercial preparations must consider the percentage dilution of the solution (g glycerin per ml) when determining the total amount to be administered.
   E. Onset of action: 20–30 min after administration.
   F. Maximum effect: 45–120 min.
   G. Duration of action: 4–5 hr.
   H. Glycerin is absorbed quickly and is metabolized by the liver.
   I. The agent is distributed in extracellular water and has poor ocular penetration.
   J. Adverse characteristics
      1. Sweet taste, which can cause nausea and vomiting. Somewhat more palatable when given chilled over ice and mixed with juice.
      2. Glycerin has a caloric content of 4.32 kcal/g. This, combined with the osmotic diuretic effect and resultant dehydration, mandates special caution when used in diabetic patients who may develop hyperglycemia and ketosis.

II. Isosorbide (Hydronol)
   A. An effective oral agent that has fewer side effects than glycerin.
   B. Administered in a dose of 1 to 1.5 g/kg body weight as a 45% (0.45 g/ml) solution.
   C. Onset of action: 20–30 min after administration.
   D. Maximum effect: 45–120 min.
   E. Duration of action: 4–5 hr.
   F. Isosorbide is absorbed quickly. It is not metabolized but is excreted unchanged in the urine. Since it is not metabolized, it has no caloric value; and it is therefore recommended over glycerine for use in diabetics.
   G. The agent is distributed in total body water and penetrates the eye.
   H. Isosorbide has an "aftertaste" but

**Table 7-5.** Oral Hyperosmotic Agents

| Agent | Molecular Weight | Dosage (g/kg) | Distribution | Ocular Penetration | Advantages | Disadvantages |
|---|---|---|---|---|---|---|
| Glycerol | 92 | 1–1.5 | Extracellular | Poor | Stable, less diuresis, poor ocular penetration | Nausea, vomiting, calories |
| Isosorbide | 146 | 1–1.5 | Total body water | Good | Stable, well-tolerated, no caloric value, rapid absorption, nonmetabolized | Penetrates the eye (slowly) |
| Alcohol | 46 | 0.8–1.5 | Total body water | Good | Stable, rapid absorption, palatable, hypotonic diuresis | Nausea, vomiting, calories, diuresis, penetrates the eye (rapidly), CNS effects |

produces less nausea and vomiting than glycerin. The agent should be administered chilled over ice.

III. Ethyl alcohol
   A. Oral administration decreases intraocular pressure. Initially there is an increase in plasma osmolarity and a hyperosmotic-induced decrease in pressure. Later there is inhibition of antidiuretic hormone, an induced hypotonic diuresis, and an additional increase in plasma osmolarity. This secondary hperosmotic effect also acts to lower intraocular pressure.
   B. Administered in a dosage of 2–3 ml/kg of the 40–50% solution (80–100 proof) or 1.0–1.8 ml/kg of absolute alcohol.
   C. Onset of action: 20–30 min after administration.
   D. Maximum effect: 45–90 min.
   E. Duration of action: 2–3 hr.
   F. Alcohol is absorbed quickly and is metabolized by the liver and thus presents a caloric problem similar to glycerine.
   G. The agent is distributed in total body water and penetrates the eye rapidly, which limits its pressure-lowering effect and duration.
   H. Adverse characteristics
      1. Alcohol can cause nausea and vomiting, and central nervous system effects. Drunkenness can occur at doses required to lower intraocular pressure.
      2. Despite its limitations, alcohol may be used in emergency situations when no other agent is available.

### Intravenous agents (Table 7-6)

Intravenous agents have a more rapid onset of action and a greater ocular hypotonic effect than oral agents.

These agents can be administered when a patient has nausea and cannot tolerate oral agents.

Adverse reactions are greater with the intravenous than the oral hyperosmotic agents.

I. Mannitol
   A. The most effective hyperosmotic agent for lowering intraocular pressure and the intravenous agent of choice.
   B. Administered in a dosage of 1 to 2 g/kg body weight of a 10% or 20% solution (10–20 g/100 ml) at a rate of 60 drops/min.
   C. Onset of action: 10–20 min after administration.
   D. Maximum effect: 30–60 min.
   E. Duration of action: 5–6 hr.
   F. Mannitol is not metabolized and is rapidly excreted unchanged in the urine.
   G. The agent is distributed in extracellular water with poor penetration into the eye.
   H. Adverse characteristics and precautions
      1. Mannitol has limited solubility, which necessitates a large volume of administration.
      2. The 20% solution should be warmed prior to administration to dissolve crystals.
      3. Administration should be through a blood filter assembly to avoid possible intravenous administration of mannitol crystals.
      4. To avoid potential overdosing, the mannitol bottle should be hung with only the desired total dose.
      5. Hypersensitivity reactions have been reported and include respiratory distress, cyanosis, and hives. Treatment consists of stopping the mannitol infusion and supportive treatment including epinephrine, diphenhydramine, corticosteroids, and aminophylline.

**Table 7-6.** Intravenous Hyperosmotic Agents

| Agent | Molecular Weight | Dosage (g/kg) | Distribution | Ocular Penetration | Advantages | Disadvantages |
|---|---|---|---|---|---|---|
| Mannitol | 182 | 1–2 | Extracellular | Very poor | Stable, rapid action, poor ocular penetration | Large volume, dehydration, diuresis |
| Urea | 60 | 1–2 | Total body | Good | Rapid action, nonmetabolized, less cellular dehydration | Unstable, penetrates the eye, slough and phlebitis |

II. Urea
   A. Administered in a dosage of 2–7 ml/kg body weight of a 30% solution.
   B. Onset of action: 15–30 min after administration.
   C. Maximum effect: 45–60 min.
   D. Duration of action: 4–6 hr.
   E. Urea is not metabolized and is rapidly excreted unchanged in the urine.
   F. The agent is distributed in total body water and rapidly penetrates into the eye.
   G. Adverse characteristics and precautions
      1. Urea solutions are unstable and require mixing just prior to administration as a 30% solution in 10% invert sugar.
      2. Old solutions of urea decompose into ammonia.
      3. Extravasation of urea solutions can produce severe thrombophlebitis and skin necrosis.
      4. To avoid potential overdosing, the urea bottle should be hung with only the desired total dose.

## Side Effects

I. Rebound increase in intraocular pressure
   A. A reversed osmotic gradient with the osmolarity of the vitreous greater than the osmolarity of the blood will result in a drawing of water into the eye and an increase in intraocular pressure.
   B. Agents that penetrate the eye are more prone to cause a rebound osmotic gradient.
   C. However, with all agents a transient rebound increase in intraocular pressure may occur if the blood osmolarity falls below that of the dehydrated vitreous body.
   D. The rebound effect is most common 2–4 hr following administration of a hyperosmotic agent.

II. Severe complications are greater with the intravenous agents.

III. Special caution is advised in the elderly and in all patients with cardiac, renal, or hepatic disease.

IV. Headache and back pain are common side effects.

V. Nausea and vomiting may be induced with the oral agents. These side effects are particularly troublesome when the hyperosmotic agent is given as a preoperative agent.

VI. All agents cause a diuresis and possible potassium depletion.

VII. Urinary retention may occur; this complication is more common in older men with prostatic hypertrophy.

VIII. Circulatory overload can occur in patients with compromised cardiac or renal status, with development of chest pain, pulmonary edema, and congestive heart failure.

IX. Cellular dehydration may cause agitation, disorientation, and vertigo.

X. Patients with decreased renal function

that precludes the removal of free water can develop profound hyponatremia with associated lethargy, seizures, and coma.

XI. Hyperosmotic agents must be used with caution in patients with renal failure. Mannitol, which is excreted by the kidneys, should be administered in a total dose of 25–50 mg. Careful observation of renal function including the measurements of osmolarity gap (the difference between measured and calculated osmolarity), electrolytes, and urine output is recommended. Treatment of mannitol toxicity in patients with renal failure consists of extracorporal hemodialysis to eliminate the drug rapidly. Peritoneal dialysis is less effective.

XII. Subdural hemorrhage due to dehydration and shrinkage of the cerebral cortex and rupture of the veins between the sagittal sinus and the surface of the brain has been reported.

# Associated Drugs and Glaucoma

## MYDRIATICS AND CYCLOPLEGICS (Table 7-7)

I. Topical mydriatic and cycloplegic medications are frequently used in the patient with glaucoma to dilate the pupil for retinal and optic nerve examination and photography, in the therapy of secondary glaucomas associated with uveitis, and postoperatively following filtration surgery.

II. These agents can result in alterations of intraocular pressure.

A. Precipitation of an attack of angle-closure glaucoma in patients with narrow iridocorneal angles. Gonioscopy performed prior to dilation will detect eyes with narrow angles and prevent this unexpected situation. Gonioscopy must be performed after a precipitated narrow-angle glaucoma attack is suspected to confirm the diagnosis.

B. The anticholinergic effect of the cycloplegics can reverse the action of

**Table 7-7.** Mydriatic-Cycloplegic (Parasympatholytic) Drugs

| Agent | Preparations | Trade Name |
|---|---|---|
| Atropine sulfate | 1% solution | Atropair (Ph) |
| | 1% ointment | Atropair (Ph) |
| | 1% ointment | Atropine Sulfate (Pd) |
| | 1% solution | Atropine Sulfate (Ag) |
| | 0.5; 1% ointment | Atropine Sulfate (Ag) |
| | 0.5; 1; 3% solution | Isopto Atropine (Al) |
| | 1% ointment | Ocu-Tropine (Oc) |
| | 1% solution | Ocu-Tropine (Oc) |
| Scolpolamine sulfate | 0.25% solution | Isopto Hyoscine (Al) |
| Scolpolamine bromide combined with phenylephrine | 0.3% with 10% solution | Murocoll-2 (Mu) |
| Homatropine HBr | 2; 5% solution | Isopto Homatropine (Al) |
| Cyclopentolate HCl | 0.5; 1% solution | Ak-Pentolate (Al) |
| | 0.5; 1; 2% solution | Cyclogyl (Al) |
| | 1% solution | Ocu-Pentolate (Oc) |
| | 1% solution | Pentolair (Ph) |
| | 0.2% solution with phenylephrine 1% | Cyclomydril (Al) |
| Tropicamide | 0.5; 1% solution | Mydriacyl (Al) |
| | | Mydriafair (Ph) |
| | | Ocu-Tropic (Oc) |
| | | Tropicacyl (Ak) |

Al, Alcon; Ag, Allergan; Ak, Akorn; Mu, Muro; Oc, Ocumed; Ph, Pharmafair; Pd, Pharmaderm.

pilocarpine therapy and therefore increase intraocular pressure.

C. The anticholinergic drugs, in particular atropine, increase pressure-independent outflow (uveoscleral outflow) and can result in a lowering in pressure.

D. Drugs with alpha-adrenergic agonist activity (e.g., neosynephrine) can decrease aqueous humor formation and therefore lower intraocular pressure.

E. Pupil dilation in patients with pigmentary dispersion syndrome releases iris pigment particles into the anterior chamber. These particles can become trapped in the trabecular meshwork and elevate intraocular pressure. The interval for the increase in pressure is 1–3 hr after dilation.

F. Patients with primary open-angle glaucoma can show a transient increase in pressure following pupil dilation independent of angle crowding, reversal of a pilocarpine effect, or pigment release. The mechanism for this response is unknown.

## Anticholinergic (Parasympatholytic) Drugs (Table 7-7)

The mechanism of action of these drugs is direct competitive antagonism with the neurotransmitter acetylcholine at muscarinic receptor sites. Binding of the drug at the receptor site prevents the presence of acetylcholine and therefore muscle contraction. The prevention of this sequence results in muscle relaxation.

### Atropine

I. The most potent direct-acting mydriatic and cycloplegic drug. Available as a 0.5%, 1%, and 3% solution and as a 0.5% and 1% ointment.

II. The onset of mydriasis is within 30 min with a duration up to 14 days.

III. The onset of cycloplegia is within a few hours with a duration up to 14 days. The onset of cycloplegia is slower and the duration of action is longer in eyes with heavily pigmented irides.

IV. Systemic side effects include flushing of the face, dryness of the mouth and skin, a rapid pulse, fever, respiratory depression, urinary retention, and irritability or delirium.

   A. The acute systemic lethal dose of a 1% solution is approximately 100 drops (10 mg) in adults and approximately 20 drops (2 mg) in children.

   B. Atropine toxicity is treated with physostigmine, 0.5–1.0 mg intravenously every 5 min for a total dose of 4 mg.

   C. The lower concentrations should be used in children. Punctal occlusion or eye lid closure for 3–5 minutes after drug administration reduces systemic drug absorption.

V. Ocular side effects include allergic lid reactions, local irritation, hyperemia, lid edema, and follicular conjunctivitis.

### Scopolamine

I. Scopolamine is similar to atropine but has a shorter duration of action.

II. Scopolamine may be substituted for atropine if an ocular allergy develops to atropine.

III. The maximum mydriasis and cycloplegia occur within 40 min with a duration of 3–7 days.

### Homatropine

I. Homatropine is similar to atropine with a shorter duration of action.

II. The onset of mydriasis is 10–30 min with a duration of 2–4 days.

III. The onset of cycloplegia is 30–90 min with a duration of 1–2 days.

### Cyclopentolate

I. The onset of mydriasis is 15–30 min with a duration up to 24 hr.
II. The onset of cycloplegia is 15–45 min with a duration up to 24 hr.
III. Adverse psychiatric reactions, particularly in children, can occur. This side effect does not appear to be dose-related but due to an individual sensitivity.

### Tropicamide

I. The shortest-acting cycloplegic agent, which has greater mydriatic than cycloplegic effect.
II. The onset of mydriasis is 20–30 min with a duration of 4–6 hr.
III. The onset of cycloplegia is 20–30 min with a duration of 4–6 hr.

## Sympathomimetic Drugs (Table 7-8)

### Phenylephrine

I. A direct-acting alpha-adrenergic sympathomimetic drug with virtually no cycloplegic effect.
II. Maximum dilation occurs 15–30 min after administration with a duration of action of 3 hr. The duration may be longer in eyes with a light iris.
III. Systemic side effects may be common following administration of the 10% solution (one drop containing 6.5–7.5 mg) with no significant adverse effects reported with the ophthalmic use of the 2.5% solution.
IV. Systemic side effects include systemic hypertension, acute pulmonary edema, myocardial infarction, and death.

### Hydroxyamphetamine

I. It is an indirect-acting sympathomimetic that displaces norepinephrine from the nerve terminal.
II. A 1% solution produces effective mydriasis in an eye with intact adrenergic innervation.
III. Onset of mydriasis is 20–40 min with a duration of 2 hr.
IV. Hydroxyamphetamine is used to differentiate a preganglionic Horner's syndrome, in which the pupil dilates since there is norepinephrine to displace, from a postganglionic Horner's syndrome in which there is little or no dilation com-

**Table 7-8.** Sympathomimetic Drugs

| Agent | Preparations | Trade Name |
|---|---|---|
| Phenylephrine HCl | 2.5; 10% solutions | Ak-Dilate (Ak)<br>Dilatair (Ph)<br>Ocu-Phrin (Oc) |
| | 2.5% solution | Mydfrin (Al) |
| | 10% viscous | Phenylephrine HCl (Ph) |
| Phenylephrine combined with scolpolamine bromide | 10% solution<br>0.3% | Murocoll-2 (Mu) |
| Phenylephrine combined with cyclopentolate | 1% solution<br>0.2% solution | Cyclomydril (Al) |
| Hydroxyamphetamine HBr | 1% solution | Paredrine (SKF) |

Al, Alcon; Ak, Akorn; Mu, Muro; Oc, Ocumed; Ph, Pharmafair; Pd, Pharmaderm; SKF, Smith Kline French.

pared to drug administration in the fellow eye.

### Cocaine

I. It is an indirect-acting sympathomimetic that prevents the reuptake of norepinephrine from the nerve terminal and therefore continued effect of norepinephrine to dilate the pupil.
II. Onset of mydriasis is approximately 20 min with a duration of 2 hr.
III. Cocaine can be used to confirm the diagnosis of a Horner's syndrome since it will not result in mydriasis secondary to insufficient norepinephrine in the nerve terminal.

## CORTICOSTEROIDS

I. A substantial percentage of the general population will develop increased intraocular pressure when treated with prolonged topical, systemic, or periocular corticosteroids. This response is related not only to the route of corticosteroid administration but also to the steroid preparation, duration of treatment, and to a genetic susceptibility for the response.
II. Patients at greater risk of corticosteroid-induced elevations in intraocular pressure include:
    A. patients with primary open-angle glaucoma.
    B. first-degree relatives of patients with primary open-angle glaucoma.
    C. patients with diabetes mellitus.
    D. patients with moderate to high levels of myopia.
    E. patients with pigmentary dispersion syndrome.
III. Corticosteroid-induced increase in intraocular pressure is related to a decrease in outflow facility.
IV. The clinical picture of corticosteroid-induced glaucoma usually presents similarly to primary open-angle glaucoma. The eye is quiet, the pressure elevated, the iridocorneal angle open, and there may be glaucomatous optic nerve cupping or visual field loss. Many cases of steroid-induced glaucoma result from the use of steroids for relatively minor conditions such as eye irritation, mild blepharitis, or contact lens discomfort. The diagnosis requires a detailed history to detect the use of steroid preparations. Discontinuing the steroid therapy usually results in return of the intraocular pressure to normal. The glaucoma usually responds to medical treatment while the steroid is discontinued; however, there are resistant cases that require filtration surgery. Argon laser trabeculoplasty is usually not successful in this type of secondary glaucoma.

### Topical Corticosteroids (Table 7-9)

I. Increase in intraocular pressure is related to the strength of the steriod preparation and to the frequency and duration of administration.
    A. Highest response is associated with the administration of dexamethasone 0.1% or prednisolone 1% eye drops. Use of these preparations four times a day for 4–6 weeks can be associated with a pressure increase in patients with a normal intraocular pressure prior to the onset of therapy.
        1. Approximately 35–40% of patients will have an increase in pressure greater than 20 mmHg with an increase of 6 mmHg or higher over baseline.
        2. Approximately 5% of patients will manifest an intraocular pressure greater than 31 mmHg with an increase of greater than 15 mmHg over baseline.
        3. Steroid-induced elevations in pressure are rare prior to 2 weeks of four times a day administration. Both the incidence and the magnitude of the pressure rise increase after this time.

**Table 7-9.** Topical Corticosteroid Preparations

| Agent | Trade Name | Preparations |
|---|---|---|
| Hydrocortisone | | |
| | Bacitracin-Neomycin-Polymxin (Pd) | 1% combined with broad-spectrum antibiotics |
| | Cortisporin ointment (BW) | |
| | Cortisporin solution (BW) | |
| | Ocu-Cort ointment (Oc) | Ocutricin ointment (Ph) |
| Prednisolone | | |
| Acetate | Pred mild (Ag) | 0.12% suspension |
| Na phosphate | Inflamase Mild (Co) | 0.12% solution |
| Acetate | Econopred (Al) | 0.125% suspension |
| Na phosphate | Ocu-Pred (Oc) | 0.125% solution |
| Na phosphate | Predair (Ph) | 0.125% solution |
| Acetate | Pred Forte (Ag) | 1.0% suspension |
| Acetate | Econopred Forte (Al) | 1.0% suspension |
| Acetate | Ocu-Pred-A (Oc) | 1.0% suspension |
| Acetate | Ak-Tate (Ak) | 1.0% suspension |
| Acetate | Predair-A (Ph) | 1.0% suspension |
| Na phosphate | Inflamase Forte (Co) | 1.0% solution |
| Na phosphate | Ak-Pred (Ak) | 1.0% solution |
| Na phosphate | Ocu-Pred Forte (Oc) | 1.0% solution |
| Na phosphate | Predair Forte (Ph) | 1.0% solution |
| Prednisolone combinations with sulfacetamide | | |
| | Blephamide (Ag) | 0.2% acetate suspension |
| | Blephamide (Ag) | 0.2% acetate ointment |
| | Cetapred (Al) | 0.25% acetate suspension |
| | Cetapred (Al) | 0.25% acetate ointment |
| | Metimyd (Sc) | 0.2% acetate suspension |
| | Metimyd (Sc) | 0.2% acetate ointment |
| | Ocu-Lone-C (Oc) | 0.2% acetate suspension |
| | Ocu-Lone-C (Oc) | 0.2% acetate ointment |
| | Poly-Pred (Ag) | 0.2% acetate suspension |
| | Predsulfair (Ph) | 0.2% acetate ointment |
| | Vasocidin (Co) | 0.2% acetate ointment |

(*continued*)

B. Certain corticosteroids (such as medrysone) show less tendency to elevate intraocular pressure. These preparations are usually less effective anti-inflammatory agents that have low penetration into the eye. However, there are patients who manifest an elevation in pressure following the use of dexamethasone 0.001% eye drops. Also, long duration administration of weaker corticosteroid preparations can be associated with delayed increases in intraocular pressure.

C. The response to topical corticosteroids is highly correlated between the two eyes of a patient. Therefore, if a possible corticosteroid-induced increase in pressure is entertained in one eye, the fellow eye can undergo a provocative test with the steroid preparation.

D. Prolonged topical administration of steroid eye drops can cause considerable systemic absorption and decreased plasma cortisol levels.

E. Prolonged use of topical steroid eye drops may cause posterior subcapsular cataract formation.

F. The most effective method of handling steroid complications during required therapy with these agents (e.g., uvei-

**Table 7-9.** (*continued*)

| Agent | Trade Name | Preparations |
|---|---|---|
| Dexamethasone | | |
| Phosphate | Ak-Dex (Ak) | 0.1% solution |
| Phosphate | Decadron (MSD) | 0.1% solution |
| Alcohol | Maxidex (Al) | 0.1% suspension |
| Phosphate | Ak-Dex (Ak) | 0.05% ointment |
| Phosphate | Decadron (MSD) | 0.05% ointment |
| Phosphate | Dexair (Ph) | 0.1% solution |
| Phosphate | Dexair (Ph) | 0.1% ointment |
| Phosphate | Maxidex (Al) | 0.5% ointment |
| Phosphate | Ocu-Dex (Oc) | 0.1% solution |
| Phosphate | Ocu-Dex (Oc) | 0.05% ointment |
| Dexamethasone | | |
| Combined with neomycin | Ak-Trol (Ak) | 0.1% acetate suspension |
| | Dexacidin (Co) | 0.1% acetate suspension |
| | Dexacidin (Co) | 0.01% acetate ointment |
| | Dexasporin (Ph) | 0.1% acetate ointment |
| | Dexasporin (Ph) | 0.1% acetate suspension |
| | Maxitrol (Al) | 0.1% acetate suspension |
| | Ocu-Trol (Oc) | 0.1% acetate suspension |
| | Ocu-Trol (Oc) | 0.1% acetate ointment |
| | NeoDecadron (MSD) | 0.1% phosphate solution |
| | NeoDecadron (MSD) | 0.05% phosphate ointment |
| Progesterone-like Compounds | | |
| Medrysone | HMS (Ag) | 1.0% suspension |
| Fluorometholone | FML (Ag) | 0.1% suspension |

Ak, Akorn; Al, Alcon; Ag, Allergan; BW, Burroughs Wellcome; Co, Coopervision; MSD, Merck Sharp Dohme; Mu, Muro; Oc, Ocumed; Ph, Pharmafair; Pd, Pharmaderm; Sc, Schering; SKF, Smith Kline French.

tis) is to titrate their administration to achieve the desired effect with the minimal amount of drug delivery.

## Systemic Corticosteroids

I. Systemic administration of corticosteroids may elevate intraocular pressure. This complication most commonly occurs following chronic, suppressive steroid treatment (e.g., renal transplant recipients, patients with collagen vascular diseases, and patients with severe asthma or atopy).

II. The complication of elevation in intraocular pressure is bilateral and occurs in approximately 2–4% of patients on chronic treatment. The time of onset of the induced pressure increase is variable and of lesser magnitude than that observed after topical steroid administration. The pressure returns to normal if the steroid is either reduced in amount or stopped.

III. The systemic and topical responses to corticosteroids differ and the side effect may be additive.

IV. Prolonged systemic steroid administration can result in posterior subcapsular cataracts. Other side effects include diabetes mellitus, systemic hypertension, adrenal gland suppression and Cushing's syndrome.

### Periocular Corticosteroid Administration (Table 7-10)

I. Periocular steroid injections are effective in delivering high concentrations of drug locally to the eye, resulting in a reduction of both systemic concentrations and potential systemic complications.
II. Subconjunctival, sub-Tenon's, or retrobulbar injections of corticosteroids may produce an elevation in intraocular pressure.
III. Persistent elevations in pressure are more common after injection of repository or "depo" preparations. These preparations should be avoided. A persistent steroid-induced increase in pressure following the administration of a depo preparation may require surgical excision of the repository corticosteroid to lower the intraocular pressure.

## SYSTEMIC MEDICATIONS ASSOCIATED WITH ANGLE-CLOSURE GLAUCOMA

I. A number of systemic medications have been associated with attacks of angle-closure glaucoma. The mechanism of this side effect is secondary pupil dilation in a patient at risk of angle-closure due to narrow iridocorneal angles.
II. The ophthalmologist should be aware of the patient's general drug regimen. Patients at risk of angle-closure should be informed that the *Physicians' Desk Reference's* warnings against using a medication in glaucoma relate to their condition. This information should be provided to the patients' other medical doctors.

### Tricyclic Antidepressants

I. This class of drugs has anticholinergic action that results in mydriasis.
II. Acute angle-closure glaucoma has been associated with administration of these compounds.
III. Commonly used agents include
   A. amitriptyline (Elavil, Amitril).
   B. protriptyline (Vivactil).
   C. imipramine (Tofranil).
IV. The action of this group of drugs may be augmented by monoamine oxidase inhibitors.

### Phenothiazine Group of Antipsychotic Drugs

I. This class of drugs exhibits both alpha-adrenergic and cholinergic blocking action with the relative action predominating in any one drug.
II. The *Physicians' Desk Reference* lists glaucoma warnings for
   A. triflupromazine HCl (Vesprin).
   B. haloperidol (Haldol).
   C. doxepin (Sinequan).
III. Acute angle-closure glaucoma has been reported with the following agents:
   A. prochlorperazine (Compazine).
   B. promethazine (Phenergan).

**Table 7-10.** Periocular Corticosteroid Preparations

| Agent | Trade Name | Concentration |
|---|---|---|
| Dexamethasone sodium phosphate | Dalalone (O'Neal, Jones, Feldman) | 4 mg/ml |
| | Decadron (Merck Sharp Dohme) | 4 mg/ml |
| | Dexamethasone Injection (Wyeth) | 4 and 10 mg/ml |
| | Hexadrol Phosphate (Organon) | 4, 10, and 20 mg/ml |
| Triamcinolone hexacetonide | Aristocort | 25 mg/ml |
| | Aristocort Forte | 40 mg/ml |
| Methylprednisolone acetate | Depo-Medrol (Upjohn) | 40 mg/ml |

### Monoamine Oxidase Inhibitors

I. This class of antidepressants has weak anticholinergic action.

II. The monoamine oxidase inhibitors' major risk is that they can potentiate the effects of other of drugs including phenothiazines, tricyclic antidepressants, antiparkinsonian drugs, and sympathomimetic agents including amphetamines and ephedrine.

III. Agents in clinical use include
- A. phenelzine (Nardil).
- B. pargyline (Eutonyl).
- C. tranylcypromine (Parnate).

### Antihistamines

I. This diverse group of compounds blocks the effect of histamine on smooth muscle as well as having an anticholinergic effect. H-2 antihistamines, which are used for their effect to reduce secretion of gastric acid, do not have a known effect on the eye.

II. The *Physicians' Desk Reference* lists glaucoma warnings for:
- A. diphenhydramine (Benadryl).
- B. orphenadrine (Norgesic).
- C. tripelennamine (Pyribenzamine).
- D. brompheniramine (Dimetane).
- E. cyclizine (Marezine).
- F. promethazine (Phenergan).

III. Acute angle-closure glaucoma has been reported with the following agents:
- A. orphenadrine (Norgesic).
- B. promethazine (Phenergan).

### Antispasmolytic agents

I. These anticholinergic agents are used to reduce gastric secretion and motility of the stomach. Secondary pupil dilation frequently occurs.

II. The *Physicians' Desk Reference* lists glaucoma warnings for
- A. methscopolamine (Pamine).
- B. propantheline (Pro-Banthine).
- C. oxyphenonium (Antrenyl).
- D. tridihexethyl (Pathilon).
- E. diphemanil (Prantal).
- F. hexocyclium (Tral).
- G. dicydlomine (Bentyl).

III. Acute angle-closure glaucoma has been reported with the following agents
- A. propantheline (Pro-Banthine).
- B. dicydlomine (Bentyl).

### Antiparkinsonian Drugs

I. Agents that replenish diminished stores of dopamine in the brain dilate the pupil due to dopamine conversion to epinephrine and norepinephrine.

II. Agents with strong anticholinergic action are used to improve clinical symptoms secondary to the disease.

III. The *Physicians Desk Reference* list glaucoma warnings for
- A. trihexyphenidyl (Artane).
- B. biperiden (Akineton).
- C. cycrimine (Pagitane).

IV. Acute angle-closure glaucoma has been reported with trihexphenidyl (Artane).

### Sympathomimetic Agents

The *Physicians' Desk Reference* lists glaucoma warnings secondary to pupil dilation with amphetamine (Delcobese, Obetrol).

## SUGGESTED READINGS

Gorin G: Clinical Glaucoma. Ophthalmology Series, Vol. 1. Marcel Dekker, New York, 1977

Kolker AE, Heatherington J., Jr: Becker-Shaffer's Diagnosis and Therapy of the Glaucomas. 5th Ed. CV Mosby, St. Louis, 1983

Shields MB: Textbook of Glaucoma. 2nd Ed. Williams & Wilkins, Baltimore, 1986

# 8

# Classification of Glaucomas

The major classification of the glaucomas relates to the configuration of the anterior chamber angle and the age at onset of the disease. Glaucomas are classified into:

1. Open-angle glaucoma
2. Closed-angle glaucoma
3. Congenital glaucoma

Each of the major classifications is subdivided into primary and secondary glaucomas based on our understanding of the pathologic events leading to the elevation in intraocular pressure. The separation into primary and secondary glaucoma, while traditional, is somewhat arbitrary. As our understanding of disease mechanisms expands, separations between primary and secondary glaucoma become increasingly artificial. The diagnosis of primary glaucoma is by exclusion and indicates our inability to recognize or detect the cause of the glaucoma.

## PRIMARY GLAUCOMAS (Table 8-1)

I. The initiating event begins in the anterior chamber angle, without an apparent or known contribution from other ocular or systemic disorders.

II. Primary glaucomas usually have a genetic basis and are typically bilateral, although the presentation can manifest itself asymmetrically.

**Table 8-1.** Classification of the Primary Glaucomas

| | |
|---|---|
| Open-angle glaucoma | Congenital glaucoma |
| Primary open-angle glaucoma | Primary congenital glaucoma |
| Ocular hypertension (preglaucoma or glaucoma suspect) | Glaucoma associated with congenital anomalies |
| Low-tension glaucoma | Aniridia |
| Associated ocular abnormalities or diseases | Sturge-Weber syndrome (oculofacial angiomatosis) |
| High myopia | Marfan's syndrome (arachnodactyly) |
| Retinal vein occlusion | Pierre Robin syndrome (microgenia and glossoptosis) |
| Diabetes mellitus | Homocystinuria |
| Retinal detachment | Lowe's syndrome (oculocerebrorenal syndrome) |
| Fuchs' corneal dystrophy | Microcornea |
| Retinitis pigmentosa | Rubella |
| Closed-angle glaucoma | Chromosome abnormalities |
| Primary closed-angle glaucoma (with pupillary block) | Rubinstein-Taybi syndrome (broad thumb syndrome) |
| Suspect | Persistent hyperplastic primary vitreous |
| Prodromal or intermittent | |
| Acute | |
| Chronic | |
| Primary plateau iris (without pupillary block) | |

**Table 8-2.** Classification of the Secondary Glaucomas Based on Disease Mechanism

- Secondary open-angle glaucoma
  - Pretrabecular block (membrane occlusion)
    - Inflammatory membrane
    - Fibrovascular membrane (neovascular glaucoma)
    - Endothelial or Descemet's-like membrane
      - Iridocorneal endothelial (ICE) syndrome
      - Posterior polymorphous dystrophy
      - Traumatic (penetrating or nonpenetrating) membrane
    - Epithelial downgrowth
    - Fibrous ingrowth
  - Trabecular block
    - Particulate block of the meshwork
      - Red blood cells
      - Ghost cells
      - Macrophages
        - Hemolytic glaucoma
        - Phacolytic glaucoma
        - Melanomalytic glaucoma
      - Neoplastic cells
        - Malignant tumors
        - Juvenile xanthogranuloma
        - Neurofibromatosis
        - Nevus of Ota
      - Pigment particles
        - Pigmentary glaucoma
        - Exfoliation syndrome (glaucoma capsulare)
        - Uveitis
        - Malignant melanoma
        - Laser iridectomy
      - Protein
        - Uveitis
        - Laser treatment
        - Lens-induced glaucoma
        - Vitreous in the anterior chamber
      - Iatrogenic foreign material
        - Alpha-chymotrypsin-induced glaucoma
        - Viscoelastic substances
    - Alterations of the meshwork
      - Meshwork swelling
        - Uveitis
        - Scleritis
        - Episcleritis
        - Alkali burns
      - Steroid-induced glaucoma
      - Traumatic angle recession
      - Intraocular foreign bodies
        - Chalcosis
        - Hemosiderosis
      - Anterior chamber cleavage syndromes
  - Posttrabecular block (elevated episcleral venous pressure)
    - Thyrotropic exophthalmos
    - Carotid-cavernous fistula
    - Retrobulbar tumors
    - Cavernous sinus thrombosis
    - Superior vena cava obstruction
    - Sturge-Weber syndrome
    - Mediastinal tumors
    - Familial elevated episcleral venous pressure
- Secondary closed-angle glaucoma
  - Anterior ("pulling") angle closure
    - Contracture of membranes
      - Neovascular glaucoma
      - Iridocorneal endothelial (ICE) syndrome
      - Posterior polymorphous dystrophy
      - Trauma (penetrating and nonpenetrating)
    - Contracture of inflammatory particles
    - Contraction of congenital angle bands
  - Posterior ("pushing") angle closure
    - With pupillary block
      - Intumescent lens
      - Subluxated lens
        - Traumatic
        - Marfan's syndrome
        - Homocysteinuria
        - Spherophakia
        - Spontaneous
      - Aphakic
        - Iris–vitreous block (intracapsular removal)
        - Iris–pseudophakic block
      - Secluded pupil associated with uveitis
    - Without pupillary block
      - Ciliary block (malignant) glaucoma
      - Aphakic forward shift of the vitreous
      - Following scleral buckling surgery
      - Following panretinal photocoagulation
      - Central retinal vein occlusion
      - Intraocular tumors
      - Iris and ciliary body cysts
      - Retrolental tissue
        - Retrolental fibroplasia (retinopathy of prematurity)
        - Persistent hyperplastic primary vitreous
- Secondary glaucoma in infants
  - Retrolental fibroplasia
  - Tumors
    - Retinoblastoma
    - Juvenile xanthogranuloma
  - Inflammation
  - Trauma

III. In primary open-angle glaucoma, the precise abnormality causing the increased resistance to aqueous humor outflow is unknown.
IV. In primary closed-angle glaucoma, there is a shallow anterior chamber that predisposes to pupillary block and angle crowding, and the acute attack.
V. In primary congenital glaucoma, there is a developmental anomaly of the aqueous humor outflow pathways.

## SECONDARY OPEN- AND CLOSED-ANGLE GLAUCOMAS (Table 8-2)

I. The factors responsible for the glaucoma are recognized.
II. These glaucomas may be unilateral or bilateral, and some have a genetic basis, while others are acquired.
III. The underlying causative factors can be used for classifying these diseases. However, this method of classification is limited since the primary causative factor is usually not completely understood.
IV. The classification by cause allows the ophthalmologist to think in terms of the underlying disorder and to begin treatment on that basis.
V. The secondary glaucomas can also be classified according to the mechanism resulting in the obstruction to outflow.

### Secondary Open-Angle

I. Pretrabecular block (e.g., a translucent membrane obstructing outflow)
II. Trabecular block (e.g., outflow blocked by red blood cells)
III. Post-trabecular block (e.g, elevated episcleral venous pressure).

### Secondary Closed-Angle

I. Anterior type (e.g., the peripheral iris is "pulled forward" by an abnormal tissue bridging the angle).
II. Posterior type (e.g. pressure behind the iris–lens diaphragm "pushes" the peripheral iris forward into the chamber angle). Pupillary block may or may not be present.

## SECONDARY CONGENITAL (DEVELOPMENTAL) GLAUCOMAS (see Tables 8-1, 8-2).

I. There is overlap in the traditional separation between primary and secondary congenital glaucoma.
II. Secondary congenital glaucomas are associated with additional ocular or systemic abnormalities not directly related to the mechanism of the outflow obstruction.

## SUGGESTED READINGS

Kolker, AE, Hetherinton, J, Jr: Becker-Shaffer's Diagnosis and Therapy of the Glaucomas. 5th Ed. CV Mosby, St. Louis, 1983

Ritch R, Shields MB: The Secondary Glaucomas. CV Mosby, St. Louis, 1982

Shields, MB: Textbook of Glaucoma. 2nd Ed. Williams & Wilkins, Baltimore, 1986

# 9

# Clinical Approach to Glaucoma

## CLINICAL APPROACH

I. The term glaucoma describes a group of diseases generally characterized by the following:
   A. An increased intraocular pressure
   B. Anatomic damage to the optic nerve manifested by disc cupping
   C. Functional damage to the visual field

II. The clinical approach to glaucoma management must consider the diverse presentations of these characteristics which define the disease.
   A. Intraocular pressure may be "normal" at times and only intermittently elevated.
   B. An elevated intraocular pressure relates to an abnormality in aqueous humor dynamics while the location of glaucomatous damage in the eye is at the optic nerve. There may be no correlation between the level of intraocular pressure and the extent of optic nerve damage in an individual patient.
   C. A normal intraocular pressure level is defined by population statistics. There is currently no method to define or measure a "normal pressure" for any given eye.
   D. In most patients elevated intraocular pressure appears to be the main reason for optic nerve damage. However, there are other factors that seem to contribute to the disease process. Many patients with elevated intraocular pressure never develop optic nerve damage while other patients with low, normal, or minimally elevated intraocular pressure may have severe damage.
   E. A large cup/disc ratio does not necessarily reflect an abnormality, while an eye with glaucoma may have a more "normal sized" cup/disc ratio.
   F. Optic disc cupping may occur prior to the onset or the progression of visual field loss.
   G. Significant damage to the optic nerve may occur in the absence of detectable alterations in the visual field. The presence of a visual field defect usually indicates rather extensive optic nerve damage.

III. The appropriate management of the patient with glaucoma depends on
   A. an accurate determination of the type of glaucoma.
   B. a clinical evaluation of the presence and degree as well as change, of glaucomatous optic nerve and visual field damage.
   C. associated ocular and general medical problems.

## INITIAL PATIENT PRESENTATION

I. The diagnosis of glaucoma may be made during a routine examination in which the patient is seen for refractive complaints, or during an examination for an ocular disease unrelated to glaucoma such as cataracts, conjunctivitis, or macular degeneration.

II. The patient may present with an ocular disease in which glaucoma is an associated finding such as uveitis or diabetic retinopathy.

III. The patient may present with complaints directly related to glaucoma such as progressive visual loss, intermittent ocular pain and visual blurring, or the appearance of halos around lights.

## GLAUCOMA WORKUP

The initial aims of a glaucoma evaluation are to place the patient into a diagnostic category, to assess the degree of glaucoma damage, and to formulate a treatment plan. The initial phase of the workup may require several examinations to provide the foundation for future care.

### Ocular History

The ocular history, supplemented by prior ophthalmic records if available, is very important in providing clues to the diagnosis and possible management of the glaucoma.

I. Important aspects of the ocular history include the following:
   A. History of ocular trauma
   B. Prior ocular surgery
   C. Symptoms relating to acute elevations in intraocular pressure
   D. History or symptoms relating to uveitis
   E. History of prolonged administration of topical or systemic corticosteroids
   F. A family history of glaucoma

II. If the patient is already receiving therapy for glaucoma, attempts should be made to obtain past medical records including copies of previous visual fields and optic disc photographs. The ocular history of a glaucoma patient should be obtained for each eye and include the following:
   A. Type of glaucoma diagnosis
   B. Date of glaucoma diagnosis
   C. Highest recorded intraocular pressure
   D. A detailed history with dates of prior and current glaucoma medical therapy
   E. History of adverse reactions to prior glaucoma agents with a detailed description of the side effects which required stopping the medication
   F. Dates and types of prior intraocular and laser surgery

### Medical History

I. A review of systems is obtained; special attention is given to a history of the following:
   A. Systemic hypertension
   B. Diabetes mellitus
   C. Blood transfusions
   D. An episode of shock
   E. Cardiovascular disease
   F. Cerebrovascular disease
   G. Thyroid disease
   H. A history of kidney stones
   I. Respiratory disease including a history of asthma

II. A listing of prior nonocular surgery is obtained.

III. The dosage and dates of current systemic medications are recorded.

IV. Drug allergies, in particular a history of sulfa allergy, are recorded.

V. The name and address of the patient's general medical physician is recorded.

### Ocular Examination

The ocular examination of a patient with glaucoma is not unique. However, there are certain physical constraints on the order in which the various tests should be performed.

Information obtained during the examination often can not be elicited in the same order in which it is evaluated. After obtaining the history, the ocular examination, under ideal circumstances, should be performed as follows:

I. Refraction to determine the best corrected visual acuity
II. Visual field examination
III. External examination including testing for an afferent (Marcus-Gunn) pupillary defect
IV. Slit-lamp examination with special attention to
   A. central and peripheral chamber depth (see Chapter 4)
   B. comparison of the chamber depths between the two eyes
   C. signs of pigmentary dispersion syndrome
   D. iris sphincter atrophy which may be a sign of the exfoliation syndrome
   E. iridodonesis and phacodonesis
   F. presence of lenticular changes
   G. signs of uveitis including cellular reaction and posterior synechiae
   H. rubeosis iridis
V. Measurement of intraocular pressure
VI. Gonioscopy

The remainder of the examination depends on the gonioscopy findings. If the iridocorneal angle is open and nonoccludable, perform the following:

   A. Dilated fundus examination for direct examination of the posterior pole and indirect peripheral ophthalmoscopy
   B. Stereo optic disc photography
   C. Dilated slit-lamp examination noting the
      1. presence of pseudoexfoliation
      2. presence of pigment deposits on the equator and posterior aspects of the lens, appearance of the anterior vitreous
      3. optic disc examination with a contact lens, the Hruby lens, or the 90 diopter lens
      4. description of the optic disc: contour and color cup-to-disc ratio, disc hemorrhages, notching, etc.

If the iridocorneal angle is narrow and possibly occludable, perform the following:

   A. Pupil dilation, if done, must be performed with care. Use an easily reversible agent, such as mydriacil, and only dilate one eye at a time. The patient is informed of possible induction of an acute attack of glaucoma. In some patients, do not dilate the pupil until a laser iridotomy has been performed.
   B. Stereo optic disc photography and slit-lamp examination are performed on the dilated eye as described above.

## SUMMARY

In summary, the approach to the glaucoma workup is as follows:

I. Does the patient have glaucoma? This is answered largely by the history, functional and anatomic status of the eye (visual acuity, pupillary response, visual field, gonioscopy, optic disc), and intraocular pressure.
II. If the patient has glaucoma, what is the classification and mechanism? This is answered by the history, general and slit-lamp examination, gonioscopy, and fundus examination.

# 10

# Diagnosis and Medical Treatment of Glaucoma

The treatment of patients with glaucoma will vary depending on the exact diagnosis. A common cause for difficulties in glaucoma management is failure to make the correct diagnosis. In some types of glaucoma, medical therapy is the primary and principal mode of treatment. In other types of glaucoma, laser surgery or conventional surgery is indicated primarily. However, medical treatment is usually required at some point in the management of the various types of glaucoma.

The choice of drugs in the medical treatment of any particular glaucoma patient depends on several factors:

1. Etiology of the glaucoma.
2. Presence of other ocular diseases.
3. Age of the patient.
4. Presence of systemic illnesses.
5. Presence of drug allergies.

Pharmacology of the drugs used in treating glaucoma has been covered in chapter 7. A general classification of glaucoma has been presented in Chapter 8. Congenital glaucoma is discussed in Chapter 13. This chapter presents the salient features of the most frequently encountered types of glaucoma in the adult patient and guidelines for their diagnosis and medical management.

## ADULT-ONSET PRIMARY GLAUCOMAS

### Primary Open-Angle Glaucoma

1. Elevated intraocular pressure ≥22 mmHg.
2. Open iridocorneal angle.
3. Glaucomatous visual field loss.
4. Glaucomatous optic disc cupping.
5. Absent findings of antecedent ocular disease.

#### Therapy

Therapy is directed to lowering the intraocular pressure to a level which is consistent with retention of visual function, usually considered to be less than 20 mmHg. However, currently there are no methods to determine what intraocular pressure level is optimum for a given eye to maintain optic nerve function. Therefore, the ultimate determinant that the treatment intraocular pressure level is being tolerated by the eye is the stability of the glaucomatous visual field loss and optic disc cupping.

##### Initiation of Therapy

I. Treatment is usually initiated with a topical agent. Except in unusual circumstances, it is preferable to institute therapy with only a single drug. This helps avoid confusion if one drug is ineffective. Treatment can be started in only one eye to allow the use of the intraocular pressure in the fellow eye as a control until effectiveness of the medication is determined. This method should not be used if there is significant glaucomatous damage in both eyes. Single eye trials are not wise when it is felt that there is a significant risk of immediate vision loss from the intraocular pressure.

II. Beta-adrenergic blocking agents are often the first line of therapy for primary open-angle glaucoma. Their twice daily dosage, high degree of effectiveness, and low incidence of side effects favor their use.

III. If beta blockers are contraindicated or have no effect on intraocular pressure, epinephrine, dipivalyl epinephrine (Propine), or pilocarpine can be used as the initial drug.

## Progression of Therapy

If the reduction in intraocular pressure to the initial drug is inadequate, additional topical drugs and, possibly, systemic carbonic anhydrase inhibitors should be added.

I. Use of multiple topical drugs

The tear lake usually retains less than a single eye drop, the second drop washing out of the cul-de-sac onto the face. Eye drops are absorbed into the eye within 3–5 min of administration. Therefore, it is important to instruct patients to wait at least 5 min between the administration of different eye drops. We also instruct patients to gently close their eyelids for 3–5 min after delivery of a drop to prevent blinking which forces drainage of the medication with the tears into the lacrimal system and into the nasal cavity. Eyelid closure increases the amount of drug entering the eye while reducing systemic absorption and, therefore, systemic side effects of the drug. These effects of eyelid closure can be achieved by external compression over the nasal area of the tear system; however, we find it easier to instruct patients on eyelid closure than nasal compression. In addition, eyelid closure is easier for patients to perform.

II. Topical agents

A. If a beta blocker is the initial agent

1. topical pilocarpine may be added as the second medication.

   The effects of pilocarpine are additive to the topical beta blocker. Since miotics may be associated with an increased risk of retinal detachment, a careful peripheral retinal examination should be performed prior to their use. Pilocarpine treatment is begun with 1% or 2% drops four times/day. Pilocarpine Ocuserts or long-acting gel may be used in patients whose intraocular pressure responds well to pilocarpine eye drops, but who have annoying visual side effects or who find four times/day dosage inconvenient. If necessary, the strength of the pilocarpine may be increased to 4% or 6%. If the response to pilocarpine is inadequate, either with initial use or a reduced effectiveness over time, then the patient can be switched to carbachol 3% three times/day. Carbachol may often be more effective than pilocarpine.

2. topical epinephrine or dipivalyl epinephrine can be used as an alternative to pilocarpine as the second medication with the beta blocker.

   These drugs are also used if pilocarpine therapy is not tolerated. However, there may be only a minimal added reduction in intraocular pressure after the addition of an epinephrine preparation to an eye receiving a beta blocker. Therefore, we initially have the patient add the epinephrine drug to only one eye, the beta blocker continued in both eyes, to determine if there is an additional benefit over the pressure reduction to the beta blocker alone.

B. If an epinephrine drug is the initial agent
   1. and there is no contraindication to a topical beta blocker, we will discontinue the epinephrine drug and begin treatment with a beta blocker and progress with therapy, if needed, as described above.
   2. and a topical beta blocker is contraindicated, topical pilocarpine is added as the second medication. The effects of pilocarpine are additive to the topical epinephrine preparation.

Maximum tolerated topical therapy consists of a beta blocker, a miotic, and an epinephrine preparation.

III. Systemic agents
   A. Carbonic anhydrase inhibitors should be used if topical therapy is inadequate or not tolerated. These agents are additive to all of the topical drugs.
   B. Acetazolamide (Diamox) is commonly used in a dosage of 250 mg four times/day or 500 mg sequels twice/day. This drug seems to be more effective but also has more systemic effects than methazolamide.
   C. Methazolamide (Neptazane), 25–50 mg two to three times/day, is preferable in many patients because it produces less systemic side effects and, therefore, is often better tolerated.
   D. Some patients have an adequate reduction in intraocular pressure following administration of lower than the recommended dosage of either carbonic anhydrase inhibitor. Lower dosage can be associated with a reduction in the systemic side effects, especially in patients with lower weights. The use of either of these agents should consider the weight of the patient, tolerance of the side effects, and the intraocular pressure response.
   E. We do not use these drugs in patients with a past history of renal stones or allergy to sulfa-containing medications. However, there is no reason to avoid long-term carbonic anhydrase inhibitor therapy in patients who tolerate these agents.

IV. Strong miotics

Cholinesterase inhibitors such as echothiophate (Phospholine iodide) should be avoided in phakic patients because they produce cataracts. These agents are often very effective in aphakic or pseudophakic patients when administered once or twice daily. However, they may be associated with an increased risk of retinal detachment. Examination of the retina is necessary prior to initiating therapy with these agents.

## Maximum Tolerated Medical Therapy

I. This is an important concept in the medical management of patients with glaucoma. This is significantly different from maximum medical therapy which would include a beta blocker, a miotic, an epinephrine compound, and a carbonic anhydrase inhibitor. Not all patients will be able to tolerate maximum medical therapy. The most medication that any single patient will tolerate constitutes the maximum tolerated medical therapy for that patient.

II. Some side effects can be controlled or tolerated with patient education (Table 10-1). For example, warning the patient of the temporary nature of the miotic associated browache will increase compliance. Patients being started on any medication should be warned of the possibility of side effects and told what to expect. Many patients will tolerate minor or slightly annoying side effects if they have been forwarned and appreciate the importance of treatment in preventing blindness.

III. Side effects can often be managed by switching to a different agent in the same class. For example, patients intolerant of acetazolamide may tolerate methazolamide. Patients with pulmonary disease may be able to use betaxolol instead of timolol.

## Overview

Diverse opinions may be found regarding which drug should be added for additional control. Pilocarpine is so universally capable of producing symptoms that it has been said that "glaucoma is a disease that has no symptoms until it is treated." No amount of reassurance will get some young patients to continue the drug. Patients with axial lens opacities may actually be visually incapacitated. While many physicians will add pilocarpine as the second drug, others prefer epinephrine or dipivalyl epinephrine, which is usually better tolerated but may be much less effective. Carbonic anhydrase inhibitors are rarely used before the trial of all three classes of topical drugs are utilized. Patients whose response to maximally tolerated medical therapy is such that progressive loss of visual function occurs, or is likely to occur, should be offered laser or surgical treatment.

## Frequency of Follow-up Examinations

I. Continued monitoring of intraocular pressure, visual fields, and the optic disc is a necessity in glaucoma therapy. The initial therapy may become ineffective with time due to tachyphylaxis, patient intolerance, or simply the inability of the recommended therapy to control the disease. Conversely, some medications (notably epinephrine) may take longer to attain an effective result.

**Table 10-1.** Intolerance to Glaucoma Therapy

| Drug | Reasons for Intolerance | Possible Solution |
|---|---|---|
| Beta blockers | Reactive airway disease, impotence, depression, cardiovascular | Use selective beta blocker, lower the dose or the frequency of administration, eyelid closure (see text) |
| Pilocarpine | Ciliary symptoms which are worse in younger patients | Start with 1% and slowly increase the dose, consider gel or Ocusert, patient education |
| | Decreased vision | Consider Ocuserts, may have to consider removing a cataractous lens |
| Propine or epinephrine | Allergy | Alternate preparation (HCl vs. borate vs. bitartrate), switch propine for epinephrine |
| | Rebound hyperemia | Patient education |
| Carbonic anhydrase inhibitors | Parasthesias | Patient education |
| | Nausea and weight loss | Methazolamide may be better tolerated |
| | Kidney stones | Discontinue medication |

II. Glaucoma follow-up evaluations should be performed two to four times a year. The frequency of visual field examinations should be based on the potential wide fluctuations which can occur in the intraocular pressure outside of the office setting. In many instances, this means we recommend a visual examination every 6 months, even in patients with "controlled" intraocular pressures. The only means to assure control of visual function is by visual field examination. More frequent examinations are determined by the patient's intraocular pressure control and the amount of glaucomatous damage. General guidelines are as follows:

A. Intraocular pressure measurements

Patients with unstable pressures, intraocular pressures which have wide fluctuation from visit to visit, and patients who require multiple medications for glaucoma control require more frequent examination than the patient with stable and low pressures (e.g., <14 mmHg) which are controlled with one medication.

B. Optic disc cupping

Patients with extensive glaucomatous cupping may require more frequent evaluation since they have a lower reserve of functioning nerve tissue. There is a clinical impression that patients with extensive glaucomatous cupping and visual field loss may be more suspectible to progressive damage and therefore require more rigorous intraocular pressure control. More frequent follow-up examinations may be required in these patients. Optic disc stability is best determined by comparing optic disc photographs obtained every year or two.

C. Visual field loss

One-eyed patients and eyes with extensive field loss extending close to fixation require more frequent visual field examinations. Testing should include central measurements to assure the status of fixation.

## Ocular Hypertension (Glaucoma Suspect, Preglaucoma)

1. Elevated intraocular pressure ≥22 mmHg.
2. Open-iridocorneal angle.
3. Normal optic discs.
4. Normal visual fields.
5. Absent findings of antecedent ocular disease.

I. Ocular hypertension (6% prevalence) does not equal primary open-angle glaucoma (0.5% prevalence).

II. Long-term studies have demonstrated that the conversion from ocular hypertension to primary open-angle glaucoma, as defined by either the onset of visual field loss or documented progression of optic disc cupping, is less than 1% per year. Therefore, if 100 patients with ocular hypertension were followed for 10 years without glaucoma therapy, only 7 to 9 patients would be expected to demonstrate intolerance of the elevated intraocular pressure and the development of either early visual field damage or progressive optic disc cupping.

III. Risk factors

These studies have been based primarily on patients with elevated intraocular pressures between 22 and 30 mmHg. Therefore, higher levels of intraocular pressure, as well as other "risk factors," may indicate initiation of medical therapy in ocular hypertension. Risk factors which may favor treatment include the following:

A. Intraocular pressure repeatedly higher than 30 mmHg
B. A family history of glaucoma, in particular glaucomatous visual loss
C. Useful vision in only one eye
D. Presence of diabetes mellitus
E. Presence of systemic vascular disease

F. Presence of an optic disc hemorrhage
G. High myopia
H. Retinal vascular occlusion by history in either eye

IV. While open-angle glaucoma is a bilateral disease, glaucomatous damage is frequently asymmetric. The patient with bilaterally elevated intraocular pressures and glaucomatous optic disc cupping and visual field loss in one eye, has open-angle glaucoma in both eyes. This patient's eye without glaucomatous damage does not have ocular hypertension. Treatment of a high intraocular pressure in this fellow eye is indicated regardless of its visual field or cup.

V. Some patients with ocular hypertension prefer treatment rather than follow-up without therapy. In addition, some patients are unwilling or unable to return for regular follow-up without treatment.

VI. Therapy

A. Initiation of therapy in ocular hypertension must consider the risk to benefit ratio (i.e., the relatively low conversion to open-angle glaucoma and the side effects and cost of the therapy).

B. A therapeutic trial with either a topical beta blocker or an epinephrine agent can be performed to test the effectiveness of the drug to lower intraocular pressure and to determine the patient's tolerance to the medication. Initially the trial should be in only one eye to allow detecting a differential intraocular pressure effect between the two eyes.

C. We rarely use miotics or carbonic anhydrase inhibitors in the treatment of ocular hypertension.

D. An acceptable aim of therapy in some patients is to partially reduce the intraocular pressure to a "safer" level and not necessarily to a level below 20 mmHg.

E. Visual fields and optic disc cupping must be followed in ocular hypertensive patients independent of the use of glaucoma therapy. We generally examine these patients twice yearly for intraocular pressure and optic disc evaluation. Visual fields are usually performed at least yearly if the intraocular pressure is <25 mmHg and twice yearly if the pressure is higher.

## Low-Tension Glaucoma

1. Normal intraocular pressure, <20 mmHg.
2. Glaucomatous visual field loss.
3. Glaucomatous optic disc cupping.
4. Open iridocorneal angle.
5. Absent findings of antecedent ocular disease.

I. Low-tension glaucoma represents the other end of the spectrum from ocular hypertension since the untreated intraocular pressure is normal but glaucomatous damage is present.

II. Low-tension glaucoma may be a variant of open-angle glaucoma.

III. Differential diagnosis includes the following:

A. A previously unrecognized primary open-angle glaucoma which is detected over time when the intraocular pressure is found to be elevated. Diurnal intraocular pressure measurements may be required to differentiate low-tension from primary open-angle glaucoma

B. End-staged ("burnt-out") open-angle glaucoma with a low rate of aqueous humor production

C. Glaucoma damage due to a previous transient elevation in intraocular pressure or to a transient episode of vascular shock

D. Anterior ischemic optic neuropathy

E. Optic nerve defects (e.g., drusen or an optic pit) resulting in a nerve fiber bundle visual field defect.

IV. Low-tension glaucoma patients who do not show progressive visual field loss or cupping probably do not require treatment.

V. Low-tension glaucoma patients may have an increased incidence of hemodynamic crises, systemic hypertension, migraine, and hypercholesterolemia. In addition, optic disc hemorrhages may be more frequent in this type of glaucoma.

VI. The management of patients with progressive glaucomatous damage is similar to that of patients with primary open-angle glaucoma. However, it is not clear that the course of low-tension glaucoma is altered much by therapy that lowers intraocular pressure.

## Primary Acute Closed-Angle Glaucoma (with Pupillary Block)

I. Acute onset of elevated intraocular pressure. Aqueous humor dynamics are usually normal prior to the onset of the acute attack.

II. Closed iridocorneal angle on gonioscopic examination.

III. Shallow anterior chamber on slit-lamp examination. The fellow eye usually will manifest a narrow and potentially occludable iridocorneal angle.

IV. The conjunctiva is hyperemic, the pupil is mid-dilated and nonreactive to light, and the cornea may be cloudy.

V. Vision is reduced and the patient may complain of seeing colored halos (the blue-green component nearest the light source) around lights due to the corneal edema.

VI. Ocular pain is usually present.

VII. The patient may also have systemic complaints secondary to autonomic stimulation, including nausea, vomiting, and bradycardia.

VIII. Many patients with primary acute angle-closure glaucoma have a past history of intermittent episodes of angle-closure symptoms.

IX. The basic ocular abnormality is an inherited anatomic predisposition, present in both eyes, to angle-closure which is manifested by the following:

A. A small anterior segment with hyperopia, a small cornea, and a well-developed ciliary body. The iris may insert anteriorly on the ciliary body.

B. A reduced anterior chamber depth with an increased diameter to the lens which is located anteriorly.

### Management of Suspects

I. Patients with asymptomatic narrow angles do not usually require medical therapy. We rarely use prophylactic pilocarpine therapy in these patients and prefer to perform a prophylactic laser iridotomy if we have the following concerns regarding the narrow-angle suspect:

A. The presence of signs or symptoms compatible with intermittent angle-closure. This includes the finding of peripheral anterior synechiae on indentation goniscopy.

B. Appositional closure of the angle for greater than 180°. This state may lead to trabecular dysfunction and progressive decrease in outflow facility.

C. The systemic use of medications which are associated with the precipitation of an acute attack (see Chapter 7).

D. A strong family history of acute angle-closure glaucoma or if the patient lives in a remote area, distant from ophthalmologic care.

II. If laser iridotomy is to be performed (see Chapter 11), a miotic should be used before treatment to facilitate the surgery. In a previously untreated eye this can be accomplished with a single drop of 2% pilocarpine 30 to 60 minutes before the laser treatment.

### Management of an Acute Angle-Closure Attack

I. The acute attack is treated medically in conjunction with the performance of a laser iridotomy. Sometimes topical agents (a beta blocker and pilocarpine) are effective in terminating an acute attack. However, the iris sphincter muscle may not respond to miotics in the presence of a high intraocular pressure. Therefore, only 1 or 2 drops of 1% or 2% pilocarpine are administered prior to the onset of intraocular pressure reduction. For this reason the primary treatment usually is a hyperosmotic agent such as intravenous mannitol or oral glycerol. Carbonic anhydrase inhibitors and beta blockers may also be effective during an acute attack in lowering intraocular pressure and permitting the miotic to function to open the iridocorneal angle.

II. Medical therapy can lower intraocular pressure without terminating the acute attack. Termination of the attack is attended by
   A. an opening of the closed iridocorneal angle and a deepening of the anterior chamber. This must be determined by gonioscopy.
   B. the pupil becoming miotic.

III. If the attack cannot be broken with medical therapy, a laser iridotomy (see page 169) or a surgical iridectomy (see page 238) should be performed.

### Management of the Fellow Eye

I. The fellow eye is at increased risk to have a spontaneous attack of acute angle-closure glaucoma, approximately an 80% risk within 5 years.

II. Prophylactic pilocarpine eye drops in the fellow eye are associated with a reduced risk of a spontaneous attack, however, the risk is still only reduced to 50%.

III. We recommend prophylactic iridectomy, preferably by laser, on the fellow eye.

### Management of Chronic Angle-Closure Glaucoma

Residual elevation in intraocular pressure following an acute attack and a patent iridectomy requires long-term medical therapy. The mechanism for the pressure increase in these cases is trabecular damage or peripheral anterior synechiae with reduced outflow facility. Treatment is similar to chronic open-angle glaucoma. However, if a significant portion of the angle is permanently closed by peripheral anterior synechiae, miotics are less likely to be effective.

#### Chronic Closed-Angle Glaucoma (Creeping Angle-Closure)

I. An insidious form of closed-angle glaucoma in which the iridocorneal angle slowly closes from the periphery to Schwalbe's line without signs or symptoms of intermittent or acute attacks of angle closure.

II. This condition may be more common in black patients and presents as an open-angle glaucoma. However, gonioscopy demonstrates synechial closure of the angle. Closure usually begins superiorly and progresses inferiorly.

III. This condition can be cured by laser iridotomy if detected early. However, medical therapy is usually required after the iridotomy. Unfortunately, many patients with this type of glaucoma are diagnosed after total synechial angle closure, and filtration surgery is the only effective method of therapy.

## Primary Closed-Angle Glaucoma (without Pupillary Block)

### Primary Plateau Iris

I. Shows gonioscopic findings of a closed anterior chamber angle with a flat iris plane as opposed to the forward bowing observed in closed-angle glaucoma with pupillary block.

II. The central chamber depth is normal in contrast to the shallow depth observed in primary closed-angle glaucoma.

III. The mechanism for angle-closure involves angle crowding. Relative pupillary block may be only a minor factor in the cause of the acute attack. This factor is eliminated by performing a laser iridotomy.

IV. Long-term treatment with pilocarpine is required after the iridectomy to prevent angle crowding and angle closure. If significant peripheral anterior synechiae are present, as a result of previous episodes of angle closure, treatment with other agents, similar to the therapy of chronic angle-closure glaucoma, may be needed.

### Aphakic Open-Angle Glaucoma

Aphakic open-angle glaucoma may be managed like chronic open-angle glaucoma in phakic patients. Echothiophate is a useful miotic in these patients because one need not worry about causing cateracts. Peripheral retinal examination is required prior to initiating therapy, and at regular intervals as long as therapy is continued since the use of strong miotics in aphakic patients may be associated with an increased risk of retinal detachment. Epinephrine compounds should be used with caution since they can be associated with a 20% incidence of reversible macular edema in aphakic patients. The risk of these side effects may be reduced in patients with an intact posterior lens capsule and posterior chamber intraocular lens implant.

## ADULT-ONSET SECONDARY GLAUCOMAS

Various conditions can cause secondary open-angle or closed-angle glaucoma. In some conditions management is in a similar manner to primary open-angle glaucoma, e.g., pigmentary and pseudoexfoliative glaucoma. Other conditions require therapy of the underlying etiology, e.g., uveitic or steroid-induced glaucoma. Many times, however, the underlying cause for the glaucoma cannot be removed. In addition, the disease process may cause alterations in outflow facility and the glaucoma persists following treatment of the underlying disease process. In these cases, continued medical therapy is required. While there are a large number of conditions which can be associated with secondary glaucoma in the adult patient (see Chapter 8), only the more frequently encountered conditions are covered in this section.

### Secondary Closed-Angle Glaucoma

Many conditions, relating to pupillary block from a secluded pupil or an anteriorly dislocated lens, result in secondary closed-angle glaucoma. In addition, peripheral anterior synechiae can result in chronic closure of the iridocorneal angle. It is important to determine whether or not pupillary block is present. If not, iridotomy will be of no benefit and is not indicated.

Ocular disorders which can lead to secondary closed-angle glaucoma include the following:

1. Rubeosis iridis (see below).
2. Ciliary body swelling, cysts, or inflammation.
3. Posterior segment tumors.
4. Scleral buckling procedures and panretinal photocoagulation.
5. Lens induced—either a swollen and mature lens or a lens which is dislocated or which is subluxated into the anterior chamber.
6. Posterior synechiae to the lens (iris bombe), e.g., uveitis, or to the vitreous humor in aphakia, or to an intraocular lens in pseudophakia.
7. Epithelial or fibrous ingrowth.

## Secondary Open-Angle Glaucoma

### Pigmentary Glaucoma

I. Pigmentary glaucoma is a bilateral disorder usually affecting young myopic men. The disease is very rare in black patients.

II. It is characterized by pigment loss (pigment dispersion syndrome) from the iris pigment epithelium. This occurs in a radial pattern, particularly in the midperiphery (Fig. 10-1). Anteriorly located packets of lens zonules rub on the back surface of the iris, causing the pigment loss.

III. Pigment is deposited in characteristic locations in the anterior segment: on the endothelial surface of the cornea, in the pattern of a base-down triangle (Krukenberg's spindle), on the iris surface, in the trabecular meshwork (see Fig. 4-2), and on the lens equator and zonules.

IV. Pigmentary dispersion syndrome can occur with or without an elevated intraocular pressure. The relative risk for the development of glaucoma in patients with pigment dispersion is unknown.

V. Pigment release into the anterior chamber can occur after pupil dilation or physical exercise. Pigment release decreases with increasing age. Pigment accumulates in the trabecular meshwork and decreases outflow facility, which results in the increase in intraocular pressure. However, the reason why some eyes develop glaucoma and others do not is unknown.

VI. Management of the condition is similar to that described for ocular hypertension and primary open-angle glaucoma.

### Pseudoexfoliation (Exfoliation) Glaucoma

I. A unilateral or bilateral (37%) disorder which increases in frequency with age, particularly after the age of 65 years. Incidence is higher among people of Danish, Scandinavian, Dutch, Syrian, Armenian, and Greek extractions. The condition is uncommon in American blacks, but it does occur. The condition, however, has an incidence of 10% in the Bantu tribe of South Africa.

II. Pseudoexfoliation is found as an incidential finding without evidence of glaucoma in 2% to 20% of elderly patients. The incidence of pseudoexfoliation in patients with open-angle glaucoma may be as high as 50%, depending on the population under study.

III. It is characterized by flakes and sheets of exfoliative material on structures of the anterior segment. The material has a close association with amyloid. The origin of the material is an abnormal epithelial basement membrane with a multifocal origin: lens, ciliary body, iris pigment, and trabecular epithelium.

IV. Exfoliative material is deposited on these structures (Fig. 10-2). Deposition within the trabecular meshwork results in reduced outflow facility and an associated elevation in intraocular pressure.

V. Pseudoexfoliation is also associated with increased pigment release within the anterior segment. A pigment line (Sampaolesi's line) can be detected anterior to Schwalbe's line on gonioscopy. Iris transillumination may reveal defects near the pupillary sphincter.

VI. Management of pseudoexfoliation glaucoma is similar to that described for ocular hypertension and primary open-angle glaucoma.

### Steroid-Induced Glaucoma

I. Topical, periocular, and systemic administration of corticosteroids can result in a secondary open-angle glaucoma in susceptible individuals (see Chapter 7).

II. Diagnosis of steroid-induced glaucoma

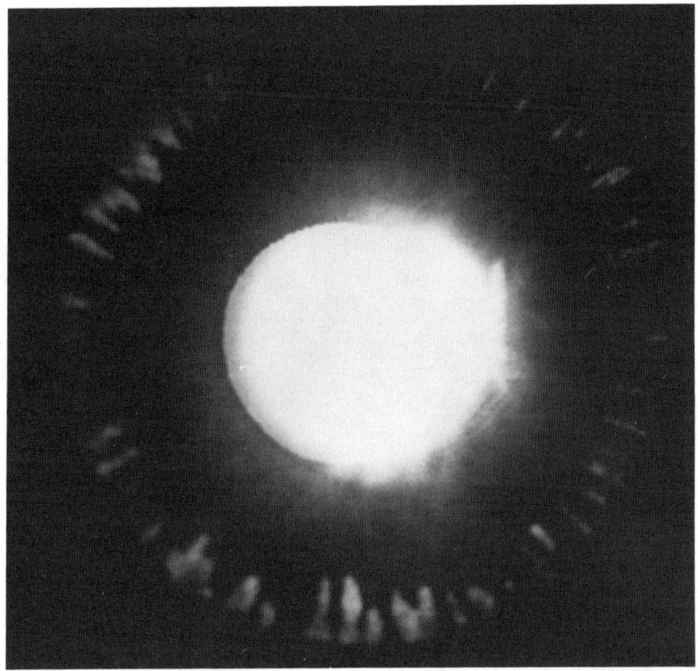

**Fig. 10-1** Radial transillumination iris defects in an eye with pigmentary glaucoma.

requires a high index of suspicion and the questioning of patients specifically about their use of steroid eyedrops, ointments, skin preparations, and pills.

III. The key to management is stopping the corticosteroid. If the drug is used for treatment of intraocular inflammation, e.g., uveitis, or postoperatively after ocular surgery, the steroid preparation should be tapered or switched to a less potent preparation such as fluorometholone (see Chapter 7).

IV. Intraocular pressure returns to baseline over a few weeks to several months after the steroid is stopped. During this period, treatment with standard antiglaucoma medications may be required to control the intraocular pressure. Steroid-induced glaucoma responds poorly to argon laser trabeculoplasty (see Chapter 11). Glaucoma resistant to standard medical management requires filtration surgery.

## Iridocorneal Endothelial (ICE) Syndrome

I. The syndrome is a spectrum of disorders which are typically unilateral and occur predominantly in white women. The condition is most often recognized in early to middle adulthood.

II. The syndrome is separated into three clinical variations as characterized by alterations in the iris.

   A. Progressive (essential) iris atrophy

      Corectopia and atrophy of the iris lead to hole formation in quadrants away from the direction of the pupillary displacement (Fig. 10-3). In addition, hole formation can occur independent of corectopia, secondary to ischemia of the iris.

   B. Chandler's syndrome

      Corectopia is mild or absent and iris atrophy is mild and limited to the superficial stroma. Corneal abnormalities are the major component of this syndrome.

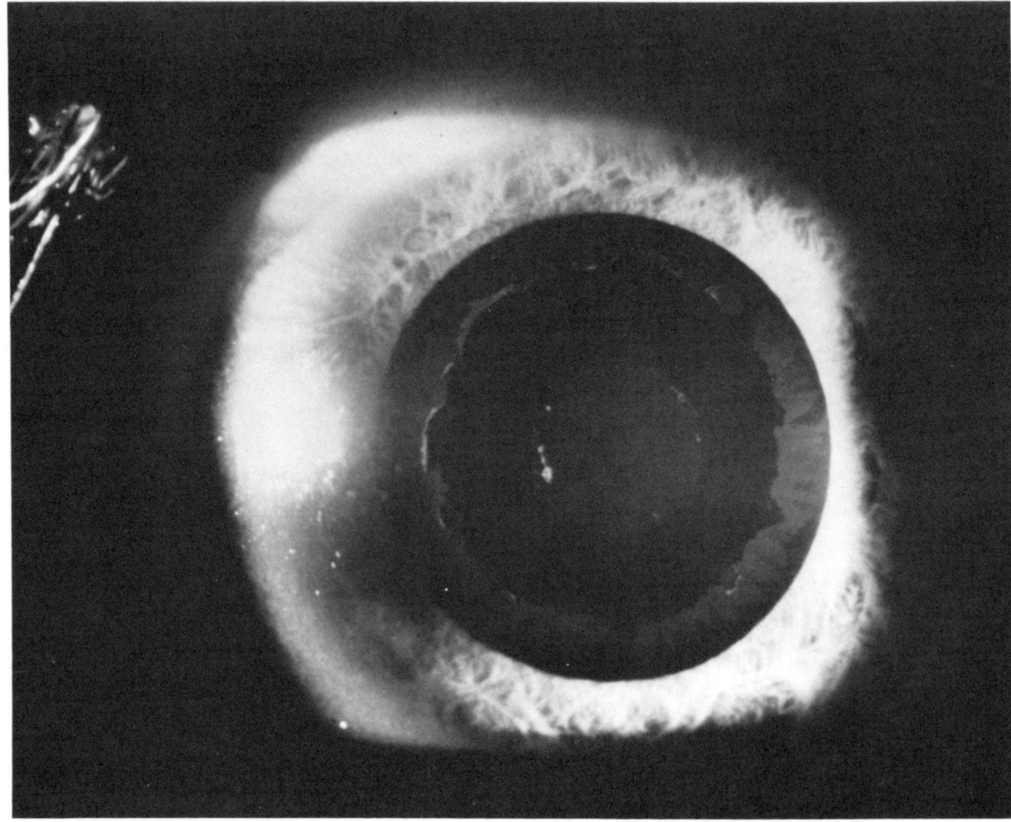

**Fig. 10-2** Pseudoexfoliation on the anterior lens capsule. Note the clear area between the central disc and peripheral zone of exfoliation material.

C. Cogan-Reese (iris nevus) syndrome

Areas of nodular or diffuse pigmented lesions appear on the surface of the iris. Iris atrophy can be mild or severe.

III. ICE syndrome also has the following additional characteristics.

A. Corneal alterations demonstrated by diffuse endothelial cell defects on specular microscopy. This is the major defect in Chandler's syndrome and can be associated with corneal decompensation with minimally elevated intraocular pressure.

B. Peripheral anterior synechiae which extend to or beyond Schwalbe's line.

C. Histologically a Descemet-like basement membrane covers portions of the chamber angle and may be associated with synechial closure.

IV. Secondary glaucoma is related to impaired outflow facility due to involvement of the angle with the Descemet-like membrane or by synechiae formation. This may develop into secondary angle-closure glaucoma.

V. Management of patients with the ICE syndrome consists of therapy of the corneal edema with topical hyperosmotic agents and bandage soft contact lens. Management of the glaucoma can usually be achieved initially with medical therapy; agents which reduce the rate of aqueous humor formation (e.g., topical beta blockers and systemic carbonic anhydrase inhibitors) being more effective

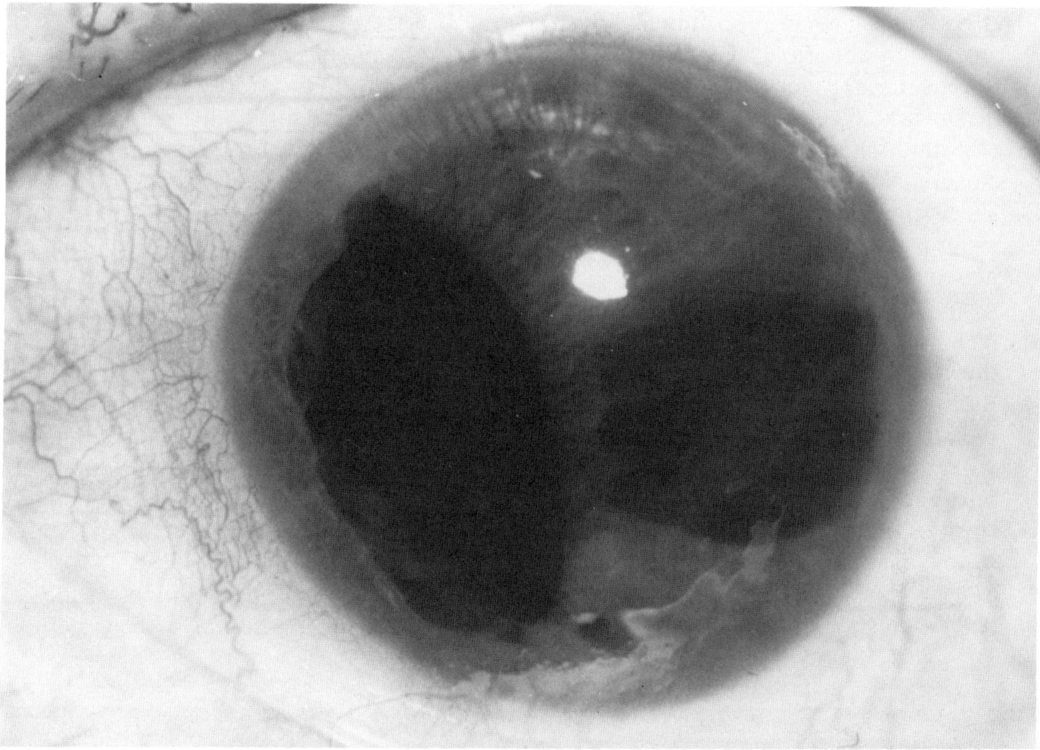

**Fig. 10-3** Iridocorneal endothelial syndrome, progressive iris atrophy. Note the melting iris hole to the right of the sphincter, the stretching of the iris with pupillary distortion to the left of the photograph, and ectropion uvea with associated peripheral anterior synechiae (counter-clockwise from 6 o'clock).

than agents which increase aqueous humor outflow. Surgical intervention is required to control the glaucoma in many eyes with this condition but has a lower success rate than primary glaucoma.

Other disorders of the corneal endothelium which may be associated with glaucoma include Fuchs' endothelioepithelial dystrophy (open-angle glaucoma) and posterior polymorphous dystrophy (autosomal recessive inheritance, angle-closure glaucoma secondary to synechial closure).

## Lens-Induced Glaucoma

I. Secondary open-angle glaucoma can result from
   A. phacolytic (lens protein) glaucoma.
   B. retained lens protein following extracapsular cataract surgery.
   C. phacoanaphylaxis.

II. Secondary closed-angle glaucoma can result from
   A. an intumescent lens.
   B. a dislocated lens either into the anterior chamber or into the vitreous. This can be secondary to trauma, Marfan's syndrome, homocystinuria, sulfite oxidase deficiency, and numerous other rare conditions.
   C. a microshperophakic lens (Weill-Marchesani syndrome).

## Neovascular Glaucoma

I. Rubeosis iridis and growth of a fibrovascular membrane over the anterior chamber angle causes neovascular glaucoma. The glaucoma is initially open-angle with abnormal blood vessels and fibrous tissue overlying the trabecular meshwork. This progresses to peripheral anterior synechiae with continued closure ("zippering") of the angle.

II. The earliest detectable finding of rubeosis iridis is the breakdown of the blood-aqueous barrier with fluorescein leakage from the iris vessels. The new vessels usually make their first appearance at the pupillary margin and progress onto the surface of the iris resulting in ectropion uvea (Fig. 10-4). Finally the vessels will grow into the iridocorneal angle and onto the trabecular meshwork.

III. Various systemic and ocular disease states can cause rubeosis iridis. The more common include the following.

A. Vascular disorders such as diabetes mellitus with the presence of diabetic retinopathy, central and branch retinal vein or artery occlusion, carotid artery occlusive disease, aortic arch syndrome, carotid-cavernous sinus fistula, and giant cell arteritis.

B. Ocular disorders such as diabetic retinopathy, chronic retinal detachment, Eales's disease, Coats' disease, sickle cell retinopathy, retrolental fibroplasia, persistent hyperplastic primary vitreous, Norrie's disease, chronic glaucoma, chronic uveitis, and sympathetic ophthalmia.

C. Intraocular tumors including retinoblastoma, malignant melanoma of the choroid, and metastatic carcinoma.

D. Postoperative conditions such as cataract extraction with or without

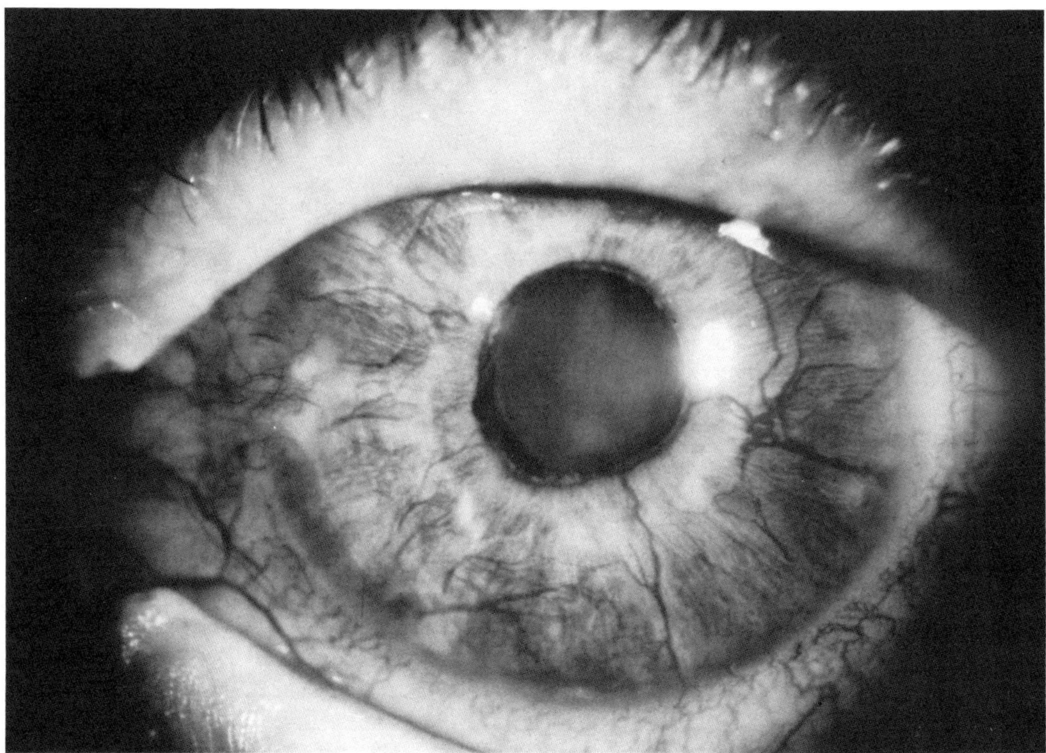

**Fig. 10-4** Neovascular glaucoma. Note the rubeosis iridis extending across the entire surface of the iris and the ectropion uvea. The iridocorneal angle was "zippered" closed for 360°.

implantation of an intraocular lens, vitrectomy, and retinal detachment surgery.

IV. Therapy

Treatment of neovascular glaucoma is directed to therapy and prevention of rubeosis iridis. Glaucoma treatment is dictated by the visual potential of the eye.

A. Panretinal photocoagulation

Neovascular glaucoma is very difficult to manage. Therefore, prevention is extremely critical to the proper management of patients with the two most common causes of rubeosis iridis, diabetic retinopathy and retinal vein occlusion. Panretinal photocoagulation in these conditions can eliminate the ischemic focus and cause regression of the rubeosis iridis. If performed at a stage prior to synechial closure of the angle, panretinal photocoagulation can prevent the severe secondary angle-closure glaucoma. The importance of treatment in central retinal vein occlusion relates to the ischemic type with areas of capillary nonperfusion that is highly associated with the development of rubeosis iridis. This is in contrast to the nonischemic form of occlusion which rarely is associated with the development of rubeosis iridis.

B. Medical management

Topical corticosteroids and atropine are administered in response to intraocular inflammation due to breakdown of the blood-aqueous barrier. Atropine also increases uveoscleral outflow, the only mechanism by which aqueous humor can exit the eye if the iridocorneal angle is totally sealed, and may therefore lower intraocular pressure. Many patients without visual potential are comfortable with this combined therapy in spite of an elevated intraocular pressure. Topical beta blockers and systemic carbonic anhydrase inhibitors are used to lower the intraocular pressure. Miotics should be avoided since they are ineffective if the angle is totally closed, may cause additional intraocular inflammation, and they decrease uveoscleral outflow. However, miotics may be effective after panretinal photocoagulation and regression of the rubeosis iridis if a sufficient portion of the angle is open.

C. Surgical management

Cyclodestructive procedures, including cyclocryotherapy, are associated with a high degree of complications when performed in eyes with neovascular glaucoma (see Chapter 12). Therefore, we only use these procedures in eyes without visual potential. Filtration surgery, either trabeculectomy or seton procedures, (see Chapter 12) are reserved for eyes with useful vision.

## Uveitic Glaucoma

I. Uveitis can cause a secondary open- or closed-angle glaucoma due to the following mechanisms.

A. Open-angle due to blockage of the trabecular meshwork by cellular debris or protein as well as a direct inflammatory effect (trabeculitis) on the outflow channels.

B. Closed-angle glaucoma due to posterior synechiae and pupillary block or peripheral anterior synechiae.

II. Various uveitic conditions associated with glaucoma include the following:

A. Glaucomatocyclitic crises (Posner-Schlossman syndrome) consisting of a unilateral elevated pressure associated with recurrent attacks of mild cyclitis. The iridocorneal angle is open and the pupil is larger, not miotic, in the involved eye. The attacks last hours to weeks. While the intraocular pressure is usually normal between attacks, this condition can be associated with later development of open-angle glaucoma.

B. Fuchs' syndrome of heterochromic cyclitis consisting of the triad of heterochromia, a mild and chronic form of cyclitis which characteristically does not respond to corticosteroids, and the late development of cataract.

C. Syphilis can be a cause of glaucoma during the active inflammatory stage. Also, in eyes with interstitial keratitis, secondary open- or closed-angle glaucoma may later develop.

D. Sarcoid uveitis frequently causes a secondary open- or closed-angle glaucoma.

E. Ankylosing spondylitis, adult rheumatoid arthritis, and juvenile rheumatoid arthritis are frequently associated with uveitis and secondary glaucoma.

F. Herpes simplex, herpes zoster, rubella, and mumps can have an associated uveitis and secondary glaucoma.

III. Management

A. Open-angle

Therapy is a balance between treatment of the inflammation and the elevated intraocular pressure. The uveitis is treated with a combination of topical, periocular or systemic corticosteroids and topical cycloplegics. The ophthalmologist must be aware of a possible steroid-induced rise in intraocular pressure. Occasionally, systemic immunosuppressive therapy is required. Topical beta blockers and epinephrine drugs and systemic carbonic anhydrase inhibitors are used to treat the glaucoma. Miotics are avoided since they increase intraocular inflammation. Argon laser trabeculoplasty (see Chapter 11) is not effective, and filtration surgery (see Chapter 12) has a lower rate of success in uveitic glaucoma.

B. Closed-angle

Pupillary block requires a laser iridotomy (see Chapter 11) or a surgical iridectomy (see Chapter 12) with the subsequent medical management of the uveitis and glaucoma as described above. Filtration surgery may be required, especially if there is extensive peripheral anterior synechiae.

## Ocular Trauma

I. Blunt trauma to the globe can result in an elevated intraocular pressure due to

A. mechanical obstruction of the outflow pathways by red blood cells (a hyphema), blood products (hemolytic glaucoma), or degenerative red blood cell products from a vitreous hemorrhage (ghost cell glaucoma). In addition, inflammatory products can obstruct the trabecular pathways.

B. lens subluxation (lens-induced).

C. direct trauma to the trabecular meshwork resulting in a tear in the ciliary body and an angle recession.

II. Penetrating injuries can cause secondary glaucoma due to

A. a flat anterior chamber resulting in permanent peripheral anterior synechiae.

B. hyphema.

C. penetration or dislocation of the lens.

D. epithelial or fibrous ingrowth.

E. sympathetic ophthalmia.

F. a retained metallic intraocular foreign body, e.g., iron (siderosis) or copper (chalcosis).

III. Chemical injuries due to acid or especially alkali compounds can cause extensive ocular damage resulting in secondary glaucoma.

A. An early pressure rise due to structural deformation of the anterior segment.
B. An intermediate phase glaucoma during the reparative phase to the chemical injury.
C. A late phase glaucoma due to permanent damage to the outflow pathways including external damage to the sclera and conjunctiva.

## SUGGESTED READINGS

Kolker AE, Hetherington J Jr: Becker-Shaffer's Diagnosis and Therapy of the Glaucomas. CV Mosby Company, St. Louis, 1983

Ritch R, Shields MB: The Secondary Glaucomas. CV Mosby Company, St. Louis, 1982

# 11

# Laser Surgery in Glaucoma

## SURGEON PREPARATION AND KNOWLEDGE OF THE LASER

I. The surgeon should have full knowledge of the operation of the particular laser used for treatment. Water-cooled lasers require the water to be turned on prior to activating the laser. The water should remain on for at least 20 min after the laser is turned off.

II. The slit-lamp optics and the laser aiming beam must be parfocal. This is checked by placing the target rod in position and setting the slit-lamp oculars at the appropriate refraction. The slit-lamp is focused on the rod. The 50 μm aiming beam should also be in focus. Lack of parfocus requires adjustment by a service representative.

III. Actual laser output may differ from that registered on the instrument panel. Power meters are available that measure laser output at the slit-beam. Low laser output requires adjustment by a service representative.

IV. Resuscitation equipment should be available in the laser operating room.

V. It is recommended that everyone in the room, with the exception of the patient and surgeon, wear safety goggles during the laser treatment.

## EXPLAINING THE PROCEDURE TO THE PATIENT

While an explanation of the laser surgical procedure is dependent upon the type of treatment being performed, general patient information includes the following.

I. The nature of the glaucomatous process, either open-angle or closed-angle, and the technique and goal of the laser treatment, either iridotomy, trabeculoplasty, or any other, should be explained to the patient.

II. The laser instrumentation is explained to the patient in an attempt to alleviate any fears. The laser is described as an intense light or energy source that has many uses including many different applications in ophthalmology, from glaucoma to retinal therapy. The clear window of the cornea, with the aid of a contact lens during treatment, permits precise focusing of the laser beam on the tissue to be treated. The patient is informed that the laser is activated for fractions of a second at a time and that numerous applications will be used. The patient is told that he or she will hear a click (depending upon the laser instrument used) and see a flash of light when the laser is activated. The patient is also told that associated pain is minimal or nonexistent. However, the patient is warned that vision will be blurred for approximately 1 hr after the treatment secondary to placement of the contact lens and the flashing of light that occurs at the time of each laser application. The patient is informed that he or she must be very still and not talk during the treatment and that the treatment can be stopped at any time if he or she becomes uncomfortable.

III. Prior to treatment the patient is informed of possible complications including inflammation and the postoperative use of topical corticosteroids. The possibility of an acute rise in intraocular pressure is explained, with the need for the patient to spend 1–2 hr in your office following treatment and the possible need for additional glaucoma therapy to treat any pressure increase. Specific complications for individual procedures (e.g. iridotomy closure) and the need for possible retreatment, the inability to penetrate the iris in one sitting necessitating an additional treatment session, the failure of trabeculoplasty to lower intraocular pressure, and other complications are also explained prior to obtaining informed consent for the treatment. The remote possibility of glaucoma surgery necessitated by the postlaser rise in intraocular pressure should be discussed.

IV. The patient is informed that his or her usual glaucoma medications will be continued after laser treatment and that steroid drops will be used for a brief period. Also, there are no restrictions on physical activity following the treatment.

## POSITIONING THE PATIENT FOR LASER TREATMENT

The patient must be comfortable in order to cooperate during laser therapy. General points for proper patient positioning at the slit-lamp include the following.

I. The patient is positioned to sit comfortably erect at the slit-lamp by adjustment of the table height and chair. The patient's stool should not have wheels.

II. The patient's head is properly centered using the chin rest to allow full excursion of the center of the slit-beam. Black marks on the chin rest frame should be aligned with the lateral canthus. With the slit-lamp on, adequate superior and inferior excursion of the slit beam to illuminate the goniolens mirrors is checked and the head repositioned if necessary.

III. The patient is instructed to keep the chin in the rest with the teeth together and to press the forehead against the instrument throughout the procedure. The importance of keeping both eyes open to reduce Bell's phenomenon is stressed. The nontreated eye is given a fixation target, either the fixation light of the slit-lamp, a portion of the slit-lamp, or the surgeon's ear or shoulder. If there is no central vision in the untreated eye, the patient is instructed to maintain a forward gaze.

IV. If the slit-lamp is restricted from sliding forward by the patient's chest, the patient's chair is moved back from the slit-lamp and the patient instructed to lean forward to insert the head into the chin rest.

## POSITIONING THE SURGEON FOR LASER TREATMENT

The surgeon must be comfortable in order to perform laser therapy adequately. General points for proper surgeon positioning at the slit-lamp include the following.

I. The height and position of the surgeon's stool is adjusted so that the surgeon sits comfortably erect at the slit-lamp. The slit-lamp oculars are properly adjusted for pupillary distance and refractive error.

II. The laser should be on but in the inactivated state. The foot switch is placed at a comfortable and convenient location for easy activation during treatment. The spot size, power setting, and duration of burst are selected prior to activation of the laser.

III. During treatment, the surgeon holds the contact lens in the left hand for treatment of the right eye and in the right hand for treatment of the left eye. This frees the other hand to adjust the slit-lamp during therapy.

IV. The contact lens is held with the surgeon's thumb and first two fingers while the other two fingers are placed gently on the patient's cheek. The wrist is held straight and the forearm as vertical as possible.
   A. The contact lens is filled with goniosolution. To avoid air bubbles, the solution is stored upside down and the initial part of the expressed solution discarded.
   B. It is important to avoid getting goniosolution and fingerprints on the front surface of the gonioprism.
   C. The patient is instructed to look up. The gonioprism is positioned so that initial contact with the eye occurs at 6 o'clock and the lens is rotated against the cornea. The lens can be used to retract the lower eye lid. Care is taken to avoid the patient's upper eyelashes.
   D. Gentle pressure on the gonioprism centered on the cornea prevents the patient from squeezing the gonioprism from the eye.
   E. Gentle pressure on the gonioprism usually expresses any trapped air bubbles. If bubbles are present and cannot be cleared, the goniolens should be removed, cleaned, and reinserted.

V. The surgeon's elbow should rest either on the slip-lamp table or on an elbow support to stabilize the gonioprism against the eye. This avoids fatigue-related tremor.

## LASER IRIDOTOMY

I. Creation of a full-thickness hole in the iris with the laser has become an acceptable and preferred alternative to surgical iridectomy. Iridotomy, whether by a laser or a surgical technique, functions by eliminating pupillary block. The term laser "iridotomy" rather than laser "iridectomy" is used in this manual.

II. The biologic response to lasers depends upon the wavelength, pulse duration, and mode of application (Table 11-1).

III. The focus of a high-density small laser spot leads to absorption and conversion of the light energy into heat by the tissue, resulting in either coagulation or disruption of the tissue.

IV. The effects of the laser beam on the iris depend on the type of laser used.

### Indications

Laser iridotomy is indicated, as is surgical iridectomy, in all cases of angle-closure glaucoma in which pupillary block is the causative mechanism. Specific indications include the following.

I. Acute angle-closure glaucoma
   A. Following medical termination of the acute attack
   B. To terminate a medically unresponsive acute attack

II. Fellow eye of a patient who has had an attack of acute angle-closure

III. Chronic angle-closure glaucoma

IV. Subacute or intermittent angle-closure glaucoma

V. Prophylactic treatment of an anatomically narrow iridocorneal angle

VI. Combined mechanism glaucoma

VII. Secondary angle-closure glaucoma including ciliary block (malignant) and aphakic pupillary block glaucoma

VIII. To aid in the diagnosis of the plateau iris syndrome.

### Contraindications

I. An uncooperative patient

Inability of the patient to sit at the slit-lamp

III. Corneal edema
   A. This limits the precise focus of the laser beam on the iris surface.
   B. It reduces the amount of laser energy delivered to the iris surface.
   C. It increases the susceptibility to laser-induced corneal burns.

**Table 11-1.** Types of Lasers

| Name | Primary Wavelength (nm) | Active Species | Use |
|---|---|---|---|
| Argon | 488.0 blue | Ar ion | Photocoagulation |
| | 514.5 green | | Photocoagulation |
| Krypton | 531.0 green | Kr ion | Photocoagulation |
| | 568.2 yellow | | Photocoagulation |
| | 647.0 red | | Photocoagulation |
| Nd:YAG | 532 green | Nd ion | Photocoagulation |
| | 650 red | | Photocoagulation |
| | 1064 infrared | | Photodisruption |
| | 1300 infrared | | Photodisruption |
| Excimer | 126 to 351 ultraviolet | various | Photoablation |
| Helium-neon | 632.8 red | Ne atom | Aiming/diagnosis |

D. The administration of topical glycerin may result in sufficient corneal dehydration and clearing of the edema to allow the safe performance of laser surgery.

IV. A flat anterior chamber

A. Contact of the iris with the cornea eliminates the normal dissipation of laser-generated heat through the aqueous humor. Corneal endothelial burns will therefore occur immediately, preventing further attempts at the laser procedure.

B. The application of pressure on the contact lens may result in sufficient deepening of the anterior chamber to allow the safe performance of laser iridotomy.

C. Contraction burns (see below) can be used, if there is sufficient chamber depth, to retract the iris from the cornea, therefore providing a deeper chamber in which to perform the laser surgery.

## Argon Laser Iridotomy

I. Argon laser iridotomy uses the heating and disrupting effect of the laser energy to create a hole in the iris.

II. The laser effects include contour changes in the iris surface and contraction of the iris stroma. Fragmentation and dispersion of the iris tissue occur.

III. The heating effect coagulates iris vessels.

### Technique

I. Topical pilocarpine 1% or 2% administered prior to the procedure places the iris under stretch and reduces the iris thickness, facilitating penetration.

II. Topical anesthesia is usually sufficient for performing the procedure. Retrobulbar anesthesia is rarely indicated; however, it may be necessary in an uncooperative patient who cannot maintain fixation.

III. Antireflective-coated iridotomy contact lens (Fig. 11-1).

A. The use of a contact lens with a plus add (e.g. the Abraham lens) is useful, and almost mandatory, for optimal success. The contact lens is filled with goniosolution. It is important to keep the anterior lens surface free of the goniosolution and fingerprints.

B. The 66-diopter planoconvex button provides convergence of the laser

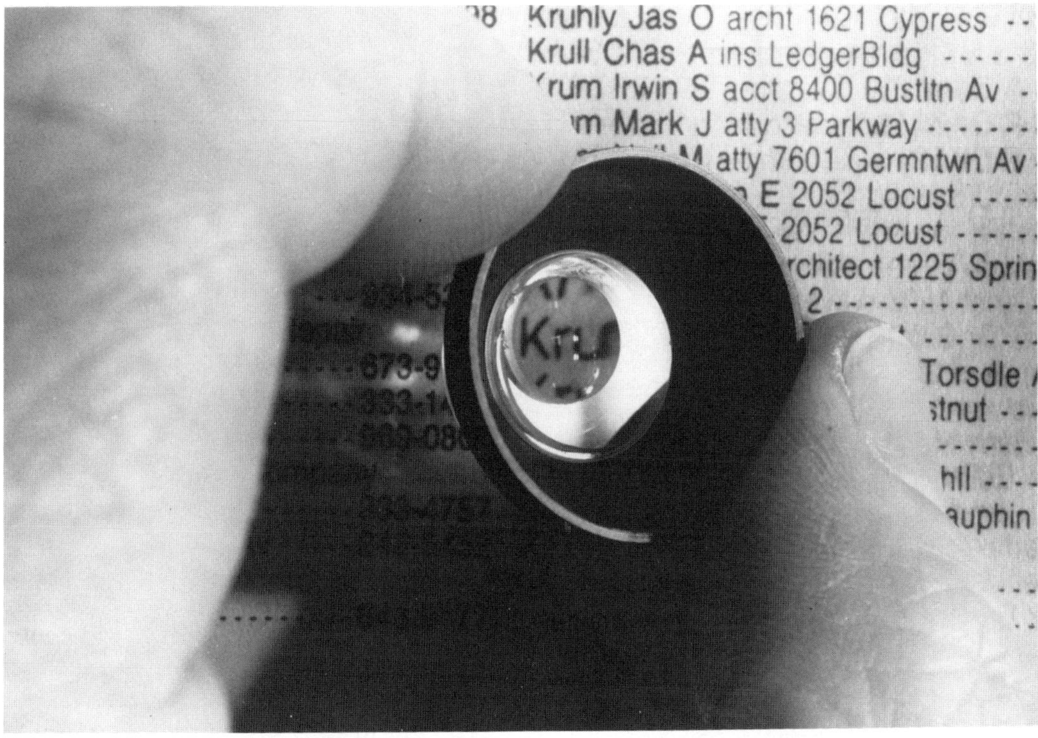


**Fig. 11-1** Laser iridotomy Abraham contact lens with off-center 66-diopter planoconvex button.

beam to a smaller spot size (the 50 μm spot is reduced to approximately 30 μm) with increased power density (energy per unit area) and increased magnification without loss of depth of focus.

C. The lens holds the eyelids open and eliminates blinking.

D. Ocular saccades and extraneous eye movements are reduced.

E. The gonioscopic solution serves as a heat sink, reducing the likelihood of corneal burns.

F. The antireflective coating reduces reflection of the laser beam and associated reduction of laser energy.

IV. Location of the iridotomy

A. While the procedure can be performed at any clock hour, the superior iris between 10:30 and 1:30 is selected so as to have the iridotomy covered by the upper lid. We prefer the area in the superior nasal quadrant with the laser aimed away from the posterior pole.

B. The 12:00 location is avoided because of possible bubble formation and migration, which can prevent visualization of the treatment site.

C. With the pupil constricted with miotics, a site between one-half and two-thirds of the distance between the pupil margin and the visible periphery is chosen. This is approximately equivalent to one half the distance between the edge of the collarette and the limbus.

D. Treatment through a corneal arcus senilis is avoided since the density of the arcus reduces the laser power across the cornea and interferes with a clear focusing of the laser beam.

E. For dark irides, select the base of an

iris crypt or a depigmented area with thinner stroma for easier penetration. In light blue or grey irides, the base of a crypt is also selected for treatment. In light-colored irides, a surface freckle that may provide improved laser absorption can be selected for treatment.

V. Laser Settings (Table 11-2)
   A. The number of required burns is dependent upon the iris color, the surgical technique, and the type of laser used.
   B. Treatment should be accomplished using the least possible energy.
   C. Laser settings are dependent upon the iris response to the delivered laser energy.
   D. The greater the iris pigmentation, the more effect a given energy level will have: blue irides require higher energy levels than brown irides to achieve a similar effect.
   E. Durations of laser exposure of 0.2 sec or less are well tolerated, while longer durations may be painful.
   F. Penetration of the iris stroma during a single burn tends to be easier with a shorter-duration, smaller spot size and higher-energy burn.
   G. Coagulation and contour changes in the iris during a single burn tend to be greater with a longer-duration, larger spot size and a lower energy level.
   H. Settings to create contraction ("Humping") of the iris:

| | |
|---|---|
| spot | 300–500 μm |
| energy | 200–400 mW |
| exposure | 0.2–0.5 sec |

   These setting have been recommended to "pull" the iris away from the lens and thin the iris for easier penetration. These applications are delivered prior to using the settings described in I and J. We rarely use this technique but prefer to procede directly with the following laser settings.
   I. Settings for "chipping" or "drilling" penetration of the iris:

| | |
|---|---|
| spot | 50 μm |
| energy | 400–1200 mW |
| exposure | 0.1–0.2 sec |

   J. Settings to perform a "punch" penetration of the iris:

| | |
|---|---|
| spot | 50 μm |
| energy | 1000–1500 mW |
| exposure | 0.02–0.05 sec |

   K. Technique for dark brown iris
      1. A brown iris may be very thick. There is a tendency for high laser energy to result in "charcoalization" or "charring," a blackening of the base of the iridotomy site due to thermal coagulative effects on the surface layers of the iris stroma. Charcoalization makes penetration extremely difficult if not impossible. The use of punch settings reduces this occurrence.
      2. The iridotomy is performed in the base of a crypt to reduce the amount of tissue that has to be penetrated.
      3. If there is lack of a tissue response to the laser or if charcoalization occurs, the surgeon should select a different site at which to perform the iridotomy.
      4. A combination of chipping and punch settings is used to perform the iridotomy in a brown iris.
   L. Technique for light-colored iris
      1. High laser settings in eyes with blue or hazel irides can disrupt the pigment epithelium prior to disruption of the iris stroma.

**Table 11-2.** Argon Laser Settings

| | Contraction | Punch | Penetration | Cleanup |
|---|---|---|---|---|
| **Iridotomy** | | | | |
| Spot size (μm) | 300–500 | 50 | 50 or 50 | 50 |
| Duration (sec) | 0.2–0.5 | 0.02–0.05 | 0.05 0.1–0.2 | 0.1–0.2 |
| Power (mW) | 200–400 | 1000–1500 | 800–1200 [illegible]00–1200 | 300–600 |
| | | Pupilloplasty | Peripheral Iridoplasty | |
| **Iris surgery** | | | | |
| Spot size (μm) | | 200–500 | 200–500 | |
| Duration (sec) | | 0.2–0.5 | 0.5 | |
| Power (mW) | | 200–500 | 200–500 | |
| **Trabeculoplasty** | | | | |
| Spot size (μm) | | 50 | | |
| Duration (sec) | | 0.1 | | |
| Power[a] (mW) | | 400–1200 | | |

[a] Power adjusted to produce blanching or a minimal bubble.

This prevents completion of a through-and-through laser iridotomy.

2. "Punch" settings can be used to create a controlled, stepwise penetration of the stroma prior to delivering laser energy to the pigment epithelium.
3. A high-energy, long-duration technique can be used.
   a) Laser is set at a 50 μm spot, 1100–1500 mW of power, and a duration of 0.5 sec.
   b) The aiming beam is focused on the iris surface and the foot switch activated until a bubble forms on the iris surface. This time is usually less than the 0.5 sec setting.
   c) The foot switch is released and the aiming beam focused on the center of the bubble.
   d) The laser is reactivated at the above settings with the bubble acting as a focusing medium.
   e) One to three shots through the bubble usually result in a complete penetration of the iris.
   f) The base of the iridotomy is enlarged with either "punch" or cleanup laser settings.

IV. Iridotomy during an acute attack
   A. Attempts should be undertaken to terminate the acute attack medically so that the iridotomy can be performed in a normotensive and noninflamed eye.
   B. Occasionally one is unable to break the acute attack and the iridotomy must be performed while the angle is still closed and the intraocular pressure elevated.
      1. Topical glycerin is used to clear corneal edema.
      2. Low-energy setting is used to avoid corneal burns.
      3. Tissue response to the laser is poor secondary to iris congestion and edema.
   C. Laser pupilloplasty or peripheral iridoplasty can be attempted to terminate pupillary block and the acute attack (Fig. 11-2).
      1. Pupilloplasty is designed to contract a small area of the sphincter and peak the pupil. A contact lens is used.

Pupilloplasty laser settings:

| | |
|---|---|
| spot | 200–500 μm |
| energy | 200–500 mW |
| exposure | 0.2–0.5 sec |

Laser burns are placed over one to two clock hours of the sphincter and posteriorly over the mid iris.

2. Peripheral iridoplasty is performed to contract the peripheral iris stroma to eliminate contact with the trabecular meshwork. The technique is also applicable in laser trabeculoplasty in an eye with a narrow angle configuration. A contact lens is used.

Peripheral iridoplasty laser settings:

| | |
|---|---|
| spot | 200–500 μm |
| energy | 200–500 mW |
| exposure | 0.5 sec |

Laser burns are placed around the circumference of the iris, as peripherally as possible.

VII. Completion of the iridotomy
   A. The anterior lens capsule must be visualized through the iridotomy to ensure a complete through-and-through iris hole (Fig. 11-3). Depending upon the optics of the laser slit-lamp, the patient may have to be moved to another instrument for this determination.
   B. Iris transillumination that indicates loss of pigment epithelium and not complete disruption of the iris stroma is a poor end point.
   C. The iridotomy should be 0.1–0.2 mm in diameter.
   D. The base of the iridotomy is enlarged with low-energy "chipping" or "punch" burns.
   E. Tissue and pigment epithelium can occlude the opening ("landsliding") at the time of enlargement. At completion of the procedure, external pressure on the contact lens is released. This permits the higher pressure in the posterior chamber to "float" residual pigment into the iridotomy, where it can be treated.

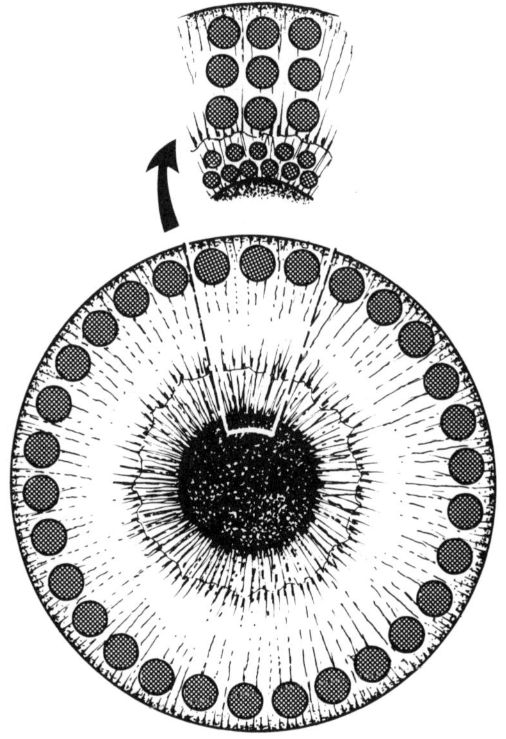

**Fig. 11-2** Laser pupilloplasty (insert) and laser peripheral iridoplasty. (From Krupin, 1984, with permission.)

## Postoperative Treatment

I. Glaucoma medications are continued.
II. Topical corticosteroids are administered four times a day for 3–5 days.
III. Intraocular pressure is measured 1–2 hr after treatment to detect and treat possible acute increases.

## Operative Complications

I. Corneal epithelial and endothelial burns (Fig. 11-4).
   A. These are rare if a contact lens is used during treatment.
   B. Epithelial burns can occur if corneal

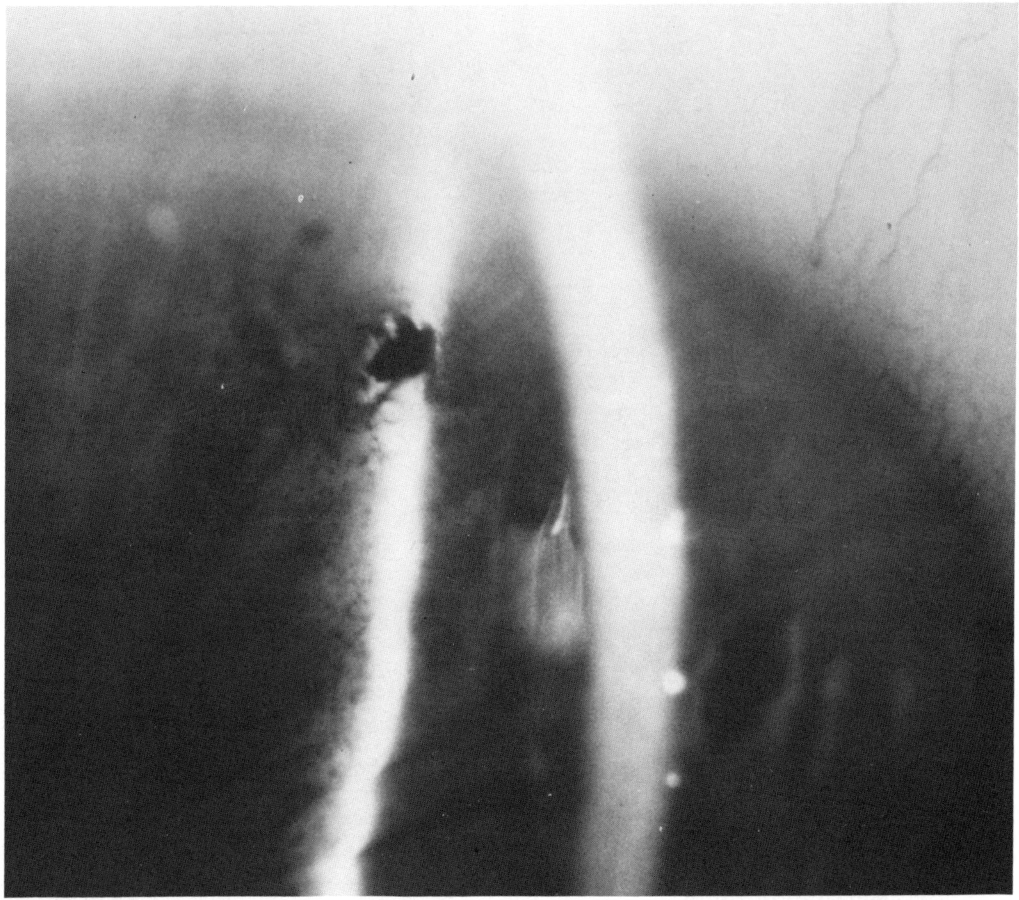

**Fig. 11-3** Laser iridotomy. Visualization of the anterior lens capsule through the iris opening is the only method of ensuring a through-and-through opening. (From Krupin, 1984, with permission.)

edema is present. These opacities may interfere with continuation of the procedure. Occasionally it is possible to treat around an epithelium burn by having the patient look to the side and aiming the laser obliquely at the treatment site.

C. Treatment of epithelial burns is similar to that for any minor corneal abrasion, with resolution within 1–7 days. However, we do not use topical antibiotics for laser burns.

D. Endothelial damage is more frequent following the use of high-energy levels and if an anterior chamber bubble is in contact with the endothelium during treatment. Endothelial burns are probably a result of thermal conduction from the iris surface.

E. Once an endothelial burn begins, a new site should be selected unless the iridotomy is extremely close to completion.

F. Endothelial damage can result in localized corneal decompensation.

II. Iris hemorrhage

A. Hyphema, a rare complication with the argon laser, may rarely occur in eyes with rubeosis iridis or uveitis or in patients receiving anticoagulant drugs.

B. Hemorrhage can be stopped by ap-

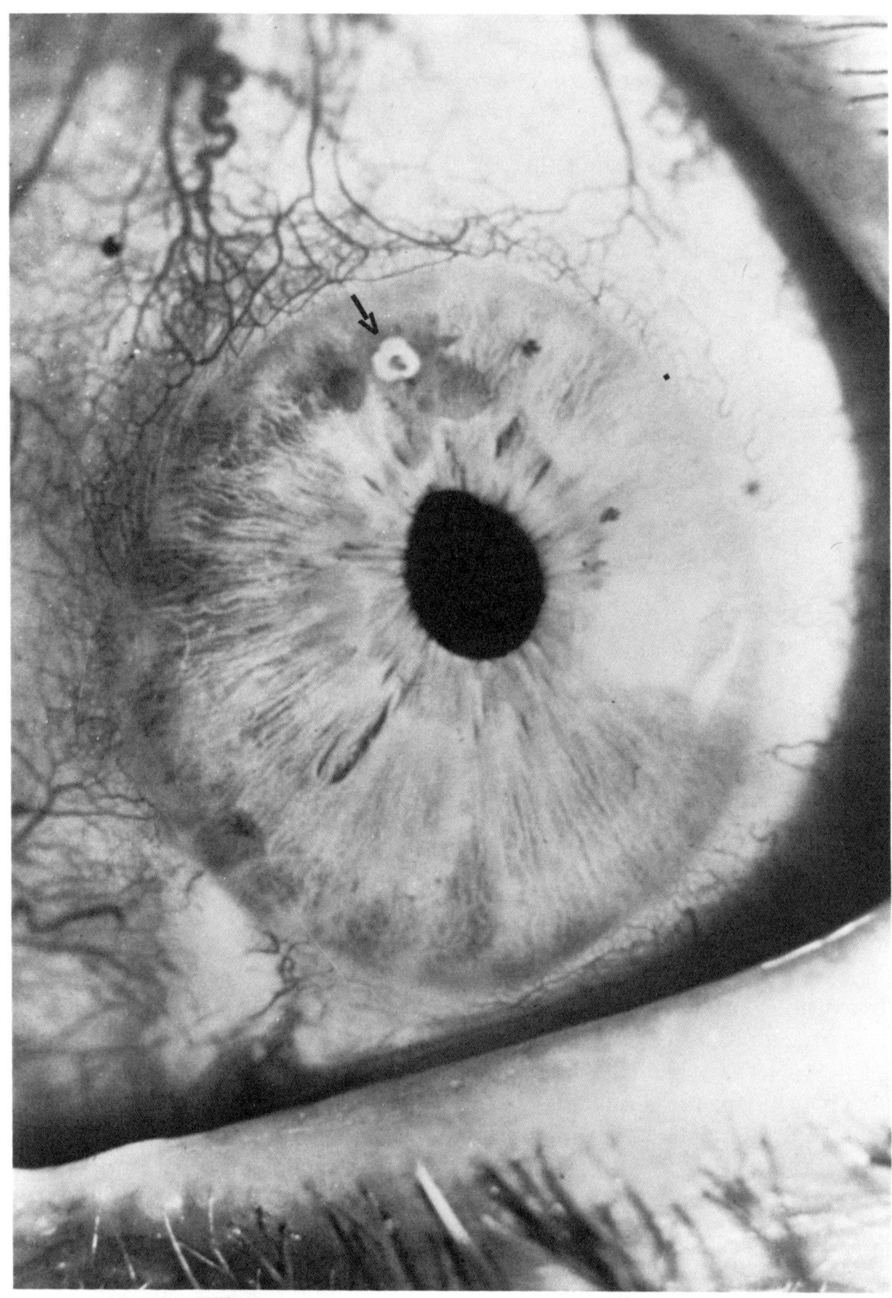

**Fig. 11-4** Corneal epithelial burn (arrow) secondary to argon laser iridotomy. Notice that the pupil is peaked towards the area of laser treatment.

plication of a larger laser spot or application of pressure on the contact lens.

C. Blood in the anterior chamber can prevent effective laser treatment. It may be best to stop the procedure. The hyphema will resolve spontaneously.

III. Laser injury to the lens

A. Localized lens opacities at the site of the iridotomy are common (Fig. 11-5).

B. The opacity represents a laser-induced subcapsular coagulation and destruction of lens protein at the site of the iridotomy.

C. The localized lens injury is nonprogressive over time. There have been no reports of rapid cataract formation following argon laser iridotomy as may occur after surgical iridectomy.

IV. Retinal burn

A. Laser energy is transmitted through the ocular media as soon as the pigment epithelium is penetrated. The laser beam is diffuse at the posterior pole if the plane of focus is maintained at the iris surface plane.

B. Retinal and macular burns have occurred following argon laser iridotomy. This complication is second-

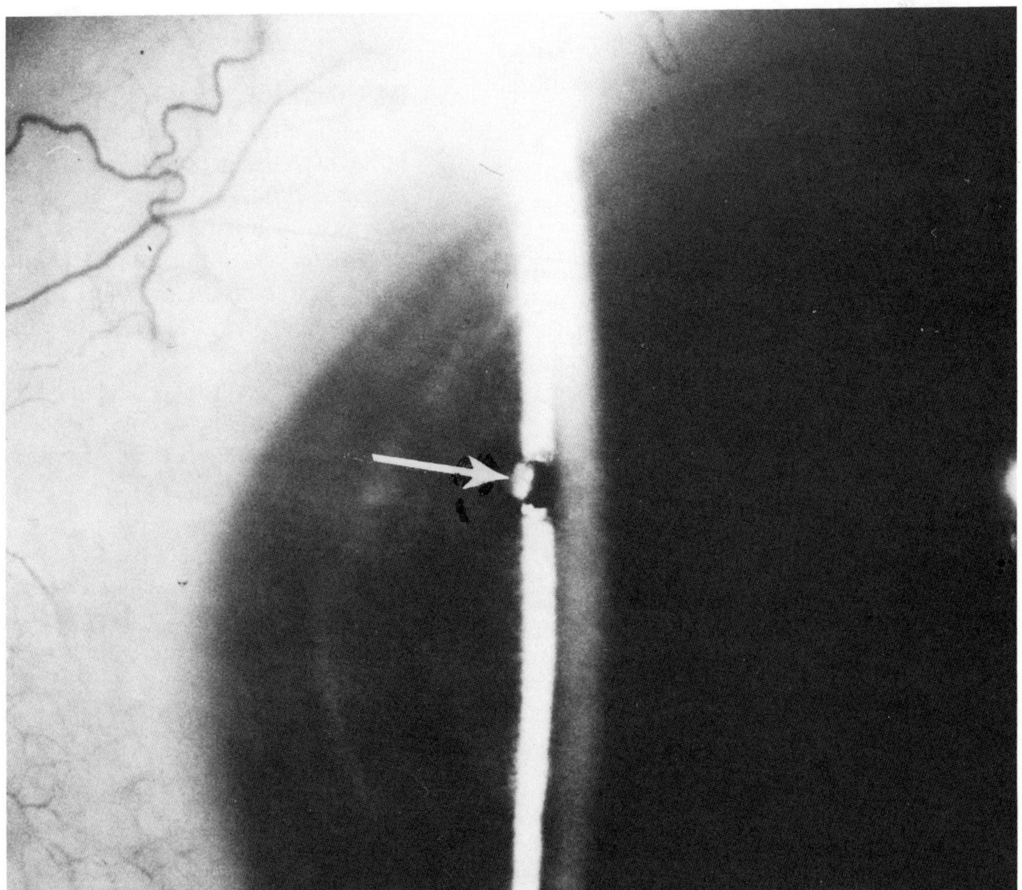

**Fig. 11-5** Argon laser iridotomy. Localized lens opacity (arrow) at the site of the iridotomy. (From Krupin, 1984, with permission.)

ary to either laser delivery posterior to the plane of the iris or to refraction by the lens so the beam is focused on the posterior pole.

C. The laser beam should be aimed away from the posterior pole to avoid injury to the macula. In addition, the beam should not be directed posteriorly through a patent iridotomy.

D. Peripheral retinal burns have not been noted to develop subretinal neovascularization.

V. Failure to penetrate the iris

A. In rare instances the iris cannot be penetrated. In some patients laser failure dictates the need for a surgical iridectomy.

B. If penetration is difficult, select another iris location and alter the initial laser settings (see above). It is not unusual to encounter difficulty in penetration at the first site while penetration is easily accomplished at a second location.

C. If penetration is impossible with the argon laser, one can terminate the procedure and treat again at a later time or the procedure can be performed with the Nd-YAG laser (see below).

VI. Pupillary distortion

A. Transient or permanent peaking of the pupil towards the iridotomy can occur. Peaking is common if the iridotomy is too close to the sphincter.

B. When permanent, pupillary distortion is generally minor and rarely noticeable cosmetically.

## Postoperative Complications

I. Visual alterations

A. Transient reduced vision and visual blurring, lasting up to 60 min, are common secondary to

1. use of the contact lens with goniosol solution.
2. retinal exposure to the laser flash.

B. Monocular diplopia can occur if the iridotomy is too large and not covered by the eyelid.

II. Acute intraocular pressure rise

A. Transient elevations in intraocular pressure are relatively common following argon laser iridotomy. Of course, it is imperative to be sure that the iridotomy is patent, that the iridocorneal angle is open, and that the pressure is not elevated due to acute angle-closure glaucoma.

B. Pressure increase may be more common following the treatment of chronic angle-closure glaucoma, but can occur following prophylactic iridotomy.

C. Peak increase in intraocular pressure is 1–2 hr after the iridotomy, with an initial increase in pressure being very rare thereafter.

D. Increase is not related to the laser parameters used during treatment.

E. Increases can be 20–30 mmHg higher than the pretreatment intraocular pressure.

F. While the increase is usually transient, there is the possibility for induced progression of optic nerve damage and possibly a retinal vascular insult.

G. A clinically significant increase in intraocular pressure has been defined as a pressure greater than 30% of prelaser measurement. This is an arbitrary value and may not be valid for eyes with extensive glaucomatous damage.

H. An elevated intraocular pressure is treated medically using a combination of the following:

1. A topical beta antagonist
2. A systemic carbonic anhydrase inhibitor
3. A systemic hyperosmotic agent

I. A rebound elevation in intraocular pressure can follow successful medical treatment; therefore, pressure should be monitored over the subsequent 24 hr.

J. In rare cases, intraocular pressure can remain elevated for longer than 24 hr after laser iridotomy.

III. Iritis

A. Inflammation and pigment release are common following laser iridotomy.

B. The inflammatory response does not appear to be related to a prostaglandin-induced mechanism. Treatment with prostaglandin inhibitors (e.g., indomethacin) does not prevent or alter the postlaser inflammatory response.

C. While inflammation is usually mild and self-limiting, use of a topical corticosteroid (dexamethasone 0.1% or prednisolone 1%), one drop four times a day for 3–5 days is recommended.

D. In rare cases a prolonged iritis can follow argon laser iridiotomy, either as a direct result of the laser treatment or due to reactivation of a previously unrecognized iritis.

1. Treatment requires prolonged administration of topical corticosteroid eye drops.
2. The prolonged iritis can result in closure of the iridotomy and return to the narrow angle condition.
3. Posterior synechiae can form, requiring the use of mydriatic agents. This requires attention to the gonioscopic appearance after pupil dilation to detect angle crowding and associated angle closure.

IV. Late closure of the iridotomy

A. There is the tendency for the argon laser iridotomy to enlarge over time. However, proliferation of iris pigment epithelium can occur after surgery, resulting in partial or total closure of the iridotomy. Partial closure with continued visualization of the anterior lens capsule does not require additional treatment.

B. Total closure of the iridotomy can occur within the first 4–6 weeks following treatment. Pigment epithelium proliferation and complete closure of the iridotomy are rare after this time.

C. Total closure of the iridotomy requires either

1. reopening the original site with the argon laser or
2. perforating a new iridotomy with either the argon or Nd:YAG laser (see below)

## KRYPTON LASER IRIDOTOMY

I. An iridotomy can be performed with the krypton laser similarly to the argon laser.

II. The krypton laser has a lower energy output than the argon laser. Therefore, the laser parameters should include a longer duration of 0.2 sec while using the 50 μm spot size. Initial power setting is 400 mW, with the power increased depending on the tissue response.

III. The remainder of the technique, operative complications, and postoperative complications are the same as for argon laser iridotomy.

## NEODYMIUM YAG LASER IRIDOTOMY

I. The Nd-YAG laser produces a sudden expansion (plasma formation) with disruption and tearing of transparent tissues. The laser delivers enormous near-infrared (1064 nm) irradiances at small spot sizes and extremely brief pulses ranging from 30 nsec to 20 psec.

II. The plasma formation consists of ionized material (a collection of ions and electrons) at the laser beam focus. The formed plasma absorbs or scatters radiation arriving later in the pulse, thereby shielding underlying tissues.

III. Important aspects in avoiding Nd-YAG laser injury to adjacent structures, such as the lens and cornea, include precise focus of the laser and the use of safe energy levels.

IV. Iridotomies performed with the Nd-YAG laser typically have a slit appearance without the more obvious pigmentary dispersion and iris contour changes noted after argon or krypton laser iridotomy.

V. The surgeon must fully understand the functioning and technical workings of the Nd-YAG laser. The greater tissue destruction with this laser results in a narrow margin of safety. The instrument must be properly aligned and focused to avoid injury to surrounding tissues.

## Technique

I. Topical pilocarpine 1% or 2% applied prior to the procedure places the iris under stretch, reducing the thickness of the iris, and decreases the number of laser burns required for penetration.

II. Topical anesthesia is usually sufficient for performing the procedure. Retrobulbar anesthesia is rarely indicated; however, it may be necessary in an uncooperative patient.

III. Antireflective-coated YAG iridotomy contact lens
   A. Specialized contact lenses constructed for the Nd:YAG laser must be used.
   B. The use of a contact lens with a plus add (e.g., the Abraham lens) is useful, and almost mandatory, for optimal success.
   C. The 66-diopter planoconvex button provides convergence of the laser beam to a smaller spot size with increased power density (energy per unit area) and increased magnification without loss of depth of focus.
   D. The lens holds the eyelids open and eliminates blinking.
   E. Ocular saccades and extraneous eye movements are reduced.
   F. The antireflective coating reduces laser beam reflection and loss of laser energy.

IV. Location of the iridotomy
   A. While the procedure can be performed at any clock hour, the superior iris between 10:30 and 1:30 is preferred in order to have the iridotomy covered by the upper eyelid.
   B. A location between one-half and two-thirds of the distance between the pupil margin and the visible periphery is chosen. This is approximately equivalent to one-half the distance between the edge of the collarette and the limbus.
   C. Treatment through a corneal arcus senilis is avoided: the density of the arcus reduces the laser power across the cornea as well as interfering with clear focus of the laser beam.

V. Laser settings
   A. With certain Nd-YAG lasers the only variables are the amount of energy used and the number of bursts per shot. Duration and spot size are constant.
   B. Setting of the Nd-YAG laser is not dependent upon the color of iris, as it is with the argon laser.
   C. Power settings between 2 and 8 mJ are used.
   D. A burst of one or two pulses per shot is sufficient to create an iridotomy. Higher numbers of pulses per shot may increase the chance of lens injury.

VI. Procedure
   A. The laser aiming beam represents the location where the Nd-YAG is focused and where optical breakdown takes place. It is sharply focused on the iris surface. This ensures delivery of the laser energy posterior into the iris stroma.
   B. The laser is armed. Discharge usually results in a full-thickness iridotomy.
   C. Additional applications can be delivered in the same area to achieve a larger opening; however, they should not be delivered directly over the lens capsule. Additional applications of the laser are most effective if delivered immediately adjacent to the iris opening, to an area of intact stroma.

## Operative Complications

I. Corneal epithelial and endothelial burns
   A. Corneal burns are rare when a contact lens is used during treatment.
   B. Corneal damage can occur if corneal edema is present.
   C. Endothelial damage can result in localized corneal decompensation.

II. Iris hemorrhage
   A. Iris bleeding is common with the Nd:YAG laser and the hemorrhage may limit visualization, necessitating termination of the procedure.
   B. The hemorrhage will usually stop spontaneously. Application of pressure by the contact lens may facilitate resolution of the bleeding. A hyphema layer is unusual and bleeding does not alter the outcome of the technique.

III. Localized lens injury
   A. Injury to the lens represents Nd:YAG laser penetration of the lens capsule.
   B. Lens injury has the potential to create a total cataract. However, we have observed lens capsule penetration and formation of a localized opacity at the site of capsule rupture with the tear sealed by a reactive mass. However, the long-term outcome of this complication is unknown.

IV. Failure to penetrate the iris
   A. Failure to create the iridotomy usually indicates either poor focus of the laser beam or the use of insufficient laser energy. Hemorrhage after laser delivery and incomplete penetration of the iris can prevent visualization and completion of the procedure.
   B. The procedure can be terminated and retreatment performed at a later time. If visualization is not limited, another site can be selected for the iridotomy.

## Postoperative Treatment

I. The patient's glaucoma medications are continued.
II. Topical corticosteroids are administered three or four times a day for 3 or 4 days.
III. Intraocular pressure is measured 1–2 hr after treatment to detect and treat possible acute increases.

## Postoperative Complications

Most complications following an Nd-YAG iridotomy are similar to those described for argon iridotomy.

I. Visual alterations

   Transient reduced vision and visual blurring may relate to use of the contact lens and the goniosol solution. Monocular diplopia can occur if the iridotomy is large and not covered by the eyelid.

II. Acute intraocular pressure rise

   This may be more common following the treatment of chronic angle-closure glaucoma, but can occur following prophylactic iridotomy. Peak increase occurs 1–2 hr after performing the iridotomy. Increase is not related to the laser parameters used during treatment and the increase is similar to that observed after argon laser iridotomy.

While the increase is transient, there is the possibility for pressure-induced progression of optic nerve damage and the possibility for a retinal vascular insult. An increase in intraocular pressure greater than 30% above baseline should be medically treated with a combination of the following:

1. A topical beta antagonist
2. A systemic carbonic anhydrase inhibitor
3. A systemic hyperosmotic agent

III. Iritis

The inflammatory response following Nd:YAG laser iridotomy is similar to that encountered after argon or krypton iridotomy. While inflammation is usually self-limiting, we treat patients with a topical corticosteroid (dexamethasone 0.1% or prednisolone 1%), one drop four times a day for 3–5 days.

IV. Late closure of the iridotomy

A. Closure of an Nd:YAG iridotomy is less common than that observed after argon iridotomy. However, late closure can occur.

B. Total closure of the iridotomy can occur within the first 4–6 weeks following treatment. Complete closure after this time is rare.

C. Total closure requires a repeat iridotomy. Reopening of the iridotomy with the Nd:YAG laser should not be performed since there is a high risk of direct injury to the underlying lens capsule.

## ARGON LASER TRABECULOPLASTY

I. The introduction of argon laser trabeculoplasty to the treatment of open-angle glaucoma has been a major advance in glaucoma surgery. The application of nonpenetrating argon laser burns to the inner surface of the trabecular meshwork is effective in lowering the intraocular pressure in many patients without the complications associated with filtration surgery.

II. Argon laser treatment to the trabecular meshwork has been described by many terms including argon laser trabeculoplasty, laser trabecular tightening, laser goniotherapy, and argon laser goniophotocoagulation of the trabecular meshwork.

III. Argon laser trabeculoplasty is currently accepted not as a replacement for medical therapy but as an auxillary or adjunctive treatment to surgery.

IV. Successful lowering of intraocular pressure following argon laser trabeculoplasty is accompanied by an increase in outflow facility. Laser trabeculoplasty does not produce a direct communication between the anterior chamber and Schlemm's canal. The rate of aqueous humor formation is not altered.

V. The sites of the laser application to the trabecular surface become scarred and apparently impermeable to aqueous humor. Scar formation and damage to the meshwork should be considered before repeating a previously failed laser trabeculoplasty.

VI. At least three possible mechanisms can occur within the trabecular meshwork in response to argon laser trabeculoplasty.

A. A mechanical effect secondary to thermal shrinkage of the collagenous components of the trabecular meshwork will act to open the intertrabecular spaces. Shrinkage can displace the trabeculum internally or can contract the tissue surrounding an individual treatment site, either of which would increase outflow facility by enlarging the surrounding trabecular spaces and possibly widening Schlemm's canal.

B. A cellular response can act to remove extracellular materials from the trabecular spaces.

C. A biochemical response secondary to laser damage to the trabecular endothelial cells may stimulate the remaining cells to increase active synthesis and turnover of the trabecular matrix.

## Indications

I. Argon laser trabeculoplasty is indicated when intraocular pressure is not adequately controlled on maximum tolerated medical therapy consisting of a beta-adrenergic antagonist, an epinephrine preparation, a miotic agent, and an orally administered carbonic anhydrase inhibitor. Inadequate pressure control implies progressive glaucomatous optic disc cupping or visual field loss in the face of maximally tolerated medical management.

II. Argon laser trabeculoplasty may also be indicated

A. in an attempt to achieve better intraocular pressure control in addition to full medical therapy.

B. as a method to eliminate poorly tolerated medications (e.g. pilocarpine) in a patient with a cataract.

III. Treatment requires that at least 180° of the iridocorneal angle be open and that there is clear visualization of the anterior chamber angle. Argon laser trabeculoplasty requires expertise in gonioscopy and the appreciation of the tremendous variability of the appearance of an open iridocorneal angle (see Ch. 4).

IV. It is important to recognize that argon laser trabeculoplasty creates sites of damage within the trabecular outflow pathways in order to achieve an overall improvement in outflow facility. These sites of damage become nonfunctioning trabecular tissue.

V. The effectiveness of laser trabeculoplasty to lower intraocular pressure is dependent upon several factors including:

A. the type of open-angle glaucoma (see Table 11-3). The procedure is less effective in some forms of secondary glaucoma.

B. the age of the patient. The procedure is less effective in young patients.

C. whether the eye is phakic or aphakic. The procedure is less effective in aphakic glaucoma. However, the response in the aphakic eye with preexisting primary open-angle glaucoma is better than the response in secondary aphakic open-angle glaucoma.

VI. The relative ease of performing the procedure and its relatively low risks suggest that laser trabeculoplasty should be attempted prior to filtration surgery, which can be performed if laser treatment is ineffective. Argon laser trabeculoplasty does not appear to alter the results of subsequent filtration surgery.

**Table 11-3.** Argon Laser Trabeculoplasty Success Rates in Open-Angle Glaucoma

| Glaucoma Diagnosis | Relative Success (%) |
|---|---|
| Phakic primary open-angle | 75–90 |
| Aphakic open-angle | 30–50 |
| Pseudophakic open-angle | 50–60 |
| Pseudoexfoliation | 80–95 |
| Pigmentary | 80–95 |
| Angle-recession | 50–60 |
| Uveitic | 5–10 |
| Postiridectomy | 50–75 |
| Juvenile onset (<40 years) | 0–15 |
| Congenital | 0–15 |
| Steroid-induced | 0–15 |

## Contraindications

I. Argon laser trabeculoplasty should not be performed when the trabecular meshwork cannot be satisfactorily visualized because of either angle closure or corneal opacities. At least 180° of open angle without peripheral anterior synechiae must be present.

II. In patients with a narrow iridocorneal angle secondary to pupillary block, a laser iridotomy is initially performed. While this can be followed with the argon laser trabeculoplasty, we prefer to only do the iridotomy and then reevaluate the patient later to determine if a trabeculoplasty is required.

III. In patients with a narrow approach blocking visualization of the trabecular meshwork, a peripheral iridoplasty immediately prior to the trabeculoplasty may be considered. For iridoplasty, a 0.5 sec duration, 200 μm spot size is used. Beginning with a power setting of 100 mW, lesions are applied through the cornea to the peripheral iris to cause iris retraction and a widening of the iridocorneal angle, which may allow performance of the trabeculoplasty. Pigment release occurs even with the lowest effective power to cause iris retraction. Therefore, iridoplasty combined with trabeculoplasty should be limited to 180°.

## Preoperative Explanation to the Patient

The indications and risks of the procedure are explained to the patient, as described previously for laser iridotomy. Informed consent is obtained. Explanations specific for argon laser trabeculoplasty include the following.

I. Glaucoma medications will be continued after the operation. While less medications may be a needed, this cannot be determined for at least 6 weeks following treatment.

II. Laser treatment will not improve vision, although it may help preserve vision by preventing further glaucoma damage.

III. Laser surgery may require 4–8 weeks to achieve its maximum beneficial effect of improving the "function of the drain in the eye."

IV. Laser surgery is 80–90% (or a more appropriate percentage depending upon the underlying type of glaucoma) effective in lowering intraocular pressure. If laser surgery is not totally effective, a microsurgical glaucoma operation will be necessary.

V. A transient intraocular pressure rise may occur following laser surgery. This does not affect the end result of the laser surgery. Eye pressure will be monitored following surgery, which requires the patient to remain in the office for at least 1–2 hr.

VI. In rare circumstances, laser surgery can result in a marked elevation in intraocular pressure and a worsening of the glaucoma. This situation may require immediate filtration surgery.

## Technique

I. Positioning of the patient and surgeon (including management of the goniolens) are performed as previously outlined for laser iridotomy.

II. Various antireflective goniolenses are available for argon laser trabeculoplasty.

A. The Goldman three-mirror gonioprism contains a dome-shaped mirror with an angle of 59° for anterior chamber angle treatment.

B. A smaller Goldmann single-mirror gonioprism with an angled 62° mirror is useful for patients with a small palpebral fissure.

C. The Ritch trabeculoplasty laser lens contains a 59° mirror designed for a face-on view of the inferior angle and a 64° inclined mirror for a face-on view of the superior angle. In addition, two additional mirrors inclined at the same angles are super-

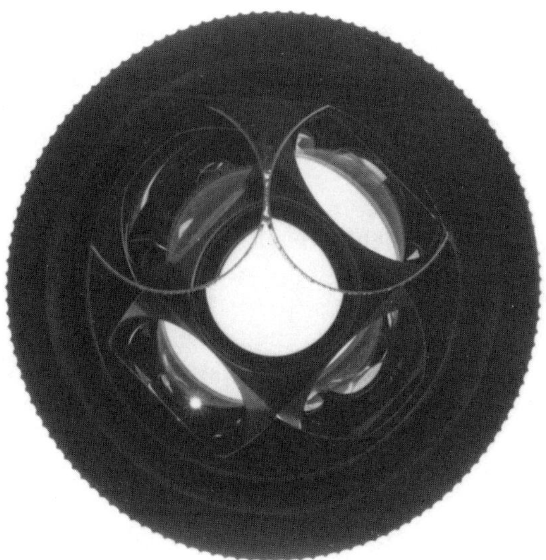

**Fig. 11-6** Ritch goniolenses for argon laser trabeculoplasty. The top two mirrors have overlying magnification buttons.

imposed with planoconvex buttons of 1.4 magnification. The magnified view decreases the spot size from 50 to 35 μm. The Ritch lens is very useful in eyes with narrow iridocorneal angles, anterior iris insertion, and lightly pigmented trabecular meshwork (Fig. 11-6).

III. Anterior chamber angle visualization

A. The gonioprism is placed on the eye with the treatment mirror at the 12 o'clock position. The patient is instructed to look straight ahead. This provides a view of the 6 o'clock angle. Four areas of the anterior chamber angle are identified: Schwalbe's line, the nonpigmented and pigmented portions of the trabecular meshwork, the scleral spur, and the ciliary body.

B. The gonioprism is rotated in 90° steps and the four areas of the angle identified in each quadrant. The surgeon should become accustomed to rotating the goniolens in one direction, either clockwise or counterclockwise, and always follow this scheme. It is very easy to become confused at the time of surgery as to what areas of the meshwork have been treated and what location of the angle is being viewed. Consistently starting with the mirror at the 12 o'clock position (inferior angle) and rotating the contact lens in one direction eliminates this difficulty.

C. It is important to identify the angle structures so as to avoid accidental treatment of the cornea or ciliary body. Pigment deposition above Schwalbe's line, known as a Sampolesi's line, can be mistaken for the pigmented trabecular meshwork and treatment can be performed accidentally to the cornea. Lack of trabecular pigmentation can result in inadvertent treatment to the ciliary body. Use of a narrow slit beam and the parallelepiped method to identify Schwalbe's line (see Ch. 4) will avoid these difficulties.

D. Difficulty in visualizing the anterior chamber structures with the patient in primary gaze can be overcome by changing fixation or the position of the goniolens on the eye.

1. The patient's gaze is directed in the same direction as the mirror. For example, to improve the view in inferior mirror (superior angle), have the patient look down in the direction of the mirror. This technique maintains an undistorted view of the angle with the light path perpendicular to the goniolens surface.
2. Shifting of the goniolens along the corneal surface toward the angle to be viewed also improves visualization. For example, to improve the view in the nasal mirror (temporal angle), the contact lens is tilted nasally. Tilting of the goniolens can result in prismatic distortion secondary to the

light path that is no longer perpendicular to the goniolens surface.

E. The minimal magnification required to visualize the anterior chamber angle structures properly is 16×. However, higher magnifications may be preferred.

## Treatment (Table 11-2)

Argon laser settings recommended in the original report by Wise and Witter were 0.1 sec duration, a 50 μm spot size, and a power setting between 1000 and 1500 mW. A total of 100–120 spots were placed posterior to the pigmented portion of the meshwork and evenly spaced over the entire 360° of the meshwork. Although the settings for spot size and duration have remained unchanged, the number of recommended spots has been reduced and the location of the treatment has been moved anteriorly. The optimal treatment parameters remain to be elucidated.

I. Spot size

A 50 μm spot setting is used. However, the actual spot size on the trabecular meshwork is altered by any induced prismatic effects from the goniolens as well as added magnification buttons incorporated into the gonioprism.

II. Duration

The duration of the laser exposure is 0.1 sec. It is important to keep the foot switch depressed for this duration since premature withdrawal will shorten the exposure time.

III. Power

A. The tissue response end-point to treatment should be blanching or minimal bubble formation. However, the lack of a visible laser response does not necessarily imply an unsuccessful result. Tissue response is directly related to the amount of trabecular pigmentation.

B. The power setting is titrated for an individual eye to achieve the minimal tissue response.

1. Beginning with the mirror in the 12 o'clock position (inferior angle), a test burn for tissue response (blanch or minimal bubble formation) is placed using a power setting of 400 mW.
2. If there is no tissue response, the power is increased by 100–200 mW steps until a response is achieved.
3. A power setting of 1200 mW is the maximum.
4. Because of the variability in trabecular pigmentation in the different portions of the angle (the greatest pigmentation is usually in the superior mirror, the inferior angle), it may be necessary to modify power settings during the procedure to achieve the minimal tissue response.

IV. Location of the beam

A. The aiming beam should be placed at the junction of the nonpigmented and the pigmented trabecular meshwork (Fig. 11-7).

B. Too anterior treatment (e.g., Schwalbe's line) can cause thermal injury to the corneal endothelium. Too posterior treatment (e.g., ciliary body) is associated with the complications of peripheral anterior synechiae, iritis, and elevated intraocular pressure (see below) and pain during treatment.

C. The aiming beam should be positioned on the area of treatment with the slit-lamp joy stick. Use of the laser beam micromanipulator is not recommended since this requires additional refocusing of the slit-lamp. Treatment of the curved surface of the trabecular meshwork with a continually changing focal distance requires continual refocusing of the

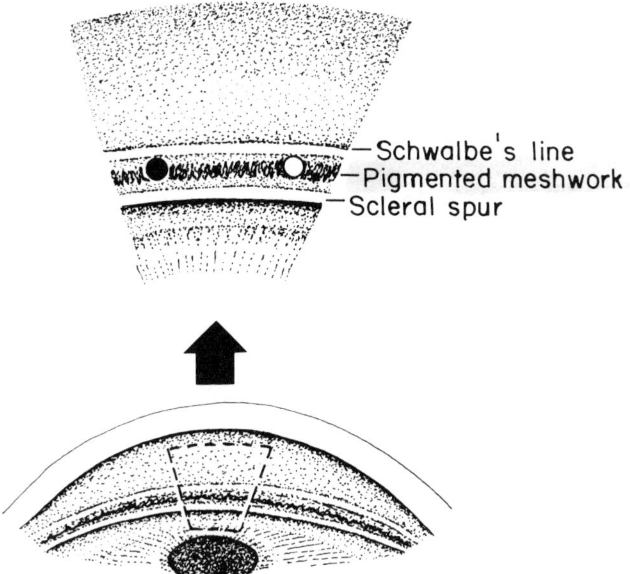


**Fig. 11-7** Argon laser trabeculoplasty landmarks in an open iridocorneal angle. The aiming beam (closed dot on the left) is placed at the junction of the pigmented and nonpigmented trabecular meshwork. Proper power settings results in a blanch (or minimal bubble) response (open dot on the right). (From Krupin, 1984, with permission.)

aiming beam before each laser application.

V. Number of applications

A. The total number of laser applications depends upon the amount of the trabecular meshwork receiving treatment during one session: approximately 50 applications for 180° and approximately 80 applications for 360° of angle treatment.

B. The mirror is placed at the 12 o'clock position and rotated either clockwise or counterclockwise with the applications evenly spaced over the area of treatment. The center portion of the gonioprism mirror should be used for treatment. This requires constant rotation of the gonioprism. Use of the edges of the mirror results in distortion of both the view and the laser beam on the trabecular meshwork.

C. If the surgeon always rotates the gonioprism in one direction, regardless of the eye being treated, there will be no question of what areas of the trabecular meshwork need to be treated if a two-stage 180° treatment schedule is used.

D. The total number of required applications for a desired lowering of intraocular pressure is unknown. The magnitude of a postoperative intraocular pressure increase may be lower following 180° than after 360° treatment. However, significant pressure increases can occur after either treatment schedule. Two separate sessions of treatment may place the patient at double jeopardy for this complication.

E. If a two-session treatment is used, the patient should be evaluated 4–6 weeks after the first session to determine if additional laser trabeculoplasty is necessary. The second treatment may not be required in many patients and can be "kept in reserve" for possible future treatment.

## Complications

I. Visual alterations

Transient reduced vision and visual blurring, lasting up to 60 min, are common secondary to

A. placement of the contact lens with the goniosolution.

B. retinal exposure to the laser flash.

II. Acute intraocular pressure rise

A. The major and possibly most dangerous complication of laser trabeculoplasty is a transient acute postoperative elevation in intraocular pressure.

B. Postoperative increases in pressure are more common with higher laser energy levels, with greater than 80 treatment burns, and with more posterior placement of the laser beam.

C. An acute rise in intraocular pressure can result in loss of central fixation ("snuff out" of central visual acuity) in patients with advanced glaucomatous visual field damage, in particular patients with field loss that splits fixation.

D. Increases as high as 25–30 mmHg above prelaser pressure can occur.

1. Approximately 50% of patients will show a postoperative pressure increase ranging from +1 to +30 mmHg.
2. Ten to 15% of patients will show a clinically significant pressure increase defined as an intraocular pressure greater than 30 mmHg, greater than a 30% increase over the mean prelaser pressure, and greater than a 10 mmHg increase over the peak prelaser intraocular pressure.

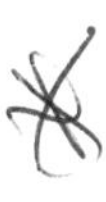

E. The peak increase in intraocular pressure usually occurs 1–2 hr following treatment. A later initial increase in pressure occurs in 2–4% of patients.

F. Increased pressure must be detected and treated medically because, theoretically, a retinal vascular occlusion or further visual field loss, including loss of central fixation, could occur.

G. Patients with a clinically significant increase in intraocular pressure should receive additional medical treatment. Intermittent therapy with carbonic anhydrase inhibitors is usually tolerated even in patients who cannot use these agents in the long term. Hyperosmotic agents are usually effective in rapidly reversing laser-induced increases in intraocular pressure.

H. Patients with a clinically significant pressure rise should be monitored over the next 24 hr since there can be a rebound elevation in intraocular pressure.

III. Worsening of glaucoma control

A. Approximately 3% of patients will show a persistent elevation in intraocular pressure, greater than prelaser pressure levels.

B. Additional medical therapy or filtering surgery is needed to obtain satisfactory glaucoma control in these patients.

IV. Iritis

A. Intraocular inflammation is common following argon laser trabeculoplasty.

B. The iritis is usually transient, mild, and easily controlled with a few days of topical corticosteroids. We routinely have patients use either dexamethasone 0.1% or prednisolone 1%, one drop four times a day for 3–5 days following treatment.

C. In rare cases, severe inflammation may occur if laser burns are inadvertently placed on the iris or if treatment is too posterior on the ciliary body.

V. Peripheral anterior synechiae
   A. Scattered, low-lying peripheral anterior synechiae extending to the scleral spur or even to the trabecular meshwork can occur.
   B. Synechiae are more common following posterior beam placement and are very rare when treatment is anterior to the pigmented meshwork.
   C. Extensive peripheral anterior synechiae that occlude the trabecular meshwork may form in rare cases.

VI. Hemorrhage
   A. Bleeding from the trabecular meshwork rarely occurs during treatment. This can happen suddenly from the point of laser application or as a slow oozing of blood through the untreated meshwork adjacent to the sites of laser application. Bleeding is most likely due to reflux of blood from Schlemm's canal.
   B. Hemorrhage can also occur following inadvertent treatment of a peripheral iris vessel.
   C. Hemorrhage is usually controlled by increasing the pressure (and therefore intraocular pressure) of the gonioprism on the cornea. If this is not sufficient, the bleeding site can be closed using low-power (200–400 mW), 200 μm spot size laser applications.
   D. Rarely will hemorrhage be severe enough to obscure visualization and thus necessitate terminating treatment.
   E. The occurrence of a hemorrhage does not have a deleterious effect on the success of the trabeculoplasty.

VII. Corneal burns
   A. Transient corneal epithelial burns can occur. No specific treatment is necessary. These defects resolve within 1 week without residual scarring.
   B. Transient, radial, spokelike corneal endothelial burns can result from inadvertent laser application.

## OTHER LASER GLAUCOMA TREATMENTS

### Incomplete Surgical Iridectomy

I. One complication of surgical iridectomy is excision of only the anterior leaf of the iris, leaving the posterior pigment epithelial layer intact. This prevents a through-and-through opening and does not relieve pupillary block.

II. Argon laser treatment is a safe and simple method to complete the iridectomy without the associated complications of reentering the anterior chamber.

III. Laser treatment is delivered to the remaining pigment epithelium. The iridectomy is easily accomplished with a 50 or 100 μm spot, a 0.1 sec duration, and a low-power setting of 200–400 mW.

### Goniophotocoagulation

I. Laser treatment of anterior chamber angle vessels (goniophotocoagulation) in combination with panretinal photocoagulation has been reported to be beneficial in patients with neovascular glaucoma.

II. Goniophotocoagulation alone does not replace panretinal photocoagulation, and, if performed, must be done in combination with retinal treatment.

III. Laser treatment alone can obliterate the angle vessels; however, the neovascularization usually continues and requires additional treatment.

IV. Individual vessels are treated as they cross the scleral spur using a 100 μm spot, 0.1 or 0.2 sec duration, and a 100–200 mW power setting.

V. The major complication of treatment is hemorrhage, which can usually be controlled by either increasing ocular pressure by applying pressure on the gonioprism or by the application of additional laser burns.

## Laser Treatment of Ciliary Processes

Various laser techniques have been used to destroy the ciliary body and reduce the rate of aqueous humor formation.

I. Transpupillary argon laser cyclophotocoagulation
   A. This technique has been performed in eyes with aphakic glaucoma.
   B. The magnitude and duration of the intraocular pressure reduction are usually very small.
   C. Probably greater than 25% of the ciliary processes must be visible and coagulated for a clinical response. This requires the presence of a large sector iridectomy. Moreover, revascularization of the ciliary processes can occur with return of a normal rate of aqueous humor formation.
   D. A contact lens is used with laser setting of 0.1–0.2 sec duration and a 50–100 μm spot. Starting with a 600 mW power setting, the beam is aimed at the ciliary process. Power is increased until a concave brown burn with pigment dispersion or bubble formation is achieved. Laser treatment that only causes a white coagulation of the processes indicates insufficient treatment.
   E. Complications include hyphema, vitreous hemorrhage, and uveitis.

II. Transscleral Nd-YAG cyclophotocoagulation
   A. The utility of the procedure is still being evaluated. Probable indications include intractable glaucoma uncontrolled with all previous therapy, where cyclocryotherapy would otherwise be used.
   B. The treatment requires retrobulbar anesthesia.
   C. The Nd-Yag laser is used in the free-running thermal mode with the beam retrofocused 3.6 mm from the aiming beam.
   D. The aiming beam is focused 3 mm posterior to the limbus. Treatment usually consists of 32 applications delivered over the entire 360°. The 3 and 9 o'clock meridians are not treated to avoid damage to the long ciliary vessels.
   E. A pulse duration of 20 msec in the thermal free-running mode is used. Energy settings between 0.5 and 4.2 J are used. Results are better with power setting between 3.5 and 4.2 J.
   F. Postoperatively the patients usual glaucoma medications are continued. The eye is also treated with topical atropine sulfate 1% twice a day and topical corticosteroids (either dexamethasone 0.1% or prednisolone 1% four times a day) are administered and tapered as the inflammation subsides.
   G. Acute postoperative intraocular pressure rises can occur. Therefore, careful monitoring of pressure must be performed and treated if necessary.
   H. Additional complications include iritis, hyphema, keratitis, corneal decompensation, and phthisis bulbi.

## Laser Treatment of Malignant Glaucoma

Laser treatment has been successful in the management of phakic and aphakic malignant (ciliary block) glaucoma. Medical therapy consisting of maximum cycloplegia and pupil dilation (topical atropine 1–3% and topical phenylephrine 5% or 10%), hyperosmotic agents to reduce vitreous volume, and agents to reduce aqueous humor formation (topical beta-adrenergic blockers and systemic carbonic anhydrase inhibitors) are administered prior to the laser treatment.

I. Argon laser shrinkage of swollen ciliary processes visible through a patent peripheral iridectomy has been a successful treatment for malignant glaucoma.
   A. Either shrinkage of the ciliary processes or alteration of the vitreal–ciliary body configuration eliminates the ciliary block. Although minimal deepening of the anterior chamber occurs immediately, full restoration of the chamber occurs in 3–5 days.
   B. Treatment requires an adequate view of ciliary processes through the surgical iridectomy. Topical glycerin is used to clear corneal edema prior to treatment.
   C. With the use of topical anesthesia and a contact lens, the aiming beam is focused on the exposed ciliary processes.
   D. Laser settings include a 100–200 μm spot, duration of 0.1 sec, and power setting between 300 and 1000 mW. Between 20 and 40 shots are delivered, with the endpoint of treatment being visible shrinkage of the processes.
   E. Postoperatively the patient is continued on topical atropine and glaucoma medications as necessary. Topical corticosteroids are used to treat the associated inflammation.

II. Nd-YAG laser treatment to disrupt the anterior hyaloid vitreous face has been successful in the treatment of aphakic or pseudophakic malignant glaucoma.
   A. With the use of topical anesthesia and a contact lens, the aiming beam is focused on the vitreous face either through the pupil or through a patent iridectomy. If the anterior chamber is flat, the laser should be focused posterior to the vitreous face to reduce the potential for corneal damage.
   B. Laser energy setting of 3–11 mJ is used.
   C. With successful hyaloid disruption, the anterior chamber will immediately deepen and loose vitreous stands may be seen in the anterior chamber.
   D. Potential complications include postoperative increase in intraocular pressure, corneal laser injury, and a retinal tear or detachment.

## Argon Laser Closure of Cyclodialysis Cleft

I. The application of argon laser energy has been used to close a planned or inadvertent cyclodialysis cleft associated with hypotony, macular edema, and optic disc swelling.

II. The cleft must be visible with an adequate anterior chamber depth to perform the laser treatment.

III. Topical anesthesia and a goniolens are used.

IV. Laser parameters include 0.1 sec duration, a 50–100 μm spot size, and power settings of 300–800 mW. Burns are directed to the area of the iris and scleral spur surrounding the cleft as well as into the depth of the cleft. Between 100 and 200 laser applications are applied.

V. Postoperatively the patient is treated with topical atropine 1% and topical corticosteroids as necessary for the associated inflammatory reaction.

VI. The effects of treatment may not be apparent until 7–14 days. A second and even third treatment session may be required.

VII. Cleft closure is associated with acute reversal of the hypotony and a markedly elevated intraocular pressure, which may require medical treatment.

## Laser Reopening of Filtration Fistulas

I. The argon and Nd-YAG lasers have been used to reopen filtration fistulas (the internal portion of the sclerostomy) that have become occluded by incarcerated tissue (iris, ciliary processes, lens capsule, or vitreous) or the formation of a pigmented or nonpigmented membrane.

II. While late failure of filtration blebs usually follows external scarring, it can be precipitated by occlusion of the internal aspect of the filtration fistula. Indications for laser treatment include a failing filtration bleb with visible occlusion of the sclerostomy. Results following laser internal revision are better in patients in whom filtration had been successfully established for at least 6 months prior to failure. Success following laser revision in eyes with early filtration failure is very poor.

III. Approximately 30–50% of filtration procedures with sclerostomy closure can be reopened with return of function following a combination of laser treatment.

### Argon Laser Internal Treatment

I. This is indicated if the internal opening is occluded by pigmented tissue. The method is unsuccessful if the fistula is occluded by nonpigmented tissue.

II. The internal sclerostomy is identified with a goniolens.

III. The argon laser is used at 0.1–0.2 sec duration and a 50 μm spot size. Applications are begun at 500 mW power and are increased accordingly. Iris incarceration is easily photocoagulated from the site. Thicker pigmented proliferative membranes require more laser energy (1000–1500 mW).

IV. Digital ocular massage should be performed immediately following treatment. Bleb elevation with decrease in intraocular pressure follows successful treatment.

V. Postoperatively the patient is instructed on how to perform ocular massage. Topical corticosteroids are used according to the extent of postoperative anterior chamber reaction as well as the external inflammation surrounding the filtration area.

VI. Potential operative complications include hemorrhage during the laser treatment. Bleeding is easily controlled either with pressure on the goniolens or the application of additional laser applications. Iritis is usually minimal and easily treated with topical corticosteroids. Acute increases in intraocular pressure, higher than the already elevated prelaser pressure, are rare.

### Argon Laser Transconjunctival Treatment

I. This is indicated in eyes that have undergone full-thickness filtration surgery that has failed, and in which pigment is visible subconjunctivally at the site of the external portion of the sclerostomy.

II. Topical anesthesia and a contact lens with a magnification add is used. The laser is focused on the subconjunctival pigmented tissue.

III. The argon laser is used at 0.1–0.2 sec duration and a 50–100 μm spot size. Applications are begun at 300 mW power and are increased up to 1000 mW with the beam directed to the subconjunctival pigment at the limbus, the presumed site of the external part of the sclerostomy. Fifty to 100 applications may have to be delivered. The endpoint is subconjunctival pigment dispersion and bubble formation. A positive response results in spontaneous enlargement of the bleb and reduction of intraocular pressure.

IV. Postoperatively the patient is instructed on how to perform ocular massage. Topical corticosteroids are used according to the postoperative anterior chamber reaction as well as to the external inflammation surrounding the filtration area.

V. Potential operative complications include laser burns to the conjunctiva. Acute increases in intraocular pressure, higher than the already elevated prelaser pressure, are rare.

### Nd-YAG Internal Treatment

I. This is indicated if the internal opening or the fistula is occluded by nonpigmented tissue.

II. The internal sclerostomy is identified with a goniolens.

III. The mode-locked laser is used with the aiming beam focused on the tissue across the internal sclerostomy. An energy range of 0.7–8.5 mJ is used and from one to four pulses delivered at each firing.

IV. Digital ocular massage should be performed immediately following treatment. Bleb elevation with decrease in intraocular pressure follows successful treatment.

V. Postoperatively the patient is instructed on ocular massage. Topical corticosteroids are used according to the postoperative anterior chamber reaction as well as the external inflammation surrounding the filtration area.

VI. Potential operative complications include hemorrhage if the occluding membrane is vascularized. Bleeding is usually easily controlled by pressure on the goniolens. While the argon laser can be used to coagulate the bleeding site, visualization is usually limited, which necessitates stopping the procedure. Retreatment can be attempted at another time using the argon laser for pretreatment before application of the Nd-YAG laser. Iritis is usually minimal and easily treated with topical corticosteroids. Acute increases in intraocular pressure, higher than the already elevated prelaser pressure, are rare.

### Laser Pupilloplasty (Table 11-2)

I. Laser energy can be used to enlarge a miotic or updrawn pupil noninvasively.

II. Pupilloplasty may be useful in glaucoma patients requiring pilocarpine therapy for intraocular pressure control who are visually hampered by the miotic pupil.

III. Pupilloplasty may be useful to enlarge a miotic pupil for retinal observation or treatment.

IV. Treatment is with topical anesthesia and uses a contact lens. The cornea must be clear and the anterior chamber of sufficient depth to avoid laser injury to the corneal endothelium.

### Argon Laser Photomydriasis

I. Laser treatment (100–200 μm spot, 0.3–0.5 sec duration, and 200–300 mW power) is directed to the entire circumference of the sphincter to cause tissue contraction.

II. A second row of larger (300–500 μm) spots is placed on the iris surface adjacent to the sphincter.

III. The effect on pupil enlargement may be temporary, with retreatment necessary.

IV. Potential complications include inflammation, iris stromal atrophy, and a postoperative increase in intraocular pressure.

### Argon Laser Sphincterotomy

I. Laser treatment is directed along a radial line starting at the edge of the pupil. Punch burns (50 μm spot, 0.01–0.05 sec duration, and 600–1200 mW power) are used to treat the superficial iris tissue. The deeper layers of the iris are then treated with very brief (0.01 sec) low-energy pulses to lessen the chance of lens injury.

II. The effect on pupil enlargement is dependent upon the ability of the pupil to expand. The effect is more permanent than pupilloplasty.

III. Potential complications include inflammation, iris stromal atrophy, and a postoperative increase in intraocular pressure.

### Argon Laser Transconjunctival Suture Cutting

I. The argon laser can be used to cut scleral flap sutures following trabeculectomy filtration surgery. This provides the surgeon the flexibility to close the scleral flap tightly at surgery and therefore reduce the incidence of a postoperative shallow anterior chamber. If necessary, the scleral flap suture(s) can be cut 2–3 weeks after surgery, when the risk of anterior chamber shallowing is low, to release tension on the flap and result in increase flow of aqueous humor and an enlargement of the bleb. A nylon suture must be used if one is to use the laser for this technique.

II. Topical anesthesia is used. The Hoskin's contact lens, which has an upper flange to retract the eye lid and a flat surface to depress the conjunctiva and help expose the suture, is placed over the bleb site.

III. Argon laser parameters include a 50 μm spot, 0.1 sec duration, and a power setting of 200–400 mW. The laser is focused on the suture, which is easily cut with a few well-directed applications.

## APRACLONIDINE

Apraclonidine (Iopidine), an alpha-adrenergic agent, has recently been approved for controlling or preventing postoperative elevations in intraocular pressure after laser iridotomy or argon laser trabeculoplasty (see above).

I. One drop of 1% apraclonidine is instilled 1 hr before and a second drop immediately upon completion of the procedure.

II. The frequency and magnitude of the postoperative pressure increase is reduced with only 2% of patients having an intraocular pressure spike ≥10 mmHg.

## SUGGESTED READINGS


Cohn HC, Aron-Rosa D: Reopening blocked trabeculectomy sites with the YAG laser. Am J Ophthalmol 95:293, 1983

Epstein DL, Steinert RF, Puliafito, CA: Neodymium-YAG laser therapy to the anterior hyaloid in aphakic malignant (ciliovitreal block) glaucoma. Am J Ophthalmol 98:137, 1984

Harbin TS: Treatment of cyclodialysis clefts with argon laser photocoagulation. Ophthalmology 89:1082, 1982

Herschler J: Laser shrinkage of ciliary processes: a treatment for malignant (ciliary block) glaucoma. Ophthalmology 87:1155, 1980

Krupin T: Anterior segment laser surgery. In Krupin T, Waltman SR (eds): Complications in Ophthalmic Surgery. 2nd Ed. JB Lippincott, Philadelphia, 1984

Krupin T, Kolker AE, Kass MA, et al: Intraocular pressure the day of argon laser trabeculoplasty in primary open-angle glaucoma. Ophthalmology 91:361, 1984

Krupin T, Stone RA, Cohen BH, et al: Acute intraocular pressure response to argon laser iridotomy. Ophthalmology 92:922, 1985

Ritch R, Podos SM: Argon laser treatment of angle-closure glaucoma. Persp Ophthalmol 4:129, 1980

Robin AL, Pollack IP: Argon laser peripheral iridotomies in the treatment of primary angle closure glaucoma. Arch Ophthalmol 100:919, 1982

Schwartz AL, Whitten ME, Bleiman B, et al: Argon laser trabecular surgery in uncontrolled phakic open angle glaucoma. Ophthalmology 88:203, 1981

Thomas JV, Simmons RJ, Belcher CD: Argon laser trabeculoplasty in the presurgical patient. Ophthalmology 89:187, 1982

Van Buskirk EM: Reopening filtration fistulas with the argon laser. Am J Ophthalmol 94:1, 1982

# 12

# Surgical Therapy in Glaucoma

## SURGICAL ANATOMY (FIG. 12-1)

### Limbus

I. The transition zone at the corneoscleral junction, known as the limbus, is the most critical millimeter in ophthalmic surgery. A knowledge of limbal anatomy is important for the proper placement of an incision that enters the anterior chamber.

II. The width of the limbal zone is normally greatest at the 12 and 6 o'clock positions. The limbus decreases to its smallest width at the horizontal meridians.

III. The anterior border of the limbus, the corneoconjunctival junction, is the ridge where the conjunctival and corneal epithelium merge at the end of Bowman's membrane.

IV. Posterior to the conjunctival ridge, the transparent and slightly blue fibers of the cornea blend with the opaque and white fibers of the sclera. This results in the gray limbal transition zone, which consists of two thin triangles of white scleral fibers enclosing the wedge of clear corneal fibers.

V. The posterior limbal border, where the clear corneal fibers stop, overlies the scleral spur and the iris root.

VI. The internal limits of the limbus are Schwalbe's line anteriorly and the scleral spur with insertion of the ciliary muscle posteriorly. The trabecular meshwork spans these limits and is 0.6 to 0.9 mm in width.

VII. The external width of the limbus is less defined due to the variable insertion of the conjunctiva, the oval shape of the cornea with its long axis horizontal, and the almost perfectly circular shape of Schwalbe's line internally. The maximum width of the limbus at 12 o'clock is 1.0–2.0 mm while the width at either horizontal side is 0.4–0.6 mm.

VIII. Location of a limbal incision into the anterior chamber is dependent on the width of the limbus and the size of the anterior segment. In addition, it is dependent on the trajectory of the proposed incision, i.e., perpendicular vs oblique.

A. In an eye with an open iridocorneal angle, a perpendicular incision at the anterior limbal border will enter the chamber through Descemet's membrane, anterior to Schwalbe's line; a midlimbal incision, at the junction of the blue and white areas, enters the chamber at Schwalbe's line or just posterior in the trabecular tissue; and an incision at the posterior limbal border

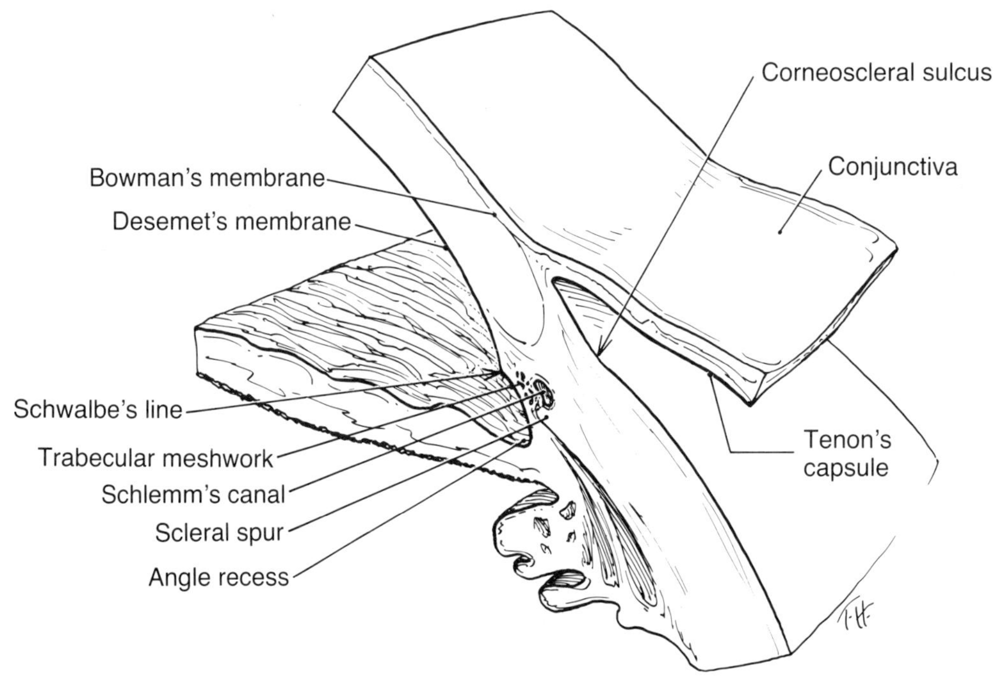


**Fig. 12-1** Anatomy of the surgical limbus.

enters the chamber at the scleral spur.

B. In an eye with a small anterior segment (e.g., hyperopia, closed-angle glaucoma), a perpendicular midlimbal incision may enter the chamber in the angle recess or even more posteriorly over the ciliary body.

C. With a truly limbal incision, clear corneal tissue is observed after cutting the external scleral fibers.

## Conjunctiva-Tenon's Capsule

I. Conjunctiva and Tenon's capsule cover the limbus. The insertion of these tissues at Bowman's membrane of the cornea defines the anterior external border of the limbus.

II. Tenon's tissue at the limbus is a fibrous connective tissue which is an extension of the posterior Tenon's capsule. The tissue is tightly adherent to the conjunctiva at the anterior insertion and to the episclera along a line approximately 1 mm behind the scleral-limbal junction. Posterior to the limbus, Tenon's capsule is weakly attached to the overlying conjunctiva and the underlying episcleral tissue.

III. Tenon's tissue tends to be denser
  A. in eyes of young patients.
  B. in eyes of black patients.
  C. in diabetics.
  D. in eyes with uveitis.
  E. in eyes with previous ocular surgery.

## Iris

I. The root of the iris inserts into the ciliary body immediately posterior to the scleral spur. This is approximately 1.5–2.0 mm posterior to the limbal zone.

II. The location of the iris root insertion is dependent on the dimensions of the anterior segment. The insertion is more anterior in hyperopic eyes and more posterior in myopic eyes.

### Ciliary Body

I. The ciliary body is attached to the sclera at the scleral spur, and consists of two parts.
   A. The anterior pars plicata which is 2–3 mm thick and extends approximately 3–4 mm posteriorly from the scleral spur.
   B. The pars plana which is located posterior to the pars plicata. This division is thinner than the pars plicata and is 4–5 mm wide. The pars plana ends at the ora serrata.

II. Ciliary processes are located on the inner surface of both divisions of the ciliary body. Processes may extend anteriorly onto the back surface of the iris.

III. The major arterial arcade lies at the iris root in the ciliary body.

## ANESTHESIA

Anesthetic mortality is similar in patients undergoing ophthalmic surgery under either local or general anesthesia. The incidence of operative complications is also similar. Preferences for general or local anesthesia vary in different regions of the United States as well as in different countries. A discussion of general anesthesia is beyond the scope of this manual.

Preoperative preparation requires cooperation and communication among the patient, the anesthesiologist, the family physician, and the surgeon. A preoperative interview and examination are required to determine the patient's physical and mental status and the risks of anesthesia. The use of medications which might effect anesthesia (e.g., systemic or topical corticosteroids, topical beta blockers, topical echothiophate iodide) as well as drug allergies must be documented. Factors which may affect the surgical outcome, such as a history of possible bleeding diatheses resulting from the use of anticoagulants or salicylates, should be obtained. Finally, an explanation of the anesthetic technique, surgical procedure, possible operative and postoperative complications, and postoperative expectations should be clearly discussed with the patient and an additional member of the family, if possible.

### Local Anesthetic Agents

Agents used for local anesthesia in ophthalmic surgery are the same as those used in peripheral nerve blocks (Table 12-1). There is a recent trend to use the longer duration agents, bupivacaine or etidocaine, which may reduce the need for postoperative analgesics and reduce eye movements after surgery. These agents can be used alone or in combination with lidocaine in order to take advantage of the rapid onset of the lidocaine and the long duration of the other agent. Prior to any injection, aspiration is performed to insure that the medication will not be injected intravascularly.

I. Epinephrine
   A. Epinephrine is frequently added to the injection solution in order to prolong the duration of the local anesthetic. Dilute concentrations of 1:200,000 (1 mg/200 ml) should be used to avoid tissue injury secondary to ischemia. However, the use of the longer duration anesthetic agents has reduced the need for the addition of epinephrine.
   B. Epinephrine can result in systemic side effects especially in patients with systemic hypertension, cardiovascular disease, or thyrotoxicosis.
   C. Retrobulbar epinephrine may reduce optic nerve blood flow and should be avoided in patients with glaucomatous optic nerve disease or a history of ischemic optic neuropathy.

**Table 12-1.** Regional Anesthetic Agents

| Agent | Concentration (%) | Maximum Dose | Onset of Action | Duration of Action |
|---|---|---|---|---|
| Lidocaine (Xylocaine) | 1–2 | 500 mg | 4–6 min | 30–60 min |
| Procaine (Novocaine) | 1–4 | 500 mg | 6–8 min | 30–45 min |
| Mepivacaine (Carbocaine) | 1–2 | 500 mg | 3–5 min | 90–120 min |
| Prilocaine (Citanest) | 1–2 | 600 mg | 3–5 min | 60–90 min |
| Etidocaine (Duranest) | 0.1–1 | 300 mg | 3–5 min | 4–6 hr |
| Bupivacaine (Marcaine) | 0.25–0.75 | 175 mg | 3–5 min | 4–12 hr |

II. Hyaluronidase
   A. The enzyme hyaluronidase is frequently added to the anesthetic solution to enhance solution diffusion through the tissues. This action is accomplished by hydrolysis of extracellular hyaluronic acid.
   B. The use of the enzyme allows a more complete and consistent block with the use of less anesthetic solution and therefore less tissue distortion.
   C. Between 7.5 and 15 turbidity reducing units (TRU) are added per milliliter of anesthetic solution.

## Akinesia of the Orbicularis Oculi Muscle

Akinesia of the eyelids is essential for all intraocular surgery to prevent squeezing of the lids and expulsion of intraocular contents. Paralysis of the orbicularis oculi muscle may be achieved by either local infiltration of the muscle or proximal infiltration of the branches of the facial nerve which supply it.

### van Lint Method

Steps 1. A sharp 25 or 27 gauge needle is inserted at the lateral orbital rim and the anesthetic solution is injected, making a small intradermal wheal.
2. The needle is advanced into the deep tissues along the inferolateral orbital margin. As the needle is withdrawn, 2–4 ml of anesthetic solution are injected.
3. The needle is redirected along the superolateral orbital margin and a similar amount of anesthetic solution is injected as the needle is withdrawn.
4. Pressure is applied to the area to promote diffusion of the anesthetic.
5. The van Lint method can be modified to reduce lid edema by placing the injections more laterally to block the facial nerve as it crosses the periosteum. The initial injection is made directly on the periosteum of the orbital rim and is followed by inferior and superior injections (Fig. 12-2).

### O'Brien Method

With this method, a facial nerve block is achieved by injection over the mandibular condyle, inferior to the posterior zygomatic process (Fig. 12-3A).

Steps 1. The condyle is palpated as the patient moves his jaw.
2. A 25 or 27 gauge needle is inserted over the condyle, to a depth of approximately 1 cm, until the periosteum is reached.
3. Anesthetic solution, approximately 2–3 ml, is injected as the needle is withdrawn.
4. The block may be incomplete due to the variable course of the facial nerve. Therefore, the following modifications have been recommended.

   After injecting over the condyle, the needle is partially withdrawn and redirected inferiorly along the posterior edge of the ramus of the mandible. Anesthetic solution is injected as the needle is withdrawn.

   The needle is repositioned anteriorly along the zygomatic arch and the anesthetic is injected upon withdrawal of the needle.

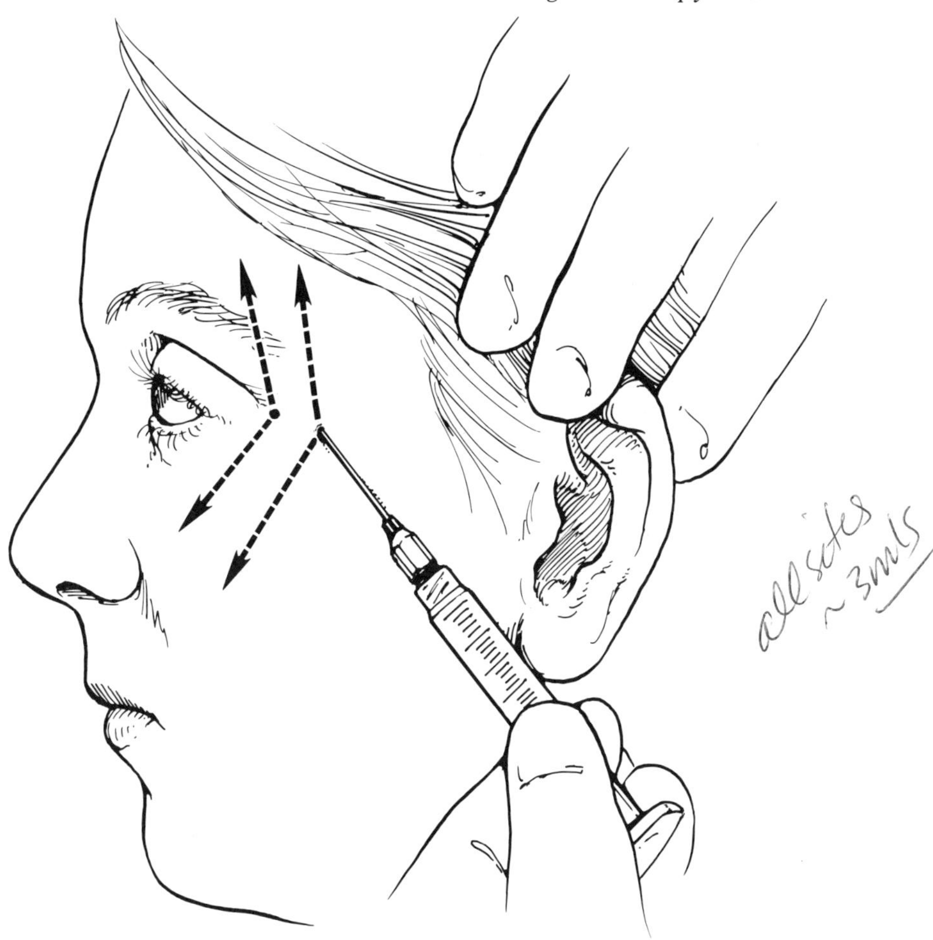

**Fig. 12-2** The van Lint technique for facial nerve block. The classic technique blocks the facial nerve at the lateral orbital rim. The modified technique (from the needle site) places the injection more lateral to avoid lid edema.

### Atkinson Method

This method involves blocking the branches of the facial nerve as they cross the zygomatic arch (Fig. 12-3B).

Steps
1. An intradermal wheal is made with a 25 or 27 gauge needle by injecting 0.5 ml of anesthetic solution at the lower margin of the zygomatic arch, below the lateral orbital rim.
2. The needle is directed superiorly and posteriorly along the zygoma (aimed just lateral to the midpoint between the tragus and lateral margin of the zygoma).
3. Between 5 and 10 ml of anesthetic is injected as the needle is withdrawn.

### Nadbath-Rehman Method

The Nadbath-Rehman method produces complete akinesia of the muscles innervated by the facial nerve by blocking the nerve at the concavity just below the external auditory meatus, between the anterosuperior border of the mastoid process and the posterior border of the mandibular ramus (Fig. 12-4). The major advantage of the technique is the consistent course of the facial nerve from the stylomastoid foramen to the postero-medial

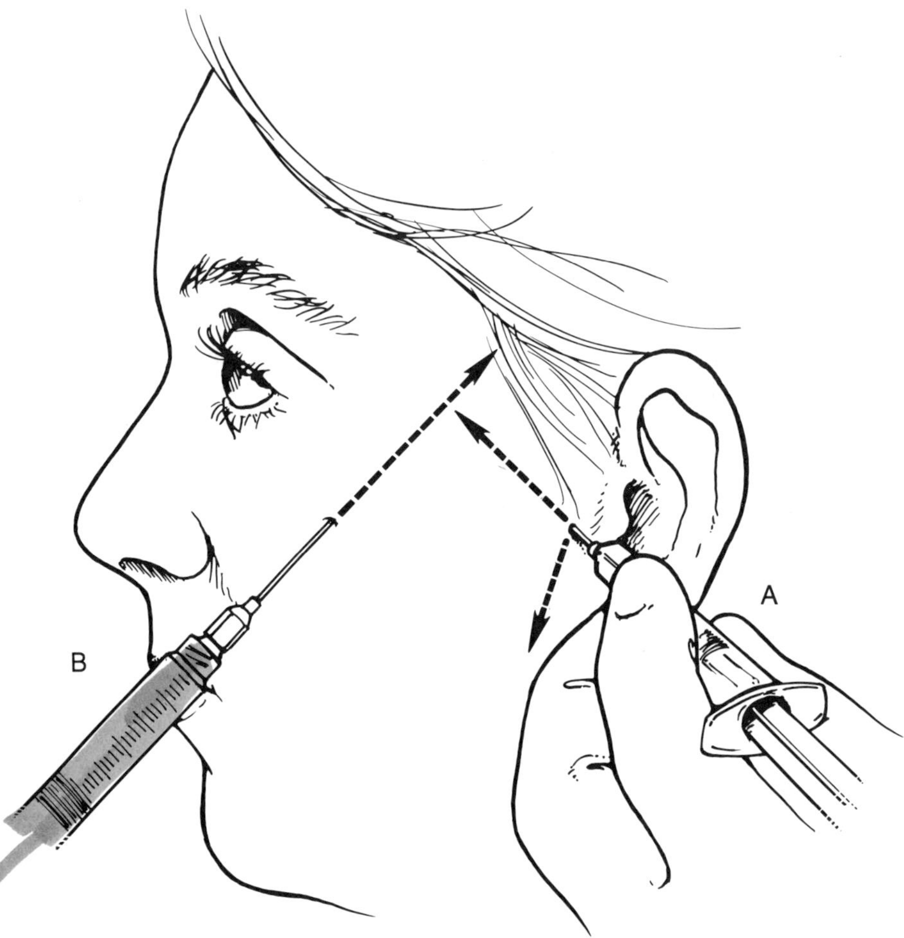


**Fig. 12-3 (A)** The O'Brien technique for facial nerve block. The injection is performed over the mandibular condyle (tip of needle). A modified technique (dotted lines) makes additional injections along the posterior edge of the mandible and anteriorly along the zygomatic arch. **(B)** The Atkinson method for facial nerve block.

surface of the parotid gland, prior to branching of the nerve. The patient must be warned that the entire side of their face will be transiently paralyzed.

Steps
1. The site is identified by palpation and confirmed by having the patient open and close his mouth.
2. A 25 gauge, 12-mm long needle is inserted into the skin and an intradermal wheal is made by injecting 0.5 ml of anesthetic solution.
3. The needle is advanced its full length perpendicularly into the tissue.
4. The plunger is withdrawn to assure the needle is not intravascular and approximately 3 ml of anesthetic solution is injected as the needle is withdrawn.

## Retrobulbar Block

Retrobulbar injection of local anesthetic provides akinesia of the extraocular muscles innervated by cranial nerves III, IV, and VI. Cranial nerve IV may course outside the muscle cone. Therefore, akinesia of the superior oblique muscle may only be partial. In addition, anesthesia of most of the conjunc-

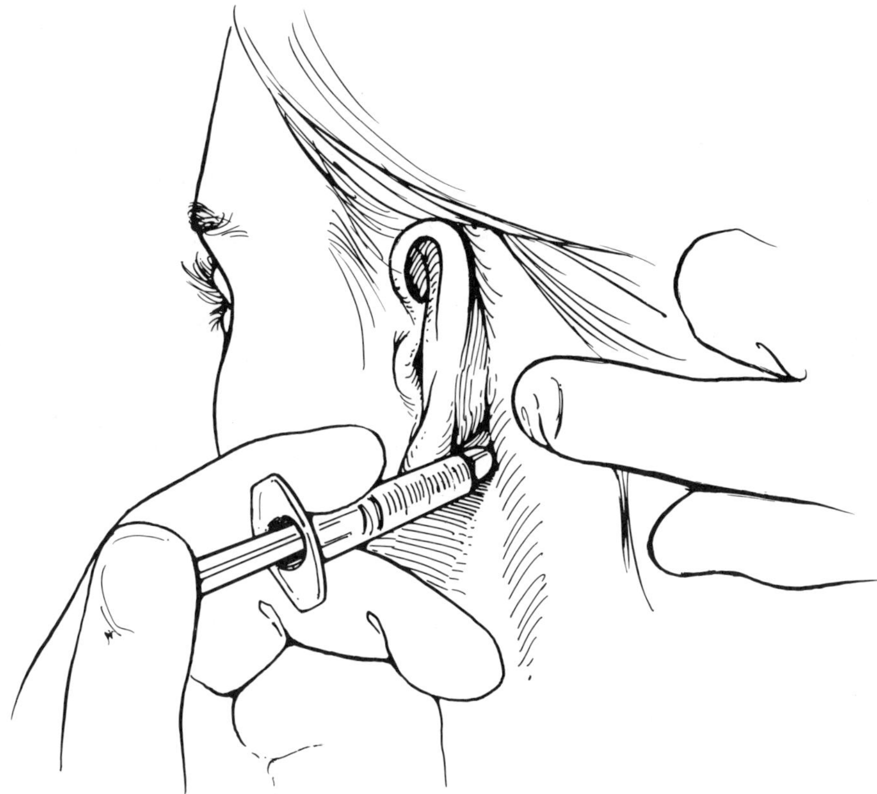

**Fig. 12-4** The Nadbath-Rehman method for facial nerve block.

tiva, the cornea, and uvea, as well as mydriasis, is achieved by blocking the ciliary nerves. Vision is reduced due to anesthetic block of the optic nerve.

### Preoperative Medications

I. Retrobulbar block can be both anxiety producing and painful to the patient.

II. Preoperative sedation, such as 25–50 mg of hydroxyzine hydrochloride (Vistaril), may help reduce anxiety.

III. A number of techniques have been advocated to lessen the discomfort and awareness of the retrobulbar injection. These methods require the presence of an anesthesiologist.

  A. Administration of intravenous methohexital sodium (Brevital), 15–50 mg, or fentanyl (Sublimaze), 0.025–0.1 mg, 2–4 min prior to the block.

  B. Administration of 50%–60% nitrous oxide (4 L/min nitrous oxide and 3 L/min oxygen) by face mask for a few minutes prior to the injection. Pure oxygen is administered after the injection to eliminate diffusion hypoxia.

### Injection

Steps 1. Traditionally the patient has been instructed to look upward and nasally during the retrobulbar injection. Recent evidence has demonstrated that this position rotates the optic nerve and posterior pole of the globe into the path of the retrobulbar needle. The optic nerve is stretched in this position which increases the chance for perforation. Therefore, it is recommended that the patient be instructed to look in primary

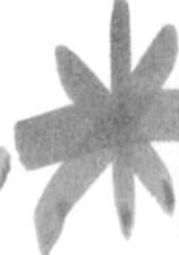

gaze (or slightly downward and outward) (Fig. 12-5).

2. A blunt needle, as advocated by Atkinson, is recommended to reduce the potential for perforation of orbital vessels or nerves. Patient discomfort with the blunt needle is diminished by first making an intradermal wheal of local anesthetic at the skin entry site with a sharp 25 gauge needle. This is done just above the inferior orbital rim at the junction of the lateral and middle thirds of the margin.

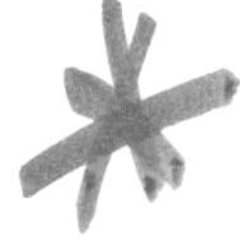

3. A 1¼-inch 23 gauge blunt needle is inserted and directed perpendicular to the skin surface, toward the midline. The bevel of the needle should face the globe to reduce chance of perforation.
4. After the needle passes the equator of the globe, it is directed upward, slightly lower than the orbital apex, towards the inferior part of the superior orbital fissure. The needle is fully inserted.
5. The syringe is aspirated to be certain that the needle is not inside a vessel. An adequate block is achieved following injection of 1.5–3.0 ml of anesthetic solution into the muscle cone.
6. If complete akinesia and anesthesia has not been achieved, it may be necessary to perform a supplemental retrobulbar injection or a transconjunctival quadrant

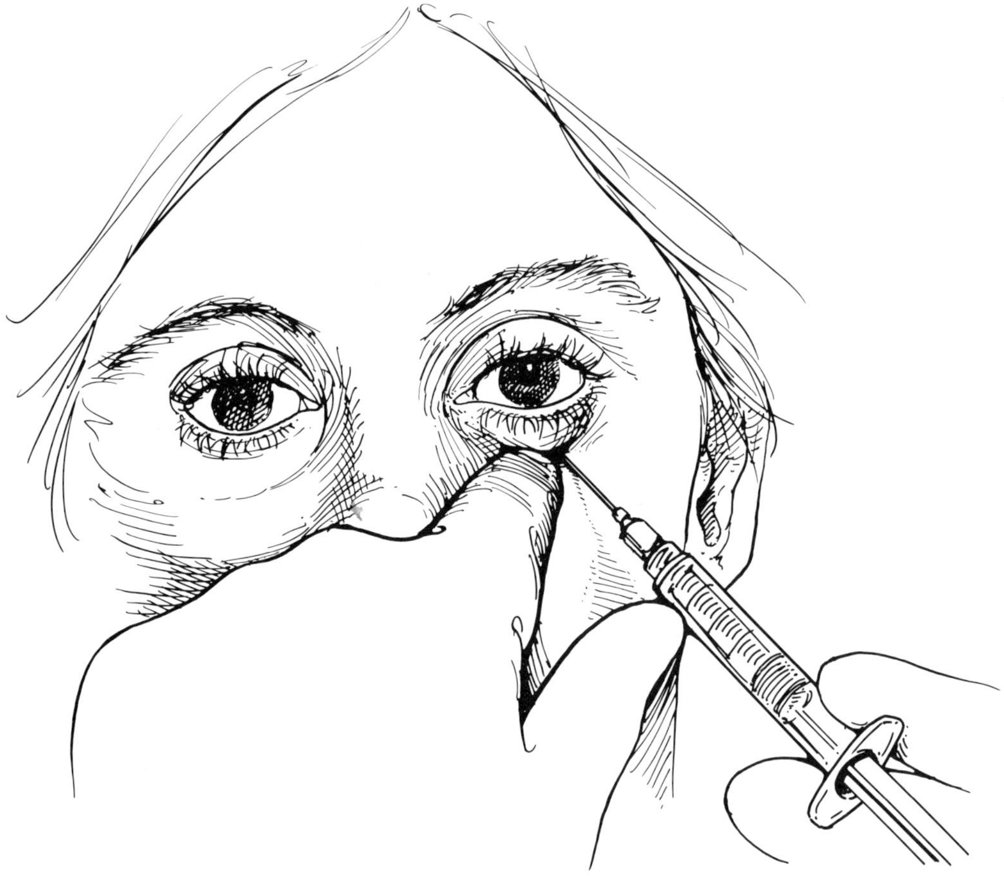

**Fig. 12-5** Retrobulbar injection with the eye in primary gaze. The index finger is palpating the orbital rim. The needle is directed slightly below the apex of the orbit.

block adjacent to the functioning extraocular muscle.

## Complications (Table 12-2)

I. Retrobulbar hemorrhage

Retrobulbar hemorrhage is the most common complication. Intraocular pressure and central retinal artery pulsations must be monitored following a retrobulbar hemorrhage for signs of an impending retinal arterial occlusion. It is to be noted that the retrobulbar injection itself results in no light perception, so that vision testing will not indicate retinal or optic nerve ischemia. If external pressure on the globe compresses the retinal arteries, a deep lateral canthotomy is performed to rapidly decompress the orbit. If this does not re-establish normal retinal blood flow, an anterior chamber paracentesis is done to decompress the globe. Failure to promptly and sufficiently treat this complication may result in total loss of vision.

A. The patient requires close monitoring for several hours following the hemorrhage. Extravasation of additional blood may precipitate an oculocardiac reflex (see below).

B. Following a retrobulbar hemorrhage, it is prudent to postpone surgery until all signs of the hemorrhage have resolved. Surgery can usually be performed 2–4 days later, preferably under general anesthesia.

Oculocardiac reflex

An oculocardiac reflex with slowing of the pulse can occur following retrobulbar injection. Bradycardia, arrhythmias, and even periods of cardiac asystole may result. Electrocardiographic monitoring will detect this complication which is treated with intravenous atropine (0.4–0.6 mg) or glycopyrrolate (0.3 mg).

III. Perforation of the globe

Perforation of the globe can occur despite using a blunted retrobulbar needle. The complication is more common in a highly myopic eye, if there is a posterior staphyloma, or following repeated anesthetic injections. The patient has immediate ocular pain following inadvertent perforation of the globe. Planned surgery should be postponed and appropriate retinal treatment undertaken.

IV. Optic atrophy and permanent loss of vision

This may occur even in the absence of retrobulbar hemorrhage. Postulated mechanisms include: direct injury to the nerve, injections into the nerve sheath with compressive ischemia, and intraneural sheath hemorrhage.

**Table 12-2.** Complications of Retrobulbar Anesthesia

| Complication | Signs and Symptoms | Mechanism |
|---|---|---|
| Retrobulbar hemorrhage | Increasing proptosis, subconjunctival or eyelid ecchymosis, pain, increased intraocular pressure | Direct trauma to the artery or vein |
| Perforation of the globe | Ocular pain, restlessness, intraocular hemorrhage | Direct trauma: myopic eye, posterior staphyloma; repeated injections |
| Optic nerve damage | Visual loss, optic disc pallor | Direct trauma to nerve or blood vessels; vascular occlusion |
| Central nervous system | Disorientation, unconsciousness, convulsions, respiratory or cardiac arrest | Excessive total drug injection, injection into subarachnoid space, oculocardiac reflex |

V. Systemic complications

Systemic complications are rare but potentially serious. These include disorientation, unconsciousness, convulsions, respiratory arrest, and cardiac arrest. Possible pathways for systemic administration of the anesthetic agent include inadvertent intravascular injection of local anesthetic or penetration of the optic nerve dural sheath with diffusion of the agent through the cerebrospinal fluid.

## RECTUS MUSCLE BRIDLE SUTURE

A bridle suture is frequently placed for stabilization of the globe. The suture should be placed beneath the tendon of the superior rectus muscle. A 4-0 to 6-0 silk suture on a blunt, noncutting needle is recommended.

### Technique

Steps 1. A lid speculum is inserted, and the eye is rotated 180° opposite to the rectus muscle to be bridled. Because the superior oblique muscle may still be functioning after a retrobulbar block, it is useful to have the patient look down while securing the superior rectus muscle.

2. Under direct visualization, the tendon is grasped 3–4 mm behind its insertion. This reduces bleeding from the anterior ciliary vessels when passing the fixation suture.
3. The needle is passed beneath the tendon and the tip is directed away from the globe in order to avoid accidental scleral perforation. The surgeon must be aware of possible muscluloscleral adhesions in eyes that have undergone previous surgery. The muscle must be free of the sclera before placing the bridle suture.

### Complications

I. Hemorrhage.

Subconjunctival or intramuscular hemorrhage can occur during suture placement. Excessive bleeding causes conjunctival and episcleral scar formation, an unwanted complication for filtration surgery. If this occurs, surgery should be postponed until the hemorrhage has resolved.

II. Scleral perforation

Signs of a bridle suture perforation are sudden hypotony and the appearance of vitreous under the conjunctiva or the muscle. Planned surgery should be postponed and appropriate retinal therapy undertaken.

III. Ptosis

There is an intimate anatomic relationship between the superior rectus and the overlying levator complex. Direct trauma during bridle suture placement or posterior infiltration of a hemorrhage into the substance of Müller's muscle can result in postoperative ptosis. If necessary, postoperative traumatic ptosis can be treated by transconjunctival levator shortening.

## FILTRATION SURGERY

### Conjunctival Flap

The conjunctival flap traditionally has been limbus-based. This type of flap was necessary in full-thickness filtration procedures that produce a direct opening into the anterior chamber at the limbus. Full-thickness filtration blebs tend to have an anterior, localized, and elevated limbal bleb. Subscleral microsurgical filtration surgery (e.g., trabeculectomy) produces a guarded opening into the anterior chamber and a posterior flow of aqueous. These procedures allow use of either a limbus- or fornix-based flap (Fig. 12-6).

The conjunctival flap is a critically important part of any filtration procedure. While the flap provides exposure to perform the surgery, the dissected conjunctival and Tenon's tissues become the site of the future filtration bleb. External tissue scarring is the primary cause of filtration surgery failure. An

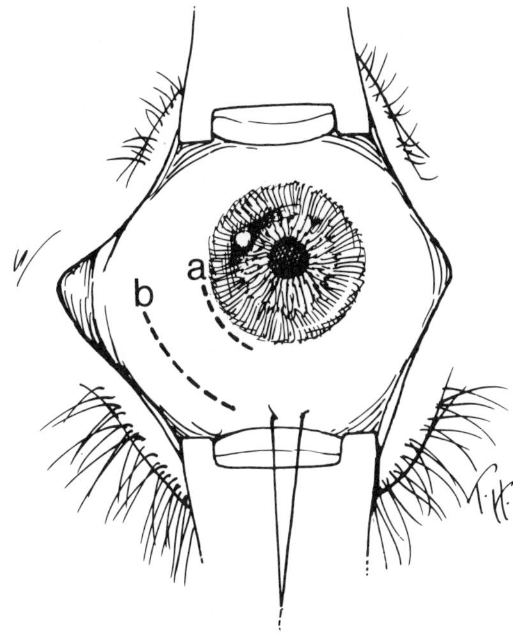


**Fig. 12-6** Location of conjunctival incision for fornix-based (a) and limbus-based (b) flap.

ideal conjunctival flap places the conjunctival incision, and therefore the sutured area of closure, some distance from the site of future bleb formation.

## Limbus-based Conjunctival Flap (Fig. 12-7)

Steps 1. The conjunctiva is grasped with a smooth forceps approximately 8 mm posterior to the limbus. A buttonhole incision is made with a scissors through the conjunctiva and Tenon's tissue to the sclera.

2. The location of the conjunctival incision is in an oblique quadrant to avoid the extraocular muscles and possible bleeding from injury to an anterior ciliary vessel. If scarring of the conjunctiva and Tenon's capsule is suspected, the tissues are distended with an injection of saline to determine a favorable site for surgery.
3. The incision is extended to a total length of 8 mm. The incision is concentric with the limbus. This circumferential incision can be performed separately for the conjunctiva and Tenon's capsule or these two layers can be incised as a single layer.
4. The edge of the flap is elevated and the tissues are dissected anteriorly by either blunt extension using dry cellulose sponges or by sharp dissection with a Beaver #57 or #67 blade or scissors if adhesions are encountered.
5. The flap is reflected at the limbus with the corneoscleral sulcus clearly visible without fibers crossing it. The surgical limbus should be clearly identified. A flat blade knife (Gill or Tooke) or a #57 Beaver blade is used to fully expose the sulcus and the anterior limit of the conjunctival insertion.

## Fornix-based Conjunctival Flap (Fig. 12-8)

Steps 1. The conjunctiva is incised at the limbus with a blunt- or sharp-tipped Wescott scissors. The change in curvature at the limbus between the cornea and the sclera must be considered in order to avoid incising the sclera when preparing the flap.

2. The blunt scissors is used to clear a plane between the sclera and episclera near the limbus and posteriorly towards the equator of the globe. The conjunctiva is incised at its corneal insertion for 7–9 mm. This incision should be placed as

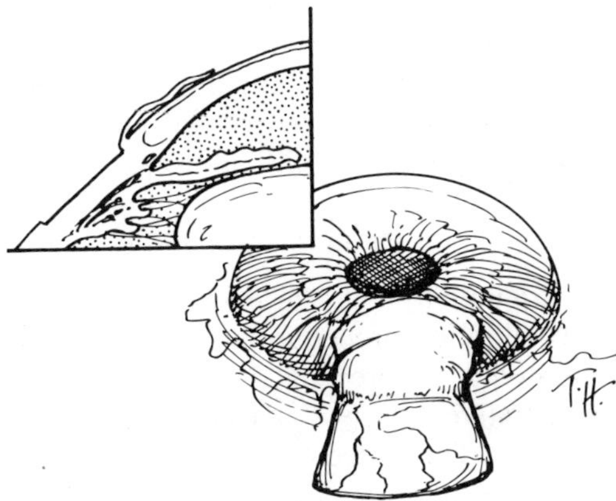

**Fig. 12-7** Limbus-based conjunctival flap reflected onto the cornea with the surgical limbus exposed.

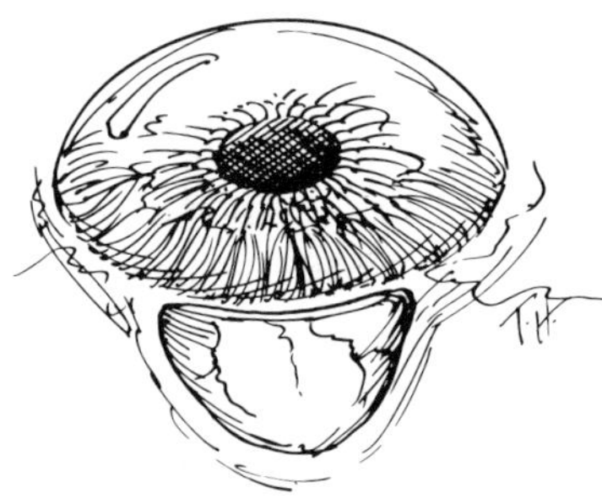

**Fig. 12-8** Fornix-based conjunctival flap with the conjunctiva retracted posteriorly exposing the surgical limbus.

anterior as possible without leaving tags of conjunctiva attached to the cornea.

3. Radial relaxing incisions can be made at one or both ends if the flap does not retract 4 or 5 mm posteriorly.

### Limbus- vs Fornix-Based Flap

I. The fornix-based flap is easier to dissect and easier to close than the limbus-based flap.

II. Buttonholes of the conjunctiva are more common with the limbus-based flap.

III. The limbus-based flap has a posterior scar line which can delimit the bleb. This does not occur with a fornix-based flap which places the conjunctival scar line at the limbus.

IV. Identification of posterior bleeding can be difficult with the fornix-based flap.

V. Wound leaks, which can occur with either type of conjunctival flap, are more common with the fornix-based method, and may be more difficult to manage.

## Iridectomy

An iridectomy must be performed as part of any filtration procedure at the site of the sclerostomy to prevent the possibility of postoperative prolapse and incarceration of iris tissue. The iridectomy in filtration surgery is not performed to prevent pupillary block, and thus each filtration procedure requires its own iridectomy. The iridectomy should be wider than the opening into the anterior chamber to prevent postoperative incarceration of tissue.

### Peripheral Iridectomy

Steps 1. The iris tissue which has prolapsed through the anterior chamber opening is grasped with a fine toothed forceps. A smooth forceps should be used if the iris must be grasped within the chamber. The iris must be grasped at least 2 mm anterior to its root to avoid inadvertent injury to the ciliary body or an iridodialysis.

2. The prolapsed iris is cut with a scissors. To have an iridectomy which is wider than the sclerostomy, the tented up iris can be excised by two scissor cuts; the iris is pulled away from the scissors for the first cut and then toward the scissors for the second cut (Fig. 12-9).

3. Massage of the cornea anterior to the anterior chamber opening usually allows the cut edges of the iris to retract into the anterior chamber. Occasionally irrigation through the chamber opening is required. Incarcerated iris tissue should be excised.

### Sector Iridectomy

A sector iridectomy may be indicated if the surgeon feels a large postoperative pupil is required for retinal examination. In addition, a sector iridectomy may be indicated in an eye with lens changes that are not significant enough for lens removal at the time of filtration surgery, but that might interfer with vision through a miotic pupil.

Steps 1. The prolapsed iris tissue is grasped with a toothed forceps. The iris is removed from the eye, using a hand-over-hand technique, until the sphincter is removed through the anterior chamber opening. This pull is from the sphincter, not from the iris root, to avoid creating an iridodialysis.

2. The iris is pulled away from the scissors for the first cut and then toward the scissors for the second cut to remove the tissue.

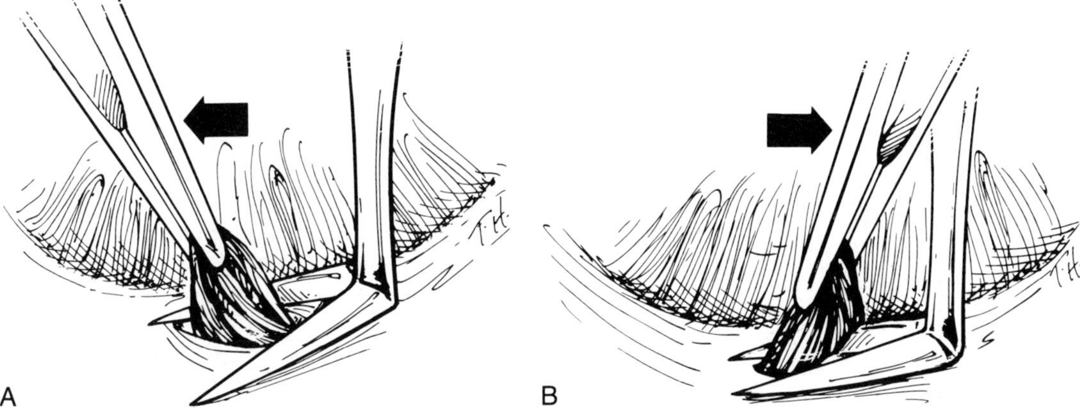


**Fig. 12-9** Peripheral iridectomy. (**A**) The iris is pulled away from the scissors for the initial excision. (**B**) The iris is pulled towards the scissors for the final excision of the tissue. This maneuver assures that the base of the iridectomy is larger than the anterior chamber opening.

3. Massage of the cornea anterior to the anterior chamber opening usually allows the cut edges of the iris to retract into the anterior chamber. Occasionally irrigation through the chamber opening is required. Incarcerated iris tissue within the sclerostomy should be excised.

## Filtering Procedures

A variety of glaucoma filtration procedures have been described. Filtration operations may be classified as full-thickness or subscleral procedures. However, all operations have a similar goal: creation of a fistula (a sclerostomy or sclerectomy) between the anterior chamber and the subconjunctival-Tenon's space. The fistula bypasses the usual drainage structures and provides a route for aqueous humor flow to the subconjunctival space (a bleb) where it can be removed via one or more of the following routes.

I. Aqueous transfer into the conjunctival or episcleral blood vessels or into newly formed aqueous-type veins.
II. Direct passage of aqueous through the conjunctiva into the tears.
III. Posterior passage of aqueous into the orbit where it can be absorbed into the venous circulation.

### Trabeculectomy (Subscleral) Procedures

Steps 1. Surgical exposure. A lid speculum is inserted after the administration of satisfactory anesthesia and akinesia. The operating microscope is positioned and a bridle suture is placed to fixate the globe.

2. Conjunctival flap. Either a limbus- or fornix-based flap is prepared (see Figs. 12-6, 12-7, and 12-8). Comparison of the two techniques demonstrates no difference in the intraocular pressure reduction and the ultimate success of the surgery. However, the character of the bleb may be different; the limbus-based flap results in a more localized, anterior, and elevated bleb which is limited by the posterior conjunctival scar line, whereas with a fornix-based flap the bleb is more diffuse and flatter.
3. Anterior chamber paracentesis. A paracentesis is usually performed through clear cornea at a location away from the area of the conjunctival incision. The corneal incision is shelved so that it is self-sealing (Fig. 12-10). Coating the knife blade with fluorescein stains the tract and makes it easier to locate during later stages of the operation.
4. Scleral flap (Fig. 12-11)
   Cauterization is lightly applied to actively bleeding vessels and to the re-

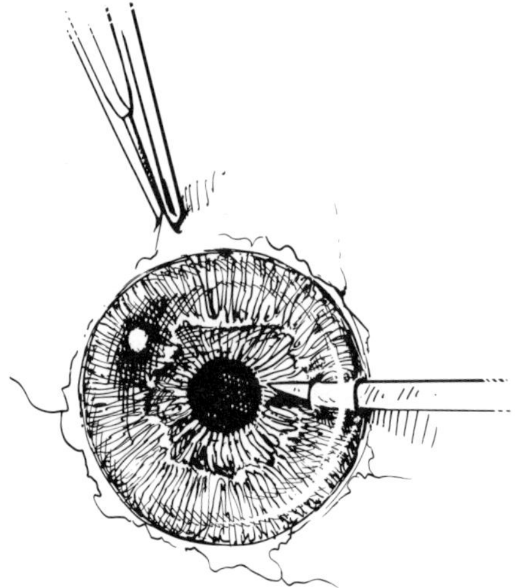

**Fig. 12-10** Paracentesis stab incision at the limbus. For the incision to be self-sealing, the plane of the blade should be flat so that the external and internal openings are at different levels. Placing fluorescein on the blade helps to mark the external entry of the shelved incision.

gion where the scleral flap will be dissected. A wet field cautery is preferred to reduce excessive heat damage to the sclera.

The corneal-based scleral flap should be one-third to one-half of the scleral thickness and can be either a triangle, square, or rectangle in shape. The flap is 4–5 mm wide at the limbus and a similar length at the sides of the square/triangle or at the apex of the triangle. The triangular flap has the advantage of producing the same length of exposure at the limbus while reducing the extent of posterior scleral dissection.

The outlines of the flap are made with a Beaver (#s 57, 64, or 69) or sharp (e.g., a super or diamond) blade to one-half to two-thirds of the scleral thickness along the two sides of the triangle or the two sides and posterior edge of the square/rectangle. These incisions should be perpendicular and cross at either the apex of the triangle or the two edges of the square/rectangle. Making the depth of these incisions greater than the planned depth of the scleral flap will facilitate the lamellar flap dissection.

The area is kept dry. Relatively high magnification is used for the lamellar dissection. The globe is fixated, and the lamellar dissection is started at a corner of the outlined scleral incisions. It is best not to fixate the scleral flap until a partial lamellar plane is dissected. The flap is then grasped and used to rotate the eye away from the surgeon. This places tension within the dissection bed and facilitates the dissection.

The lamellar dissection is carried forward toward the limbus. The surgeon must remember that the curvature of the globe changes abruptly at the limbus. Therefore, the lamellar plane is redirected as the cornea is reached. The dissection is made 1–2 mm into

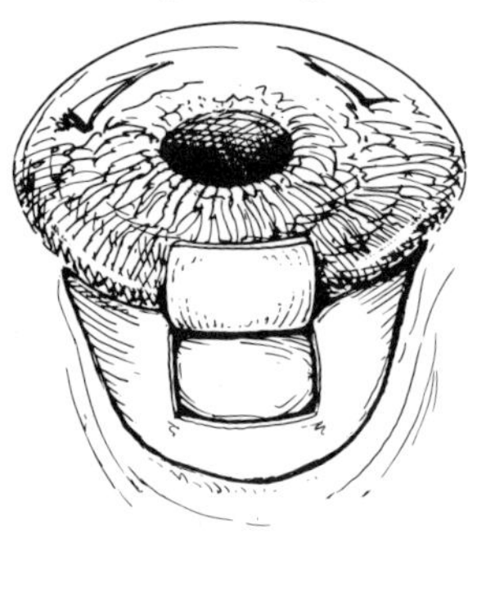



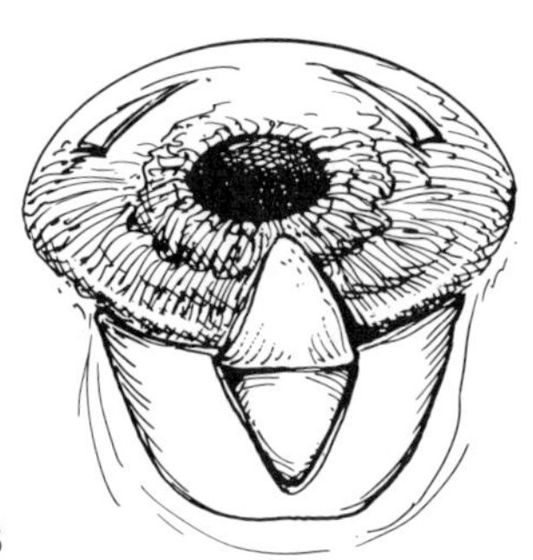



**Fig. 12-11** Alternative choices for scleral flap; **(A)**, square or rectangular; **(B)**, triangular.

clear cornea with the iris visible through the base of the dissection bed.

5. Excision of the internal block

The scleral flap is elevated and used to rotate the globe away from the surgeon. This fixates the globe and exposes the corneal-scleral lamellar bed. A traction suture is often helpful in retracting the scleral flap.

Many methods can be used to excise the internal block. The primary concern with all methods is to avoid damage to intraocular structures (e.g., the lens and iris). The block should be excised anterior to the scleral spur in order to avoid damage to the ciliary body, which can result in hemorrhage, and possible vitreous loss.

We prefer to incise the anterior edge and both sides of the block prior to cutting the posterior scleral-side of the block (Figs. 12-12A, 12-12B). This permits better visualization and control of the location of the posterior side of the block and prevents a posterior incision over the ciliary body. Instillation of a viscoelastic agent through the paracentesis prior to dissecting the block may deepen the iridocorneal angle and provide additional area between the iris and the corneoscleral tissue to be removed. This can facilitate excision of the internal block.

After the anterior incision has been made into the anterior chamber, radial incisions are made with either a microblade or Vannas scissors at the lateral extent of the proposed block. One blade of a Vannas scissors is placed into one of the radial incisions and slid anteriorly, parallel to the limbus, to incise the corneal side of the block.

Alternatively, the anterior corneal or posterior scleral side of the incision can be made using a microblade. The Vannas scissors is then used to create the two side incisions which can be either radial resulting in a rectangular block or at greater than a 90° angle resulting in a romboid block.

The block is rotated posteriorly exposing the internal aspect of the scleral spur and root of the iris. The posterior scleral side of the block is excised with the internal blade of the scissors under direct visualization (see Figs. 12-12C, 12-12D). If iris prolapses into the sclerostomy, a small iridotomy usually will allow it to fall back out of the way.

The scissors and microblade should always be held in a vertical orientation so that the edges of the block are cut squarely and not shelved. If a posterior shelved incision occurs, the shelf should be trimmed to create vertical edges to the sclerostomy opening.

Alternative means to perform the anterior chamber opening within the bed of the scleral flap include

*Cautery*. Heat can be used to separate the lips of the sclerostomy, thereby performing the anterior chamber entry, in a similar manner as used in full-thickness filtration surgery. An adjustable disposable cautery unit is recommended. Heat is applied anterior to the scleral spur resulting in retraction of the corneal-scleral tissues. The retraction should be of uniform depth across the dissection bed, to the level of Descemet's membrane. The anterior chamber should be entered with a microblade which is used to extend the opening across the entire length of the cauterized bed (see below).

*Posterior lip excision*. A posterior lip sclerectomy can be used to create the anterior chamber opening. A scratch incision is made into the chamber and posterior punch excisions are made using a microsurgical punch (see below).

*Trephination*. A trephine entry can be performed within the bed of the scleral flap (see below).

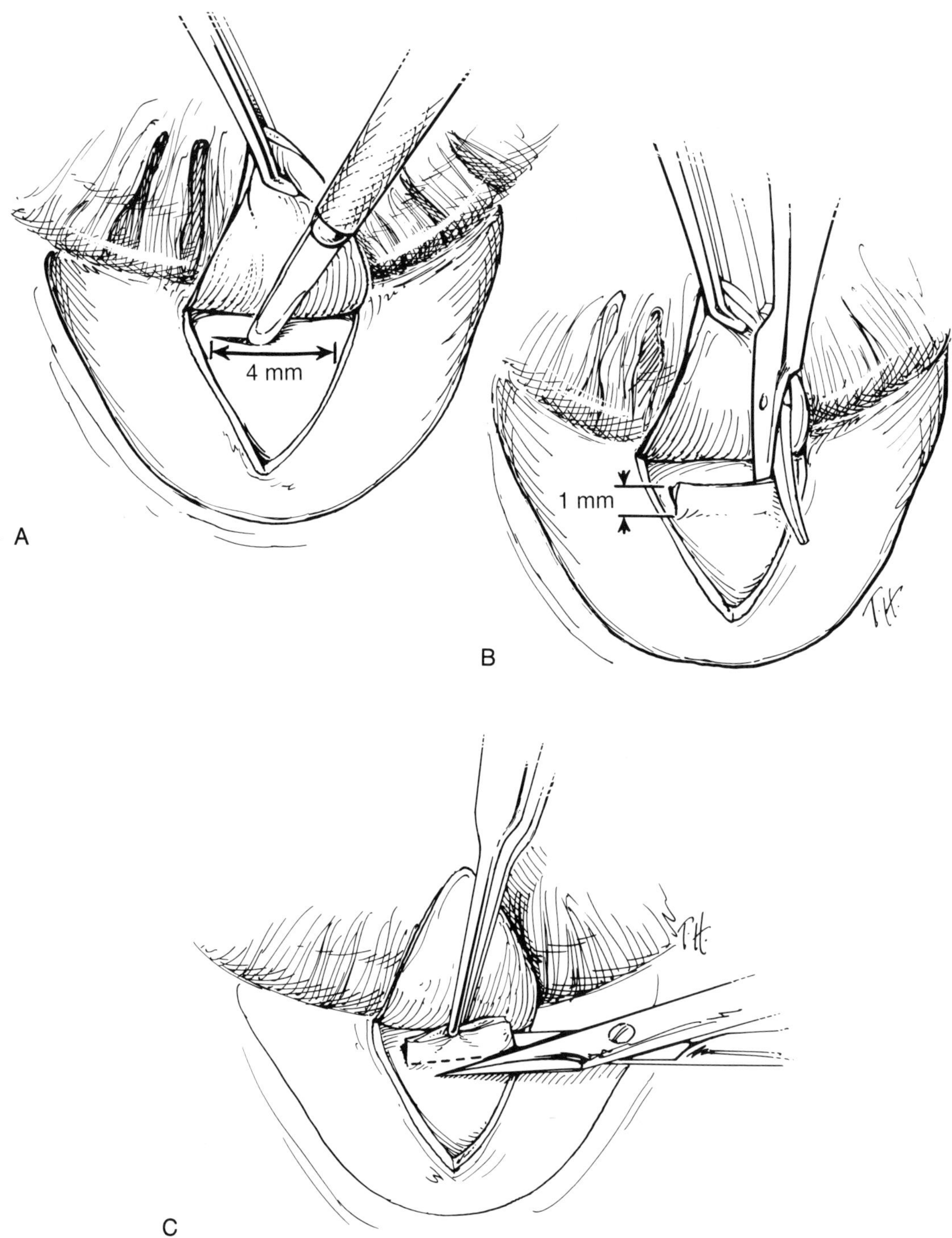


**Fig. 12-12** Excision of trabeculectomy block. (**A**) Knife incision of anterior edge of block. (**B**) Vannas scissors used to cut sides of the block. (**C**) The block is rotated posteriorly and the scleral side is cut with a Vannas scissors excising the tissue block. (*Figure continues.*)

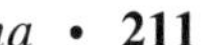

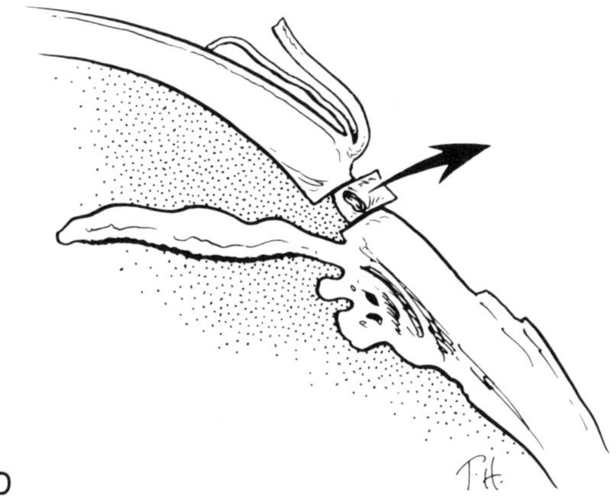


**Fig. 12-12** (*Continued*). **(D)** Side view of excised trabeculectomy block.

6. Iridectomy. A peripheral or sector iridectomy is performed (see page 206) following completion of the sclerostomy.
7. Closure of the scleral flap
   The scleral flap is closed with 10-0 nylon sutures placed at the apex of the triangular flap or at the corners of a square/rectangle flap (Fig. 12-13). We prefer to tie these sutures tight in order to create a radial pull on the flap which we believe is the method by which the scleral flap provides resistance to aqueous flow.
   The suture knot may be buried beneath the scleral flap by placing the posterior bite through the scleral side prior to passing the needle through the scleral flap. These bites should be of equal length on the scleral and flap sides (approximately 0.5 mm long) to avoid unequal tension and a "buckling" effect.
   The tightness of the closure is evaluated by reforming the anterior chamber with balanced salt solution through the paracentesis tract. Adequacy of filtration is evaluated in the following manner:

   1. By the rate of flow at the scleral flap edges by holding cellulose sponges at the flap edge.
   2. The ability of the anterior chamber to remain formed.
   3. The amount of pressure on the syringe which is required to reform

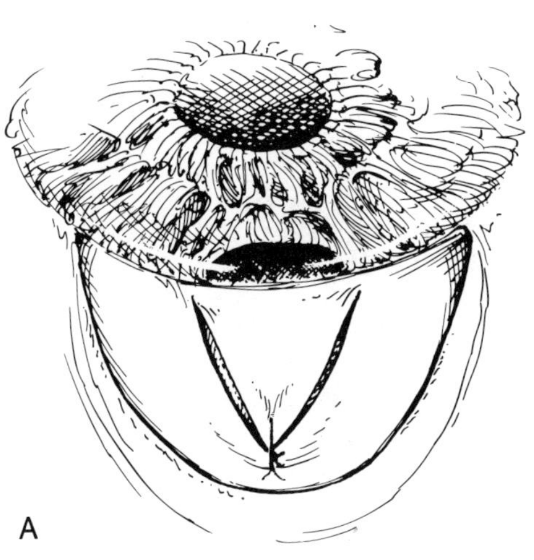


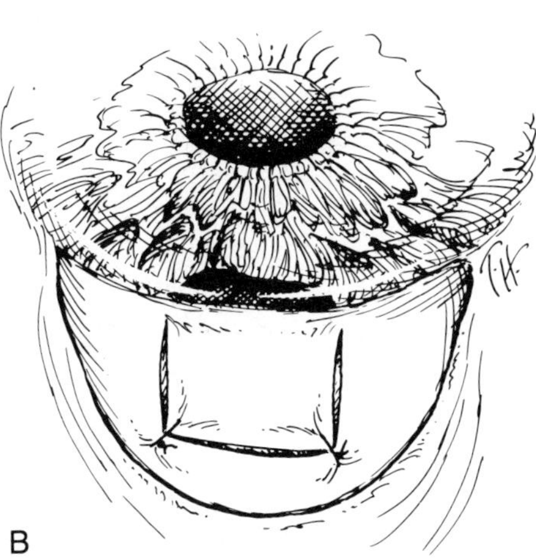


**Fig. 12-13** Closure of scleral flap. **(A)** One suture at the apex of a triangular flap. **(B)** Sutures at the posterior corners of a rectangular flap.

the chamber and then result in flow across the scleral flap.

If flow across the scleral flap is extensive and the anterior chamber shallows, additional sutures are placed across the flap.

If the globe is firm after reformation of the anterior chamber and the flow across the scleral flap is thought to be inadequate, the sutures should be loosened or removed and replaced. In addition, cautery may be applied to the edges of the scleral flap or to the sclera adjacent to the flap to gape the wound and increase flow at the edges. Incisions may be made on the edge of the flap to relax tension of the flap. Finally, if flow is still restricted, the scleral flap should be raised again and the internal block inspected and enlarged if necessary.

The ideal situation is free flow of fluid across the edges of the scleral flap with the anterior chamber remaining formed.

Releasable sutures which are externalized and loosened by adjusting a slipknot or cutting the suture have been described. We do not perform these techniques since transconjunctival release of the scleral flap suture has been made technically feasible and safe using the argon laser and a Hoskins contact lens (see below).

8. Closure of the conjunctival flap

   Limbus-based flap

   Tenon's tissue may be closed as a separate layer using a running or interrupted 8-0 or 9-0 vicryl or chromic suture. We do not find this separate closure necessary, and include Tenon's closure with the conjunctiva.

   The flap closure must be watertight. Meticulous closure is obtained using a 8-0 to 10-0 nylon or absorbable suture. A tapered and noncutting needle is preferred to avoid tearing the conjunctiva and creating holes larger than the diameter of the suture. A running suture with intermittent locking throws is used for closure with the bites approximately 1 mm from the free edge of the conjunctiva.

   Fornix-based flap

   The epithelium at the limbus and peripheral rim of the cornea must be removed. This is performed with a flat blade, a cellulose sponge, or low energy cautery. The epithelium must be removed in order for the free edge of the conjunctival flap to become adherent.

   The bridle suture is removed and the free edge of the conjunctiva is advanced to the limbus. The free edge of the flap is closed with wing sutures of 8-0 to 10-0 nylon or absorbable suture material on a cutting needle.

   One side of the flap is closed by passing the needle through the limbal or corneal tissue which is adjacent to one side of the incision area. The needle is removed from the tissue and the free edge of the conjunctiva advanced to the point of suture exit, the point where it will be attached. The needle is passed through the free conjuctival-Tenon's tissue edge and the suture is tied. This should advance this side of the conjunctival closure anteriorly onto the cornea (Fig. 12-14A).

   The second side of the flap is closed by passing the needle through the limbal or corneal tissue at the other side of the incision area. After removing the needle, the free edge of the conjunctiva is brought to the point of the suture attachment. This should advance the entire edge of the flap onto the cornea, anterior to the scleral flap, with the free edge under tension against the cornea (Fig. 12-14B). Corneal indentation along the conjunctival edge is desirable.

9. Reformation of chamber and enlargement of bleb

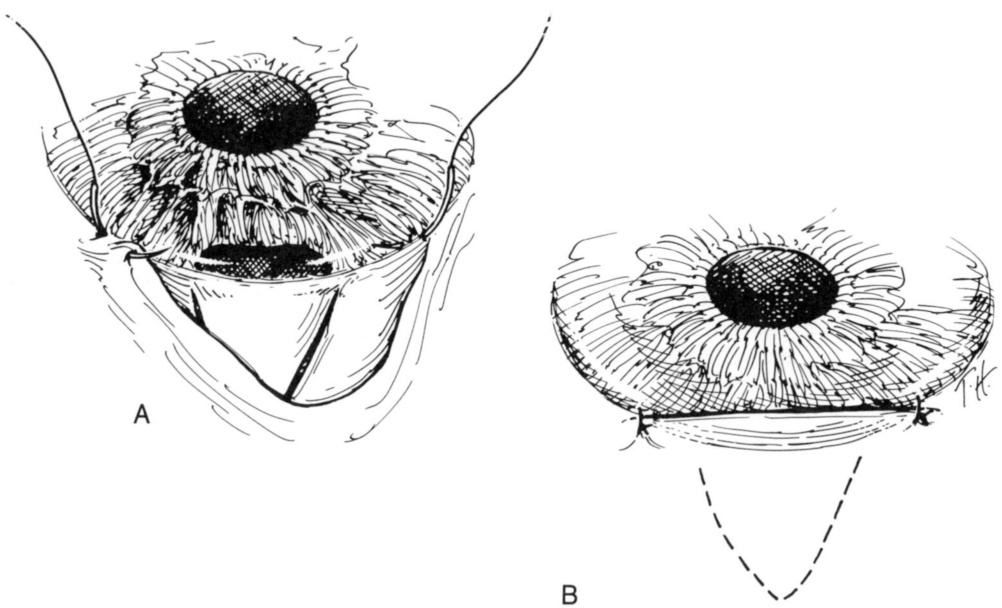


**Fig. 12-14** Closure of fornix-based conjunctival flap. **(A)** The suture is initially passed at the edge of the peritomy, at the site of the conjunctival insertion to the cornea. The second pass of the suture, through the cut edges of the conjunctiva, should advance the edge onto the cornea. **(B)** The conjunctival edge is advanced onto, and taught against, the cornea.

The chamber is reformed through the paracentesis tract with balanced salt solution. Fluid should exit the chamber via the flap into the subconjunctival space, resulting in formation of a bleb.

The suture line of the limbus-based flap and the free edge of fornix-based flap at the limbus are inspected for leakage of fluid. Additional sutures are placed across the sutured edge of the limbus-based flap as needed. Leakage of the fornix-based flap may be from areas of incomplete closure at either wing end. These defects are closed with interrupted sutures. In addition, leakage can occur along the limbal edge of the flap due to inadequate tension from the wing sutures. Additional sutures may be required to tighten and further advance the conjunctival edge against the cornea. Occasionally radial sutures are required to attach the free conjunctival edge to the cornea.

The ideal condition is an anterior chamber which remains formed with the fluid creating a large conjunctival bleb without leakage of fluid.

The anterior chamber can be reformed with viscoelastic materials. The use of these materials may help maintain the anterior chamber for the first few days after surgery. However, many studies have not shown added benefit with the use of these agents. Viscoelastic materials will not freely exit through the scleral flap and therefore cannot be used to expand the bleb to determine if the conjunctival wound is fluid tight, an extremely important step in the operation. We will place viscoelastic agents into the chamber only after we are certain that the conjunctival incision is properly closed.

10. Operating room care

    In the operating room topical atropine (1%) is delivered to help assure adequate pupillary dilation. Atropine also assists in moving the iris-lens diaphragm posteriorly which may reduce the risk of a flat anterior chamber or malignant (ciliary block) glaucoma (see below).

Subconjunctival corticosteroids may be administered at the conclusion of surgery. We use short-acting agents, avoiding the depot steroids. This injection is made into the cul-de-sac opposite from the surgical area.

Subconjunctival antibiotics may be given at the conclusion of surgery. Subconjunctival gentamycin may increase the postoperative conjunctival reaction. Therefore, we usually administer a topical antibiotic in the operating room and use subconjunctival antibiotics only if the surgery is complicated, including a reoperation.

## Full-Thickness Procedures

Full-thickness filtration procedures produce a direct communication from the anterior chamber to the subconjunctival space. Postoperative complications occur more frequently with full-thickness filtration procedures than with subscleral filtration surgery. However, intraocular pressure may be lower, and the long-term success may be greater, following full-thickness surgery.

Steps

1. Surgical exposure. Following the delivery of satisfactory anesthesia and akinesia, a lid speculum is inserted and a bridle suture is placed to fixate the globe.
2. Conjunctival flap. A limbus-based conjunctival flap should be used for full-thickness filtration surgery. The unguarded limbal anterior chamber opening precludes the safe use of a fornix-based flap; postoperatively, the flow of aqueous humor will be at the area of the conjunctival closure. The corneoscleral sulcus is clearly defined as described on page 195.
3. Anterior chamber paracentesis. We usually perform a paracentesis in full-thickness surgery to have better control of the anterior chamber during surgery. The incision is made in clear cornea, away from the area of the conjunctival incision. The blade is coated with fluorescein to stain the shelved corneal incision.
4. Anterior chamber entry

   Scleral cautery (Scheie procedure)

   Two rows of cautery are made in the limbal region for a length of 3–4 mm. The cautery should be hot enough to cause retraction of the tissue but not hot enough to cause charring.

   A groove is made in the midlimbal region through the area of cautery application, using a sharp blade.

   A trough-like wound is formed by alternately cutting with the blade and applying more cautery to the posterior edge of the incision (Fig. 12-15A). The lateral sides and anterior edge should not be cauterized to prevent the formation of conjunctival buttonholes.

   The process of alternating cautery and cutting is continued to create a trough of uniform depth and to the level of Descemet's membrane (Fig. 12-15B). The trough should be the same length internally and externally in order to assure an adequate area for the internal opening.

   The anterior chamber should be entered with the blade with the entire opening completed without removing the blade. This reduces the chance of iris prolapse and of hitting the lens. However, once the chamber has been entered with the cautery, it is difficult to apply further cautery because the escaping aqueous humor cools the adjacent tissue. The entire length of the sclerotomy is then completed either with a blade or fine scissors.

   Posterior or anterior lip sclerectomy

   A mid- to posterolimbal incision is made with a shelved entry into the anterior chamber. The incision is extended 4–5 mm using corneal scissors.

   A posterior lip sclerectomy is per-

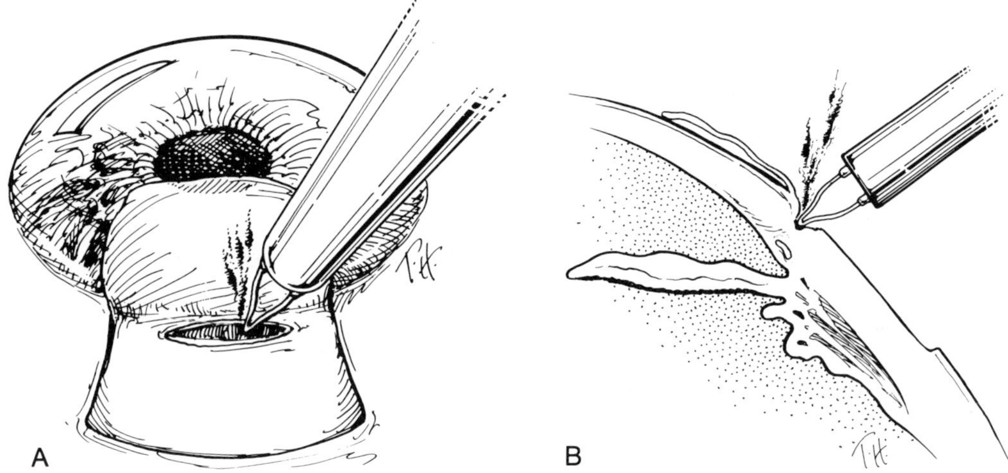


**Fig. 12-15** Thermal sclerostomy. (**A**) Application of cautery to the posterior lip of the incision. (**B**) Cautery is applied to the depths of the incision, to Descemet's membrane.

formed by taking one to three bites of complete scleral thickness through the posterior wound margin using a 1.0 or 1.5 mm Holth, Walser, or Gass punch (Fig. 12-16). Too posterior of a punch can damage the ciliary body.

An anterior lip sclerectomy is very similar except that the incision is placed more posterior with the an-

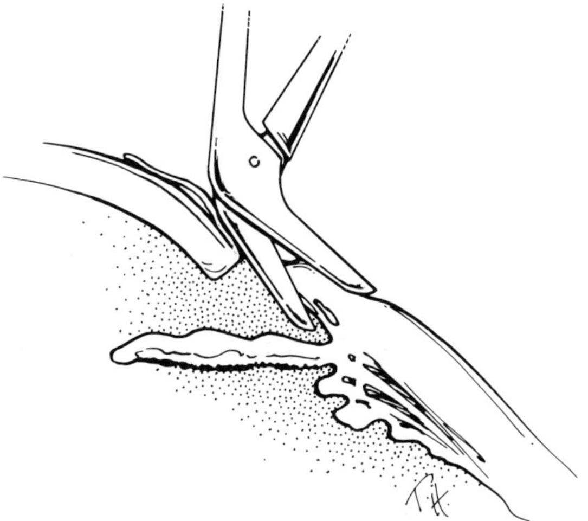

**Fig. 12-16** Posterior lip sclerectomy.

terior chamber entered in front of the scleral spur. Punch excisions are performed from the anterior lip of the wound.

The total size of the sclerostomy is 1 mm wide by 3–4 mm long.

Trephination. While highly successful, trephination is rarely recommended as a full-thickness glaucoma procedure because it is very difficult to perform for the occasional surgeon and is associated with increased complications of lens injury, incomplete tissue removal, incarceration of tissue in the wound, and vitreous loss.

A 1.5 mm diameter trephine is used to remove a button of corneoscleral tissue at the limbus.

The trephine is centered on the limbus in eyes with deep anterior chambers. In an eye with a shallow chamber, this procedure is contraindicated because it can result in entry into the chamber over the ciliary body.

The trephine is rotated with a slight bevel forward so that the anterior edge enters the chamber first (Fig. 12-17A).

The trephine is removed when the

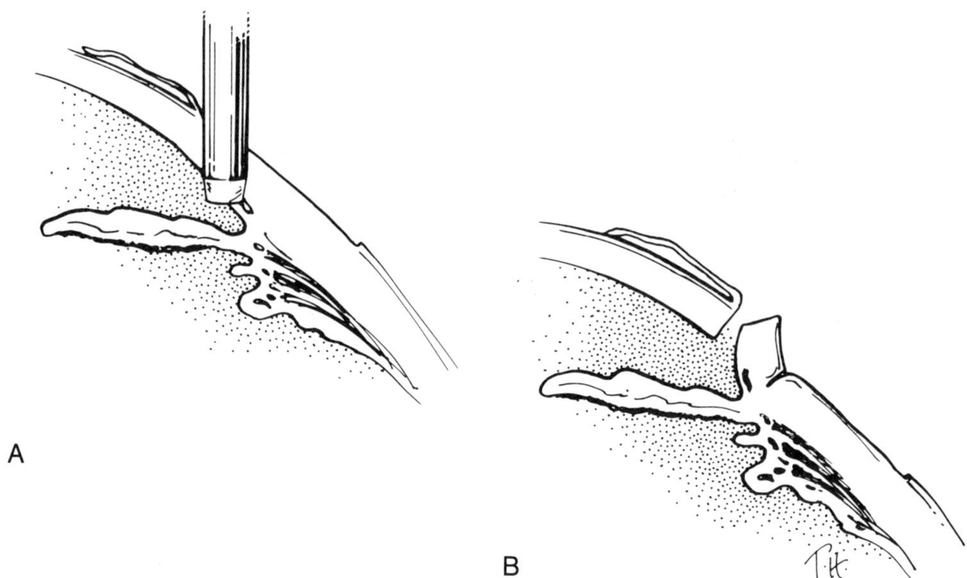


**Fig. 12-17** Limboscleral trephination. **(A)** Trephine button partially excised. **(B)** The excision is completed by cutting the posterior attachment with a scissors.

pupil peaks or the iris moves. The scleral button is excised with a fine scissors (Fig. 12-17B).

5. Iridectomy. A peripheral or sector iridectomy is performed as described above.
6. Closure of the limbus-based conjunctival flap. The conjunctival flap is closed, as previously described for trabeculectomy, using a running or interrupted 8-0 or 9-0 vicryl or chromic sutures. The closure must be water-tight.
7. Reformation of chamber and enlargement of bleb

   The chamber is reformed through the paracentesis tract with balanced salt solution. Fluid should exit the chamber via the flap into the subconjunctival space; this results in formation of a bleb. We feel this step is extremely important in full-thickness procedures and may result in a lower incidence of postoperative flat anterior chambers.

   The suture line of the conjunctival flap is inspected for leakage of fluid. Additional sutures are placed across the sutured edge as needed. The ideal condition is an anterior chamber which remains formed with the fluid creating a large conjunctival bleb without leakage of fluid.

   The anterior chamber can be reformed with viscoelastic material, as previously discussed (see page 213).
8. Operating room care

   Topical atropine (1%) is administered at the completion of surgery to help assure adequate pupillary dilation. Atropine also assists in moving the iris-lens diaphragm posteriorly, which may reduce the occurrence of a flat anterior chamber or malignant (ciliary block) glaucoma (see below).

   Subconjunctival corticosteroids may be administered at the conclusion of surgery. We use short acting-agents, avoiding the depot steroids. This injection is made into the cul-de-sac opposite from the surgical area.

   Subconjunctival antibiotics may be given at the conclusion of surgery. Subconjunctival gentamycin may increase the postoperative conjunctival reaction. Therefore, we usually administer a topical antibiotic in the operating room and use subconjunctival antibiotics only with complications or reoperation.

## Special Considerations During Filtration Surgery

### Tenonectomy

I. Tenon's layer is especially thick in young patients and black patients. This tissue is believed to be the major source of fibroblasts, which are involved with postoperative healing and scarring.

II. Prospective studies have shown no benefit of performing a tenonectomy during the time of primary filtration surgery. However, we feel that tenonectomy may be beneficial in the high-risk patient including young, black patients and patients whose eyes have experienced previous filtration surgery failure.

III. Tenon's tissue is removed at the time of preparation of the conjunctival flap with removal dependent on the type of flap.

   A. Limbus-based conjunctival flap

      1. The conjunctiva is incised as described above without incising the underlying Tenon's tissue that is attached to the sclera. The conjunctival flap is dissected anteriorly to the limbus. Tenon's tissue is then dissected from the sclera in the exposed area up to the limbus. The tissue is excised.

      2. The conjunctival flap, including Tenon's tissue, is incised and dissected as previously described. Tenon's tissue is then dissected from the underside of the conjunctival flap. The cut edge of the conjunctiva is grasped with a smooth forceps with tension of the flap towards the surgeon. An assistant uses a fine toothed forceps to grasp Tenon's tissue from the underside of the flap with the tissue fixated away from the conjunctiva, towards the sclera. The combination of conjunctival-Tenon's fixation causes a plane of separation in which a blunt tipped Wescott scissors can be used to separate Tenon's from the underside of the conjunctiva. The scissors always should be visualized through the conjunctiva to avoid producing an inadvertent buttonhole.

   B. Fornix-based conjunctival flap

      The flap is performed as described above. Tenon's tissue is dissected from the underside of the conjunctival flap in a manner similar to the above description for the limbus-based flap. The cut edge of the conjunctiva is grasped with a smooth forceps with tension of the flap away from the surgeon; an assistant uses a fine toothed forceps to grasp Tenon's tissue from the underside of the flap with the tissue fixated away from the conjunctiva, towards the sclera; a blunt tipped Wescott scissors is used to separate Tenon's from the under-side of the conjunctiva with the scissors visualized through the conjunctiva to avoid buttonhole formation.

### Vitrectomy in Aphakia

Filtering surgery in aphakic eyes with vitreous in the anterior chamber has a low rate of success. Vitreous may have an adverse role in promoting scarring or mechanically occluding the internal sclerostomy. An anterior vitrectomy is performed using automated instrumentation placed through the sclerostomy opening into the anterior chamber to remove forwardly displaced vitreous.

### Compression Shell

I. Simmons has designed a compression shell (Fig. 12-18) to be placed over the bleb in the early postoperative period to encourage formation of a diffuse bleb as well as to support the anterior chamber by temporarily increasing resistance to aqueous flow. The device is made from hard polymethylmethacrylate and con-

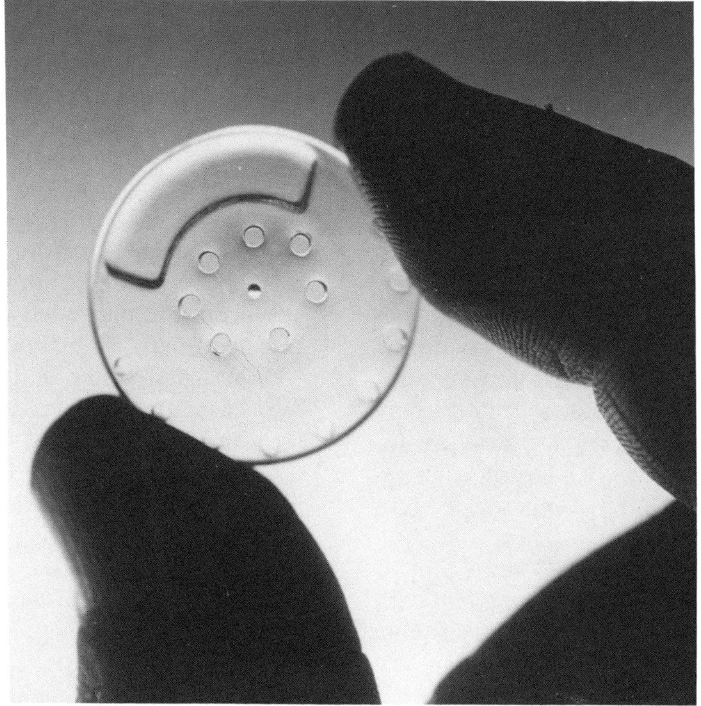

**Fig. 12-18** Simmons shell. The circumferential ridge is placed over the area of the bleb (or an area of conjunctival leakage). The holes are provided for tear circulation and oxygen delivery to the cornea.

tains an internal platform which is placed over the fistula tract.

II. The shell was originally designed to be fixated to the globe with two inferior episcleral sutures at the time of surgery and the eye bandaged. However, many surgeons have not found suture fixation to be necessary. The shell is left in place for three days.

III. The shell compresses the filtration area, partially restricting flow and thereby minimizing complications associated with hypotony, a flat anterior chamber, and choroidal effusion.

IV. The major difficulties with the shell are patient discomfort, corneal trauma, a limited visualization of the anterior chamber, and the inability to measure intraocular pressure. However, long-term intraocular pressures are reported to be low, with diffuse blebs, following use of the shell.

V. The shell has also been used as a patch to seal leaking filtration blebs (see page 224).

### Antimetabolites

I. The chemotherapeutic agent 5-fluorouracil (5-FU) is reported in experimental and pilot clinical studies to increase the rate of filtration success in eyes with a poor surgical prognosis. Specific indications include prior filtration failure, aphakia, neovascular glaucoma, and uveitic glaucoma.

II. 5-FU inhibits fibroblast proliferation and associated scar formation. However, the agent also prevents growth of other cells, including the epithelium of the conjunctiva and cornea.

III. 5-FU (10 mg/ml solution) is administered as a subconjunctival injection of 0.5 ml given at a site away from the surgical area. Injections are made using a 30-gauge needle and topical anesthetic drops. While the frequency of injection has been recommended as twice a day for the first postoperative week and daily for the second postoperative week, 5-FU has been reported to be effective following less frequent administration: daily to every other day for 7–14 days after surgery.

IV. 5-FU retards all healing processes, including healing of the conjunctival incision. Therefore, meticulous closure must be performed using a nonabsorbable suture, e.g., 10-0 nylon. In addition, a nontraumatic (e.g., vascular) tapered needle is used to prevent creating large holes in the conjunctiva which will not heal in the presence of 5-FU.

V. While the individual injections are well tolerated by the patient, the frequency of office visits can be burdensome.

VI. Complications associated with 5-FU include the following:
   A. Conjunctival wound leaks, either at the wound edge or pin point defects away from the suture tract, frequently occur and can result in a shallowing of the anterior chamber. Spontaneous healing will not occur as long as the 5-FU is continued. If possible the defect can be sutured, patch glued, or pressure patched with or without a compression shell (see below). We have not had much success in treatment of these defects while the 5-FU is still administered and therefore we stop the medication at least temporarily.
   B. Corneal epithelial defects. Superficial punctate defects occur in all eyes receiving 5-FU and are of no consequence. However, epithelial defects, some which can be very large, can occur. These defects usually mandate stopping the medication since they will not heal while the 5-FU is administered.
   C. The blebs following 5-FU administration are very localized, ischemic and thin walled. Late bleb leaks may be more frequent following use of this medication.
   D. The frequency of postoperative suprachoroidal hemorrhage is increased in eyes treated with 5-FU.

## Postoperative Management

### Postoperative Examination

I. Frequency

Postoperative examination and management of the patient undergoing filtration surgery is extremely important to the surgical success. We routinely admit patients to the hospital following surgery for appropriate management during the critical few days after surgery. The frequency of examinations during the first 3–4 weeks varies depending on the postoperative course. It is not unusual to require examinations daily or every other day during the early postoperative period.

II. The following observations are made at the time of each postoperative examination:
   A. External examination for the presence of lid edema and chemosis that usually relates to an allergy to topical atropine but can be an early sign of postoperative infection.
   B. The height, extent, and description of the bleb including the presence of limbal micro- or macrocysts, limbal scalloping of the conjunctiva, injection, and ischemia. If a wound leak is suspected (e.g., low pressure, flat anterior chamber), a Seidel test is performed.
   C. The anterior chamber is examined for

1. corneal clarity and the presence of epithelial defects.
2. chamber depth with a shallow chamber graded as follows:

Grade 1 peripheral iris touching the cornea.
Grade 2 central iris-cornea touch to the pupil margin.
Grade 3 lens-cornea apposition.

3. chamber reaction (hyphema, cells, protein, hypopyon).

D. The intraocular pressure is measured in both the operated as well as the contralateral eye, especially if preoperative carbonic anhydrase inhibitors have been discontinued.

E. The posterior pole is examined for appearance of the disc (possible hemorrhages, edema), the macula (possible edema), and the presence of choroidal detachment.

### Cycloplegia

I. Topical cycloplegics are administered for the following functions:
   A. Tightening of the lens-iris diaphragm by paralysis of the ciliary muscle
   B. Stabilization of the blood-aqueous barrier resulting in reduced anterior chamber protein and cells
   C. Patient comfort by eliminating ciliary spasm.

II. Topical agents include twice a day atropine 1%, homatropine 5%, or scopolamine 0.25%.

III. Topical mydriatics (neosynephrine 2.5% or 5%) can be intermittently administered in addition to the cycloplegic agents. These may facilitate chamber deepening.

IV. Therapy with these agents is started at the time of surgery. Their administration is directed by the degree of intraocular inflammation. These drugs usually are continued for 2–6 weeks after surgery.

### Corticosteroids

I. Corticosteroids are administered postoperatively to reduce intraocular and extraocular inflammation and associated scar formation.

II. We begin corticosteroid therapy at the conclusion of surgery by performing a subconjunctival injection of dexamethasone phosphate 2–4 mg or triamcinolone acetate 20–40 mg. Depot steroid injections are avoided since they can be associated with a later steroid induced elevation in intraocular pressure.

III. Topical corticosteroids are started after the first postoperative day examination. We use dexamethasone (0.1%) or prednisolone (1%) solutions which are administered very frequently (every 1–2 hours) if the anterior chamber reaction is severe or four times/day if the degree of inflammation is minimal to moderate. Dexamethasone ointment can be administered at bedtime.

IV. The topical corticosteroids are reduced as the inflammation subsides. We routinely have patients use steroids for a minimum of 6 weeks and occasionally for up to 10–12 weeks following filtration surgery. The frequency of administration is slowly reduced as the anterior chamber reaction subsides. The stronger steroids are switched to weaker corticosteroids (e.g., prednisolone acetate 0.125% or medrysone) when there is no anterior chamber inflammation. This allows continued external steroid therapy to reduce bleb inflammation.

V. Occasionally we use oral corticosteroids during the early postoperative period if there is extensive intraocular inflammation. In addition, oral steroids are administered if there is an extensive or prolonged choroidal detachment. It is our clinical impression that systemic steroids may reduce the duration of a choroidal detachment, possibly by reducing inflammation associated with this condition. Prednisone 60–100 mg daily is administered for 5–7 days if there are no systemic contraindications. If there are any medical concerns, the patients general medical physician is contacted prior to starting this treatment. This dosage of prednisone does not require a tapering regimen and can be discontinued acutely.

### External Ocular Pressure ("Digital Massage")

I. External pressure on the globe raises the intraocular pressure and forces more aqueous humor through the sclerostomy site into the subconjunctival area.

II. External ocular pressure can break external adhesions in the bleb and result in an increased area of external filtration. In addition, the maneuver can disrupt early scar formation at the edges of a scleral flap by causing misalignment of the flap edge.

III. Several methods are available for performing the technique.

   A. In the early postoperative interval we prefer to apply focal pressure under direct visualization at the slitlamp. A moistened cotton-tipped applicator, a muscle hook, or the end of a scleral depressor is applied to the conjunctiva overlying the edges of the scleral flap or on the cornea just anterior to the base of the scleral flap. This deforms the edge of the flap and does not cause marked elevation in intraocular pressure.

   B. External pressure can be applied by the ophthalmologist or the patient by pressing firmly through the lid against the globe. It is not important if this pressure is directed to the cornea, the superior, or the inferior portion of the globe. We instruct patients to close their eye, place one or two fingers on the eye lid and feel their globe, and then press the globe posterior into the orbit. Constant pressure is held for approximately 10 sec and then released. We have patients repeat this process for 5 to 10 times per session.

   C. Patients are instructed on home use of digital pressure if their intraocular pressure is consistently in the high teens and is lowered following massage in the office setting. We measure intraocular pressure before and following digital massage to assess the effect of the maneuver. In addition, the appearance of the bleb is noted before and after digital pressure is applied. The duration of effect should also be measured. We instruct patients who are performing the maneuver at home not to apply digital pressure on the day of their office visit. At that time, the pressure is measured, the patient performs the maneuver, and the intraocular pressure is remeasured. Depending on the measured response, we may also perform digital pressure ourself and measure any additional effect. Digital pressure is continued if the bleb is of limited size, the intraocular pressure is in the high teens, and only if there is a reduction of intraocular pressure and increase in the size of the bleb.

## Trabeculectomy versus Full-Thickness Filtration Surgery

I. The rates of intraocular pressure control are similar following trabeculectomy and full-thickness filtration surgery. However, the mean intraocular pressure is in the mid to low teens following full-thickness surgery, as compared to the mid to upper teens with trabeculectomy procedures.

II. Long-term success appears to be similar between the two procedures. However, recent uncontrolled studies have raised the question that the long-term success rate may be higher following full-thickness surgery. Success with full-thickness surgery may be greater in black or young patients and in eyes with various types of secondary glaucoma, e.g., uveitic and aphakic glaucoma.

III. Trabeculectomy produces less postoperative complications (see below) than full-thickness filtering procedures. Postoperative shallow or flat chambers, hypotony, and ciliary detachment are more common in full-thickness procedures.

IV. Full-thickness blebs tend to be cystic in contrast to more diffuse and posterior blebs following trabeculectomy. Postoperative bleb leakage and infection and endophthalmitis are more frequent following full-thickness surgery.

V. There is a lower rate of visual loss due to cataract development after trabeculectomy than after full-thickness procedures.

## Complications of Filtration Surgery

The most frequent complication following filtration surgery is failure of the procedure; 10%–20% of primary surgeries fail in eyes with primary glaucoma. The failure rate is much higher in repeat operations and in eyes with aphakia and other types of secondary glaucoma.

Many complications can occur after any intraocular procedure and are not unique to filtration surgery. This section discusses management of the common and specific complications relating to glaucoma filtration surgery.

### Operative

I. Conjunctival buttonhole
   A. The presence of a large buttonhole during the early stages of the operation is best managed by repairing the defect and selecting a new surgical site. Attempts to repair a large conjunctival defect are associated with increased postoperative scarring and a lower rate of filtration success.
   B. A small buttonhole noted during surgery can be repaired using a 10-0 or 11-0 nylon suture on a tapered atraumatic vascular needle. The defect is closed with an interrupted, running, or mattress suture. If a limbus-based conjunctival flap has been used and the buttonhole is near the limbus, a small peritomy can be made excising the buttonhole. The corneal epithelium is removed and the conjunctiva is sutured to the cornea using 10-0 nylon interrupted or mattress sutures.

II. Disinsertion of scleral flap
   A. Avulsion of the scleral flap during a subscleral procedure can occur especially if the flap is very thin or if the corneal part of the lamellar dissection does not follow the curvature change of the cornea but is directed too anteriorly.
   B. If the sclerostomy has not been performed, the surgery is converted to a full-thickness procedure, either a posterior lip or thermal sclerostomy. If in this instance a fornix-based conjunctival flap has been used, extra care must be given to insure adequate conjunctival closure.
   C. If the sclerostomy has already been performed, an attempt should be made to protect and reduce the size of the opening into the anterior chamber. Excessive filtration can occur because the subscleral sclerostomy is much larger than that produced during a full-thickness procedure. The scleral flap can be repaired if it is only partially avulsed or an attempt can be made to reap-

proximate the flap with 10-0 or 11-0 nylon sutures. Tenon's tissue or partial thickness donor sclera can be sutured to the scleral flap site. Finally, a 9-0 or 10-0 nylon suture can be placed across the center of the sclerostomy and tied to reduce the size of the opening.

III. Dissection into the suprachoridal space

Inadvertent entry into the suprachoroidal space can occur during dissection of the scleral flap. While this has been recommended by some surgeons as a combined cyclodialysis-trabeculectomy procedure, this complication can be associated with bleeding, prolapse of ciliary body, and vitreous loss. This is managed by early recognition of the pigmented uveal tissue and changing the direction of the scleral flap dissection to be more superficial.

IV. Hemorrhage

A. Hyphema

1. A hyphema can occur when performing the iridectomy as a result of cutting an iris vessel, an inadvertent iridodialysis, or from traumatizing the ciliary body including amputation of a ciliary process. Predisposing factors include drug-induced clotting disorders and possibly systemic hypertension. Bleeding is more common if the internal sclerostomy is performed too far posteriorly. Therefore, entry into the anterior chamber should be performed as far anteriorly as possible, preferably in clear cornea.
2. Bleeding from a ciliary process or the iris often stops after a few minutes of gentle pressure with a cellulose sponge. Balanced salt solution can be instilled into the anterior chamber through the paracentesis tract to irrigate the blood through the sclerostomy opening. In addition, air or a 1:100,000 solution of epinephrine (the cardiac, nonpreserved preparation) can be introduced through the paracentesis in an attempt to stop the bleeding. Intraocular cautery can be dangerous and should be avoided unless the bleeding does not stop. The iris should not be cauterized. A bipolar cautery is used after identifying the bleeding site.

B. Suprachoroidal expulsive hemorrhage

1. An expulsive hemorrhage can occur during a filtering procedure or in the first few days after surgery. This rare complication may be more common in eyes with uncontrolled glaucoma which have had numerous failed attempts at filtration surgery, patients with systemic vascular disease, and in highly myopic eyes. Reduction of intraocular pressure and control of systemic hypertension prior to surgery may decrease the likelihood of this complication.
2. The patient experiences acute pain, the eye becomes firm, the anterior chamber shallows, and a dark mass is seen in the pupil. Intraocular contents can escape from the wound.
3. Once the diagnosis is made, rapid action is necessary to close the incision and to save the eye.
   a) If a combined cataract-filtration procedure (see below) is being performed, the preplaced sutures are pulled up and tied. Additional sutures are placed to close the wound and include suture closure of the filtration procedure sclerostomy. Closure is performed as quickly as possible while intermittently gently re-

positing the prolapsed tissue with an iris spatula.

b) Decompression of the globe may be necessary to close the surgical wound. A posterior stab incision is made through the sclera over the mass, or if the mass is not seen, in the inferior temporal quadrant. The stab incision is easily performed, in spite of an open wound, since the globe is very firm. If blood does not drain through the incision, a second one is made in another quadrant.

c) In summary, attempts are made to soften the eye, excise or reposit prolapsed tissues, reform the anterior chamber, and repair the wound. Prognosis for recovery of vision is poor even in patients without loss of uvea or retinal tissue. Repeat suprachoroidal hemorrhage is not uncommon.

4. Detachment of Descemet's membrane
   a) Detachment of Descemet's membrane can occur at the paracentesis site or at the site of entry into the anterior chamber. Small scrolls of Descemet's membrane probably do not have to be repaired; however, large detachments can lead to a localized area of corneal decompensation.
   b) A large scroll is replaced against the cornea by injecting air or viscoelastic material into the anterior chamber. The scroll is then reattached to the cornea using a 10-0 nylon suture with the needle first passed through the region of attached Descemet's membrane and then through the area of the scroll.

## Postoperative

I. Hypotony and flat anterior chamber
   A. A low intraocular pressure with a flat, or shallow, anterior chamber following filtration surgery may be due to
      1. excessive filtration.
      2. a ciliochoroidal detachment with reduced aqueous humor formation.
      3. a conjunctival wound leak.
   B. A shallow postoperative anterior chamber depth is graded as described on page 220.
   C. Wound leak
      1. A defect in the conjunctiva may have been undetected at the time of surgery or may have developed as a dehiscence postoperatively.
      2. A leak can usually be detected by Seidel testing.
         a) Topical anesthesia is applied to the eye.
         b) Concentrated fluorescein is applied to the eye either as an impregnated strip or as a 2% drop.
         c) The eye is examined at the slit-lamp with a cobalt blue light. The concentrated fluorescein is a dark orange color. Aqueous leakage appears as a flow of green fluid.
         d) With a flat anterior chamber there may be insufficient aqueous humor to leak through the wound defect. Cautious external pressure on the globe may be required to demonstrate the site of aqueous leakage. Examination also is performed

in different positions of gaze which may influence aqueous humor flow through the defect.

3. Conservative medical therapy consisting of a pressure patch and application of an ophthalmic ointment is sometimes sufficient in the management of a small conjunctival wound leak. In addition, aqueous humor suppressants (e.g., topical beta blockers or systemic carbonic anhydrase inhibitors) can be administered to reduce aqueous flow through the area of defect.
4. With a thin cystic bleb, a Simmon's compression shell can be successful in mechanically compressing the area of defect. This can result in reformation of the anterior chamber and sealing of the wound leak. The shell is placed on the cornea with the internal platform located over the defect. The shell is not sutured to the globe. The eye is patched and re-examined 12–24 hours later. If the shell is successful in compressing the area of leakage, the anterior chamber will be deeper. The shell is left in place for an additional 2–4 days with the eye patched between examinations. Topical antibiotic ointment is instilled.
5. Tissue adhesive can be used to seal a small leak, allowing the defect to heal beneath the glue. However, tissue adhesive is very irritating and is poorly tolerated when applied directly to the defect. We have found the following method useful in applying the glue while providing a protective plastic covering to prevent ocular irritation (Fig. 12-19).
   a) A piece of plastic is cut from a surgical drape in a circular or oval shape which is 2–3 mm larger than the area of conjunctival leak.
   b) A thin layer of ointment is placed on a flat spatula. The piece of plastic is placed on the spatula, held in position by the ointment. A thin layer of tissue adhesive is then placed on the central two-thirds of the plastic.
   c) The area of leaking conjunctiva is identified and dried with a cotton tip applicator or a cellulose sponge. The plastic patch with the applied glue is placed over the defect with pressure applied with the spatula. After the tissue glue polymerizes, the spatula is removed, leaving the plastic glue patch in place.
   d) The eye is patched with ophthalmic ointment. The patch usually remains in place for 2–4 days. During this time the conjunctiva can heal beneath the patch to close the defect.
6. A small conjunctival wound leak near the limbus can sometimes be covered with a bandage contact lens. The management after placement of the contact lens is similar to that described using the Simmon's shell.
7. A wound leak which does not respond to the above therapies requires repair by suture closure. We have placed 8-0 vicryl and 10-0 nylon sutures with tapered, noncutting needles at

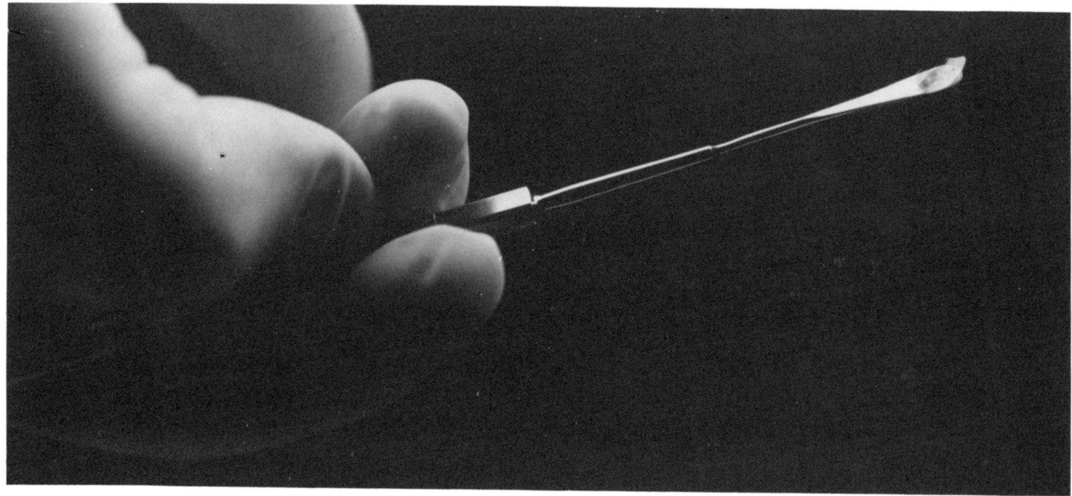

**Fig. 12-19** Spatula with tissue adhesive glue patch.

the slit-lamp across a localized conjunctival defect. Similar repair can be performed in the operating room. If simple closure techniques are unsuccessful, major bleb revision is necessary.

II. Flat anterior chamber without a wound leak
   A. Excessive filtration is common during the early postoperative period. This usually resolves within 5–10 days. Conservative management using a light pressure patch or an external scleral shell to tamponade the scleral flap is usually effective. Aqueous suppressants can be administered to reduce aqueous production and allow conjunctival scarring to occur, and therefore limit the amount of potential filtration.
   B. Choroidal detachment with aqueous humor shutdown can be the cause or result of excessive filtration. A prolonged state of hypotony is associated with choroidal detachment.
   C. Complications associated with postoperative hypotony and a flat anterior chamber, which are indications for surgical intervention, include corneal decompensation, cataract formation, and bleb failure. The formation of peripheral anterior synechiae are not an indication for surgical intervention since the filtration procedure was performed because outflow facility was already inadequate.
   D. When surgical intervention is indicated, repair should include the following:
      1. The original paracentesis tract is identified, if possible, or a new corneal tract incision is made. This may be quite difficult in a hypotensive eye and great care must be taken to avoid stripping Descemet's membrane or injury to the iris or lens. The anterior chamber is reformed with balanced salt solution.
      2. A Seidel test is performed to be sure the conjunctival wound is water tight. Additional sutures are placed as necessary.
      3. Since most eyes have a choroidal detachment, we prefer to

drain the detachment in order to allow a more rapid recovery of aqueous humor formation. Sclerotomies are performed in the inferior nasal and temporal quadrants, 5–6 mm from the limbus. These incisions are 2–3 mm in length and concentric to the limbus. A partial thickness incision is performed and a 4-0 to 6-0 suture on a spatula needle is placed across the wound and looped out. This allows spreading of the incision and a controlled scratched entry into the suprachoroidal space (Fig. 12-20). Suprachoroidal fluid is straw-colored. As the fluid is drained, additional balanced salt solution is placed into the anterior chamber. The sclerostomy incisions do not have to be closed and the preplaced traction sutures are removed after drainage has been completed.

4. The anterior chamber is finally filled with additional salt solution or with viscoelastic material to keep the chamber formed until the ciliary body and choroid reattach and aqueous humor production is re-established.
5. Subconjunctival antibiotic and corticosteroid injections are given at the conclusion of surgery. Topical atropine and corticosteroids are given postoperatively.

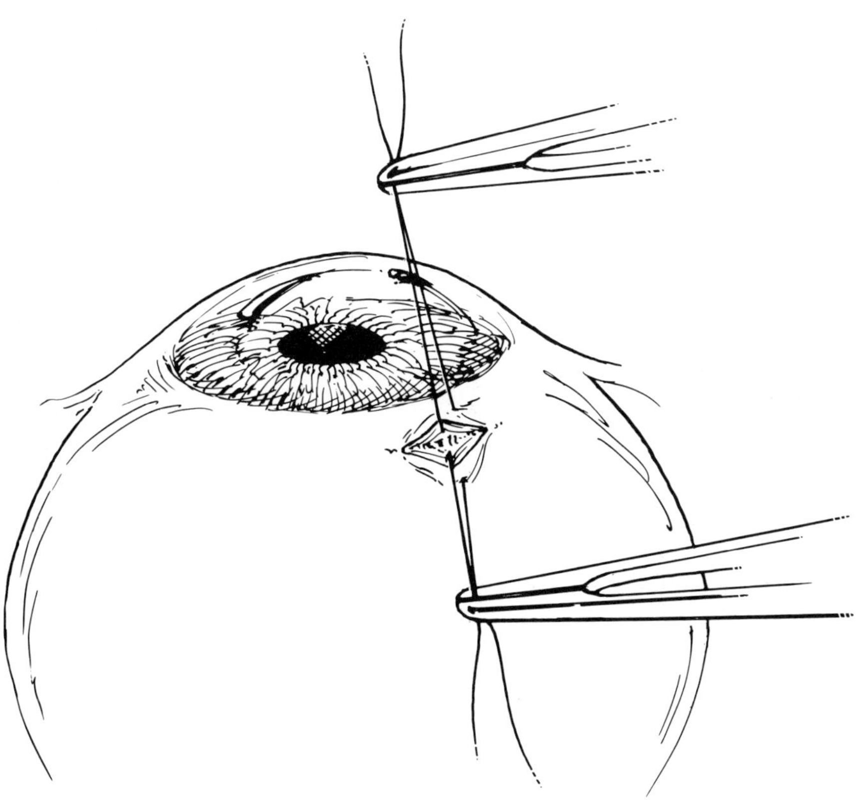

**Fig. 12-20** Posterior sclerotomy incision for drainage of choroidals. The incision is parallel to the limbus and held open by a suture placed across and then looped out of the incision.

III. Malignant glaucoma (ciliary block or aqueous misdirection)

A. This is a rare complication consisting of a flat anterior chamber with an elevated intraocular pressure in the presence of a patent iridectomy that eliminates the possibility of a pupillary block. Aqueous humor appears to flow posteriorly into the area of detached vitreous and forces forward the iris-lens diaphragm in the phakic eye, the iris-anterior vitreous plane in the aphakic eye, or the iris-intraocular lens implant in the pseudophakic eye.

B. The condition is more common in eyes with chronic angle-closure glaucoma. If the condition develops in one eye it may be more common in the fellow eye.

C. Medical treatment is successful in about 50% of the cases and includes the following:

1. Administration of a systemic hyperosmotic agent.
2. Maximal mydriasis achieved with topical atropine (1% or 4%) and phenylephrine (10%). If this therapy is effective in treating the attack, atropine must be continued permanently.
3. Topical beta blocker and systemic carbonic anhydrase inhibitor administered to lower the intraocular pressure.

D. Argon laser treatment of visible ciliary processes through the iridectomy can be successful in the management of phakic malignant glaucoma (see Chapter 11).

E. Nd-YAG laser treatment to the anterior hyaloid face may be successful in aphakic or pseudophakic malignant glaucoma (see Chapter 11).

F. If conservative treatments, including the use of laser treatment, are not effective, a pars plana vitrectomy in the phakic eye or a limbal vitrectomy through the anterior chamber in the aphakic eye is required. The vitrectomy should remove central vitreous as well as the pocket of posterior fluid. We prefer to perform the vitrectomy using automated instrumentation rather than placing a needle into the vitreous cavity and aspirating vitreous with a syringe. The anterior chamber is reformed following the procedure. Occasionally there is the need to perform a lensectomy in combination with the vitrectomy in the phakic eye.

IV. Endophthalmitis and bleb infection

A. Early postoperative endophthalmitis can occur following any intraocular surgical procedure including filtration surgery.

B. Even with a successful filtering operation late bacterial infection of the bleb or endophthalmitis can occur. Infections are more common if there is a thin cystic bleb; this is more common following a full-thickness than a subscleral filtration procedure. Additional risk factors for infection include the presence of diabetes mellitus, malnutrition, blepharitis, or a compromised immune system. Use of a contact lens in face of a thin bleb may increase the risk of late bleb infection.

C. Patients with a functioning filtration bleb should be instructed to report immediately if ocular injection, discharge, irritation, or photophobia occur. Patients living a great distance from an ophthalmologist should be given a topical broadspectrum antibiotic to be used every 30–60 minutes until medical care can be obtained.

D. The earliest signs of bleb infection are injection around the bleb and a milky discoloration of the contents of the bleb. This can progress to a bleb abscess or to endophthalmitis with a hypopyon.

E. Management is related to the type and stage of infection.

1. If confined to the anterior segment, an anterior chamber tap is performed for Gram stain, culture, and determination of antibiotic sensitivity. Topical and periocular antibiotics may be adequate.
2. If there are findings indicating involvement of the vitreous, a vitrectomy is performed with the contents used for Gram stain, culture, and determination of antibiotic sensitivity. Intravitreal, periocular, systemic, and topical antibiotics are administered.
3. Topical and systemic corticosteroids are administered 24 hours after the initiation of antibiotic therapy to reduce scarring in an attempt to preserve the filtration site.

V. Cataract

Cataract formation occurs in approximately one-third of eyes following filtration surgery. Few cases occur immediately after surgery and are related to direct surgical trauma to the lens. Most cases occur months to years later and may be related to either hypotony, a prolonged postoperative flat anterior chamber, drug therapy including the use of topical corticosteroids, inflammation, the patient's age, or the presurgical state of the lens. This complication of filtration surgery may alter the surgical management of the glaucoma patient who requires filtration surgery in which lens changes are present preoperatively (see below).

VI. Transient elevation in intraocular pressure

A. An increase in intraocular pressure 3–4 weeks after trabeculectomy is common. This elevation is usually transient, and associated with the presence of active filtration with a diffuse and ischemic bleb. This transient state is of no concern to the long-term functioning of the procedure.

B. The increase in pressure may be associated with a Tenon's capsule cyst, a fibroblastic overgrowth which results in a tense, opalescent, injected, and thick-walled bleb. A Tenon's cyst usually occurs within the first or second postoperative months. While there is still a direct communication between the cyst and anterior chamber, aqueous flow is limited across the wall of the cyst and the intraocular pressure is elevated. In most cases, the Tenon's cyst will resolve within 2–4 months. Therefore, conservative management with the addition of glaucoma medications is indicated. A weak topical corticosteroid, e.g., prednisolone acetate (0.125%) or medrysone, and possibly digital massage may decrease the time course. While bleb revision has been performed by simple needle incision into the cyst wall, this maneuver usually produces only a transient effect.

C. Approximately 5%–10% of eyes with a Tenon's cyst will not show spontaneous resolution. In these eyes, either the cyst is excised in toto or a repeat operation is performed at another location. Repeat operations should consider modifications of the original technique;

e.g., if a fornix-based conjunctival flap was initially performed, a limbus-based flap should be done on repeat surgery, with surgical excision of Tenon's tissue; and the postoperative use of pharmacologic agent to modify scar formation, e.g., 5-FU.

VII. Excessive size of bleb
   A. Occasionally a bleb can become so large that it creates a foreign body sensation. A dellen may develop anterior to the bleb. In some eyes topical application of artificial tears or bland ointments may eliminate symptoms.
   B. Any attempt to reduce the size of the bleb should be made only if symptoms persist and the bleb is stable or enlarging in size at least 3–4 months after filtration surgery. A number of techniques have been reported to reduce the size of the bleb; these include the application of cauterization, cryotherapy, photocoagulation, and trichloroacetic acid. Results are inconsistent and often disappointing secondary to production of excessive scarring and bleb failure. We prefer using cryotherapy with limited transconjunctival applications at the lateral extent of the bleb. One or two 30-second applications at minus 60° are delivered.
   C. A bleb can overlie the cornea resulting in irritation and a cosmetic problem. This can be repaired by reflecting the corneal portion of the bleb with a flat spatula and excising the excess tissue with a scissors. The conjunctiva is closed with 10-0 nylon sutures.

VIII. Internal closure of the sclerostomy
   A. Internal closure of the sclerostomy is frequently the cause for bleb failure. Closure can be secondary to the incarceration of iris, vitreous, the lens, or ciliary processes, or to the formation of a pigmented or nonpigmented membrane. Gonioscopy must be performed to detect this condition.
   B. Laser therapy, either argon or Nd:YAG, can be successful in clearing the internal sclerostomy of an occluding membrane, vitreous, or iris/ciliary process tissue (see Chapter 11).

## MANAGEMENT OF COEXISTING CATARACT AND GLAUCOMA

Management of a visually significant cataract in an eye with glaucoma consists of one of three approaches: cataract surgery alone, filtration surgery initially followed by later cataract removal, and combined cataract-filtration surgery. Indications and preferences vary among surgeons as to which approach to take. It is important to realize that cataract extraction in an eye with glaucoma is a more complicated and difficult operation than cataract surgery in a nonglaucomatous eye.

### Cataract Removal In An Eye With Glaucoma

I. Special considerations include the following:
   A. An eye which has received long-term miotic therapy has poor pupillary dilation, frequently has posterior synechiae between the iris and lens, and the iris is usually very immobile and rigid. Cataract removal requires surgical enlargement of the pupil and lysis of the posterior synechiae. The rigid iris demands special attention at the time of intracapsular lens removal or nucleus removal in extracapsular surgery.
   B. Bleeding may be more common in eyes receiving long-term glaucoma therapy. In addition, lens zonules may be abnormally weak, especially in eyes with pseudoexfoliation.

C. The preferred method of cataract surgery in an eye with glaucoma is an extracapsular extraction. Glaucoma does not preclude the use of a posterior chamber intraocular lens implant, but does make the use of an anterior chamber intraocular lens implant ill advised. If the lens is dislocated, we perform an intracapsular removal with a vitrectomy if needed.

D. Postoperative increases in intraocular pressure are common following cataract removal especially if a viscoelastic agent is used. Glaucomatous eyes with low outflow facility may be more prone to pressure rises. A glaucoma-damaged optic nerve may not tolerate postoperative rises in intraocular pressure.

E. Postoperative loss of central fixation has been reported as a complication in the immediate interval following cataract surgery in eyes with glaucoma. While the incidence of this dreaded complication is unknown, it has only occurred in eyes which had preoperative visual field loss splitting fixation.

F. Postoperative intraocular inflammation usually is more severe, frequently resulting in a fibrinoid exudate. Intensive and prolonged corticosteroid therapy is usually required.

G. Short-term postoperative visual recovery is usually slower in eyes with glaucoma. Aphakic cystoid macular edema may be more frequent (incidence as high as 10%). Glaucoma patients should be informed of this prior to surgery.

H. In spite of these difficulties, cataract removal, in particular extracapsular extraction with a posterior chamber lens implant, in the eye with glaucoma usually results in improved visual acuity. In addition, intraocular pressure control usually is not worsened by an uncomplicated cataract extraction. Postcataract glaucoma control may even be improved, with intraocular pressure control achieved with the same or even reduced numbers of medications.

II. Indications

Cataract surgery alone is recommended if the glaucoma is under good medical control and the cataract is causing a sufficient visual handicap for the patient. The indications are similar to those in the nonglaucoma patient. However, the impact of the glaucoma damage to the optic nerve and to the visual field must be considered in the over-all decision process.

III. Technique

The following technique for cataract surgery is used for an eye with a small and fixed pupil which does not dilate secondary to long-term miotic therapy. Surgery can be performed under general or local anesthesia. We usually admit patients to the hospital following completion of the surgery. Admission is necessary due to the higher frequency of complications including postoperative rise in intraocular pressure.

Steps 1. A 4-0 or 5-0 silk bridle suture on a noncutting needle is passed as described on page 204.

2. A limbus- or fornix-based flap is prepared to expose the surgical limbus. We prefer the fornix-based flap since it is technically easier to perform and to close, and the conjunctiva is not in the surgical field during the procedure.

3. A limbal groove is prepared and preplaced sutures are used. The anterior chamber is entered for a length of 2–3 mm through the groove and a peripheral iridectomy is performed. The chamber is deepened with a viscoelastic substance and a blunt dialysis spat-

ula is inserted through the iridectomy and passed under the iris towards one horizontal meridian. The spatula is rotated toward the 6 o'clock meridian to separate synechiae between the iris and lens as well as synechiae at the pupil margin. The spatula is removed and the sweeping technique is repeated in the other direction.

4. Further pupil enlargement is achieved by performing a sector iridectomy or multiple sphincterotomies. We prefer converting the peripheral iridectomy into a sector iridectomy and also performing a sphincterotomy at the 6 o'clock position of the pupil. The sector iridectomy does not have to be repaired at the end of surgery.
5. A viscoelastic material is injected behind the iris to further mechanically dilate the pupil.
6. The above maneuvers usually provide sufficient pupil enlargement to perform the anterior capsulotomy in a relatively closed eye. Occasionally the limbal wound must be enlarged to perform these maneuvers and the capsulotomy is then done in an open anterior chamber filled with the viscoelastic substance.
7. The capsulotomy should be at least 5–6 mm in diameter. An iris retractor can be used to push the iris peripherally to assist in performing the capsulotomy, or the capsulotomy needle can be placed beneath the iris with the anterior capsule opened without direct visualization. Lens zonules may be weak. Therefore, excessive pressure on the lens is avoided. The excised portion of the anterior capsule is removed. The lens nucleus is engaged with the capsulotomy needle and gently dislocated.
8. The incision is enlarged for removal of the lens nucleus. Routine nucleus expression in a glaucomatous eye is associated with a higher incidence of complications, including vitreous loss. In the glaucomatous eye, in contrast to a routine nonglaucomatous cataract removal, the anterior capsulotomy opening is usually smaller and the iris is rigid, and the lens zonules may be weak. Therefore, only the bare minimum of pressure necessary to have the superior pole of the nucleus tilt up into the wound is applied. This is achieved by gentle pressure on the scleral side of the wound at 12 o'clock with counter pressure at the 6 o'clock limbus. Once the superior pole of the nucleus is in the wound, the nucleus is hooked, pressure on the globe is released, and the nucleus is pulled or rotated out of the eye. This method is in contrast to the usual technique of pushing the nucleus out of the eye. With a sector iridectomy, the anterior capsular flap may be carried into the wound or even out of the eye at the time of nucleus removal. The surgeon must be sure that the capsular tag is free prior to removing it from the eye. If the tag is still attached to the anterior capsule, removal will result in zonular dehiscence and probable vitreous loss.
9. The incision is closed and the lens cortex is removed by irrigation and aspiration. The surgeon should avoid the temptation of excessive aspiration superiorly in face of a sector iridectomy with unobstructed visualization of the superior capsule. This can be associated with dehiscence of the capsule and vitreous loss. If vitreous loss occurs, we perform an anterior vitrectomy, being sure that formed vitreous is not present in the anterior chamber or in the limbal wound. We do not use anterior chamber lens implants in eyes with glaucoma. The indications for using a posterior chamber intraocular lens implant with capsular rupture or vitreous loss are similar in glaucomatous and nonglaucomatous eyes.
10. The wound is closed except for the needed length for insertion of the posterior lens implant. We presently prefer a lens with a 7 mm diameter optic which does not have positioning holes. Due to the potential for weak zonules (see above), we place the lens in the sulcus and not in the capsular bag; capsular bag placement may be more often as-

sociated with postoperative lens displacement. The lens is rotated so the haptics are horizontal, out of the area of the iridectomy.

11. Viscoelastic material is irrigated from the anterior chamber prior to closure of the wound. The conjunctiva is closed. Subconjunctival corticosteroids and antibiotics are injected. Topical corticosteroids are administered starting on the morning after surgery. The pupil is intermittently dilated. The patient's preoperative glaucoma medications are withheld until the first postoperative examination.
12. Postoperative management includes careful monitoring of intraocular pressure during the first 24–48 hours after surgery. Treatment of a pressure rise includes the use of systemic hyperosmotic agents, topical beta blockers, and systemic carbonic anhydrase inhibitors. Routine glaucoma therapy is reinitiated depending on the level of the intraocular pressure. A visual field is performed approximately 1–2 months postoperatively.

## Two-Stage Filtration Cataract Surgery

I. Management of a cataract in the patient with glaucoma can be addressed in a two-stage approach, managing each problem separately. The glaucoma is initially controlled by performing a filtration procedure. Three to six months later the cataract is removed (see below).

II. The disadvantage to this approach is the time interval between filtration surgery and cataract removal and the obvious need for two procedures. The combined procedure eliminates both of these concerns.

III. Advantages to this approach may include decreased operative complications. The prognosis for each procedure may be better when performed individually than when performed together. However, evidence for this statement is based on limited clinical impressions.

## Combined Filtration/Cataract Surgery

I. Combined surgery addresses the visual problems relating to the cataract at the same time as glaucoma control is achieved. The need for two operations is eliminated and the postoperative recovery occurs during the same interval for both procedures.

II. Combined procedures offer the opportunity for long-term surgical control of the glaucoma. In addition, the combined filtering procedure may protect against immediate postoperative increases in intraocular pressure.

III. Disadvantages include the increased risk of operative or postoperative complications. Also, it is unclear if the rate of filtration success is greater or lower if the filtering procedure is performed separately, as in the two-stage management, or if the two procedures are combined. The surgeon must make this decision based on personal experience.

IV. We prefer to do combined surgery in our patients with uncontrolled glaucoma and a significant cataract.

### Combined Trabeculectomy/Cataract Removal

Steps
1. A limbus-based conjunctival flap is preferred to a fornix-based flap.
2. The trabeculectomy scleral flap is created and dissected into clear cornea.
3. The corneoscleral groove for the cataract surgery is performed to both sides of the scleral flap and a paracentesis entry may be performed away from the surgical site.
4. Entry is made into the anterior chamber through the base of the scleral flap dissection. At this stage, the trabeculectomy can be completed followed by the iris surgery for pupil enlargement, and the capsulotomy (Fig. 12-21). Alternatively, only the anterior chamber incision is performed for the iridectomy and capsulotomy with the trabeculectomy block excised later.

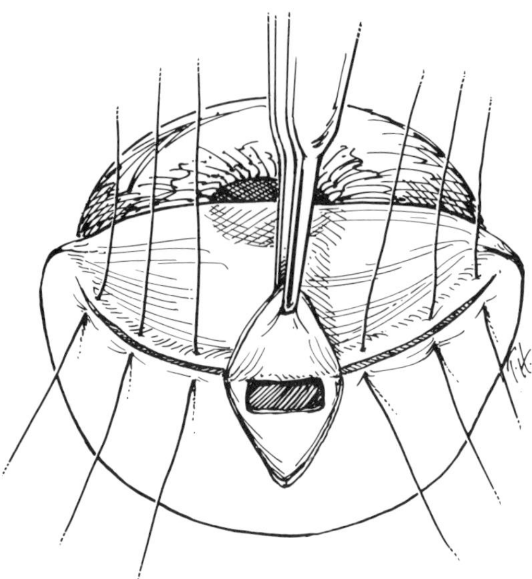

**Fig. 12-21** Combined trabeculectomy and cataract extraction.

5. The wound is completed on both sides of the scleral flap and the nucleus is removed, the wound is partially closed for irrigation and aspiration of lens cortex, and the posterior chamber lens implant is inserted. We prefer placement of the lens implant in the ciliary sulcus rather than in the capsular bag for reasons discussed above. The cataract portion of the wound is closed.
6. The trabeculectomy scleral flap is closed with 10-0 nylon suture and the conjunctiva is closed with 8-0 suture. The anterior chamber is reformed through the paracentesis tract or through the cataract portion of the wound.

## Combined Posterior Lip Sclerectomy/Cataract Removal

Steps 1. Extracapsular cataract surgery with the posterior chamber lens implant is performed as usual except the corneoscleral incision is made posteriorly with a long and beveled shelf. We recommend that the conjunctival flap be limbus-based.
2. A 3–4 mm length of the incision is not closed and is used for placement of the posterior lip excision. A 10-0 nylon suture is placed on either side of this area and looped out of the wound. The posterior lip sclerectomy is performed followed by an iridectomy at the site. The 10-0 nylon sutures are tied, completing the wound closure. The conjunctiva is closed with an 8-0 suture.

## Cataract Surgery in An Eye with a Functioning Filtering Bleb

I. Cataract removal in an eye with a functioning filtering procedure can be associated with up to a 50% incidence of subsequent failure of the bleb. The rate of failure is similar following intracapsular and extracapsular cataract removal. Intraoperative and postoperative complications may be similarly encountered as previously described in cataract patients on long-term miotics.

II. We perform extracapsular removal with insertion of a posterior chamber lens implant in eyes with a functioning bleb.

III. Cataract surgery can be performed via
   A. a corneal incision anterior to the bleb. This avoids manipulation of the conjunctiva and allows the surgeon to operate superiorly—the normal location for cataract surgery. The anterior location of the corneal incision requires a longer cord length for the cataract removal. Also, attention must be given to the more anteriorly located posterior lip of the wound during nucleus delivery. The corneal sutures are removed 4–6 months after surgery. Suture-induced corneal estigmatism may limit vision during this interval. However, the long-term degree of astigmatism is similar to cataract surgery performed through a limbal incision.
   B. a conjunctival incision to one side of the bleb. While conjunctiva is manipulated, it is distant from the area of external filtration. This requires that the filtration surgery had been performed at either a nasal or temporal location. Cataract surgery is

performed in a near normal superior location.

C. an inferior 6 o'clock location. This places the cataract wound distant from the filtration bleb. However, cataract surgery is now performed at a location which is not routine for most surgeons.

## CYCLODIALYSIS

I. Cyclodialysis consists of creating a separation of the ciliary body from the scleral spur. This results in a direct communication between the anterior chamber and the suprachoroidal space.

II. A successful procedure probably reduces intraocular pressure by increasing uveoscleral outflow. Detachment of the ciliary body and chronic inflammation may also result in reduced aqueous humor formation.

III. Cyclodialysis is rarely performed as the primary surgical glaucoma procedure in an eye with a favorable prognosis. Decreased use of this procedure relates to its unpredictable results and high rate of complications when performed in a phakic eye.

IV. Indications include the following:
   A. As a primary procedure in secondary aphakic glaucoma with extensive peripheral anterior synechiae.
   B. As a combined cyclodialysis procedure at the time of cataract surgery in an eye with uncontrolled glaucoma. However, we prefer to manage the coexistence of cataract and glaucoma as previously discussed.
   C. As a technique in eyes which have not responded to other surgical procedures.

V. Technique

Steps 1. The conjunctiva is incised 5–7 mm posterior to the limbus in a superior quadrant between the insertions of two rectus muscles. Surgery should not be performed in the horizontal meridians to avoid the long posterior ciliary vessels and the anterior ciliary vessels which enter the globe 1–2 mm anterior to the rectus muscle insertions.

2. A paracentesis incision is made in clear cornea at a distant area from the surgical site.
3. A scleral incision 3–4 mm in length is made 3–4 mm posterior to the limbus, immediately posterior to the scleral spur. The incision is initially made to approximately one-half of the scleral thickness, and a 4-0 to 6-0 suture is passed across the incision and looped out. The ends are used for traction to separate the incision while it is deepened until the choroid is exposed (Fig. 12-22). It is important to incise the entire thickness of the sclera; remaining fibers can prevent passage of the spatula.
4. A 1-mm wide blunt cyclodialysis spatula is introduced into the suprachoroidal space. The heel of the instrument is pressed down, lifting the inner surface of the sclera with the tip of the instrument. The tip of the instrument must stay close to the inner surface and not be depressed since this can perforate the ciliary body or the iris root, leading to hemorrhage, vitreous loss, iridodialysis, or a cataract and broken zonules in a phakic eye.
5. The ciliary body is detached as follows:
   The spatula is passed parallel to the limbus for 1½ clock hours and then rotated into the anterior chamber (Fig. 12-22B). Little or no resistance should be encountered as the tip of the instrument enters the chamber. The spatula is rotated and pulled towards the incision, detaching the ciliary body. It is important that the spatula is parallel to the plane of the iris as it is rotated into the chamber. This avoids damage to the corneal endothelium and Descemet's membrane as the ciliary body is depressed from the scleral spur. The instrument is removed and the process repeated in the opposite direction.
   An alternative technique is to create the ciliary body separation using multiple forward thrusts of the spatula into the chamber.

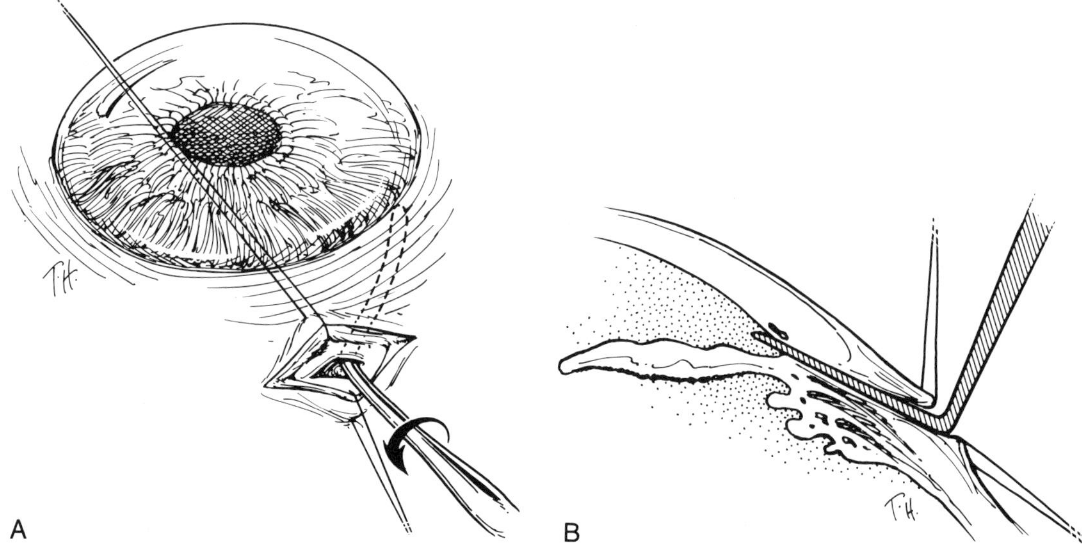


**Fig. 12-22** Cyclodialysis. **(A)** The circumferential incision is held open with a looped-out suture to ensure that the choroid is exposed. The cyclodialysis spatula is inserted into the suprachoroidal space and rotated toward the anterior chamber. **(B)** The spatula is against the inner scleral surface as the tip enters the chamber.

A cleft 3 to 4 clock hours in size is more than sufficient to control intraocular pressure. An iridectomy is not performed.

6. The preplaced suture is tied and the anterior chamber reformed through the paracentesis. The conjunctiva is closed with a 6-0 to 8-0 running suture.
7. Subconjunctival antibiotics are given at the conclusion of surgery and the eye is patched.
8. Postoperatively, topical corticosteroids are administered. Echothiophate iodide (0.125%) is given twice a day to produce maximum miosis in an attempt to keep the cleft open.

VI. Operative complications

A. Hemorrhage

Brisk bleeding can occur as the spatula separates the ciliary body and enters the chamber. The anterior chamber is filled with air through the paracentesis tract. In addition, the spatula is inserted into the wound and turned sideways to allow blood to exit from the eye. Postoperatively the patient's head is turned away from the side of the cleft so that blood does not accumulate in the surgical area. Blood in the cyclodialysis site predisposes to scarring and closure.

B. A spatula positioned too anterior can strip Descemet's membrane while a position too posterior may tear the ciliary body or iris, injure the lens in a phakic eye, or rupture the hyaloid face and possibly cause vitreous loss.

VII. Postoperative complications

A. Chronic hypotony is a common postoperative complication. This may lead to an extensive choroidal detachment, papilledema, and macular edema. Partial closure of the cleft may be required if visual acuity is reduced. Closure can be attempted using laser treatment directed to the cleft (see Chapter 11), external diathermy, penetrating diathermy with or without a lamellar scleral flap, cryotherapy, and external plombage. Occasionally, the cleft has to be repaired by direct suturing: a lamellar scleral flap is dissected over the area of the dialysis, multiple radial incisions are performed in the scleral bed to drain suprachoroidal fluid, and the scleral spur or ciliary body is sutured with 10-0 nylon to the sclera.

B. Other complications include cataract formation and chronic iridocyclitis.

## SETON PROCEDURES

I. Various types of foreign materials and devices have been used during glaucoma filtration surgery in eyes with a poor surgical prognosis, e.g., neovascular glaucoma, uveitic glaucoma, glaucoma in aphakia, and eyes with previously failed filtration surgery. A detailed description and the surgical insertion of these devices are beyond the scope of this manual.

II. Four different devices are currently used. These have the following in common:

A. Placement of an open tube into the anterior chamber that functions as the effective sclerostomy. In eyes with peripheral anterior synechiae and a sealed iridocorneal angle, the tube permits access to the anterior chamber and a drainage pathway for aqueous humor from the eye.

B. An external explant sutured to the sclera in the region of the equator of the globe. The anterior chamber tube is attached to the explant. The explant becomes encapsulated but usually provides a sufficient drainage area for aqueous humor to transfer across the bleb and subsequent reduction in intraocular pressure. The posterior site for filtration also may be important in eyes with prior surgery and conjunctival scar formation in the region of the limbus.

III. Posterior open-tube shunts

A. Molteno implant

Molteno implant consists of an open silicone rubber tube attached to a thin acrylic episcleral plate, 13 mm in diameter. One or multiple plate implants are attached to the sclera with the anterior edge of the plate 8–10 mm from the limbus.

B. Schocket procedure

This operation, an anterior chamber tube shunt to an encircling band, places an open Silastic tube into the chamber. The tube is sutured into the grooved portion of a #20 silicone encircling band which is sutured grooved-side against the sclera for 360° 10–12 mm behind the limbus.

IV. Posterior valved-tube shunts

A. Krupin-Denver long-glaucoma valve implant (Fig. 12-23)

The open silastic anterior chamber tube has a pressure-sensitive and unidirectional slit-valve at the external end. The opening pressure is approximately 11 mmHg and the closing pressure is approximately 9 mmHg. The valve end is sutured within the grooved portion of a #220 silastic explant which is attached to the globe, grooved-side down, for 180° to 360° in length. The valve limits aqueous humor flow through the device.

B. One-pieced valved silicone explant (Hitchins and Joseph)

The open silicone rubber anterior chamber tube has a slit in the side of the external portion of the tube which functions as a valve with an opening pressure between 4 and 20 mmHg. The tube is attached with adhesive to a rubber strap which is 9 mm wide, 1 mm thick, and 85 mm

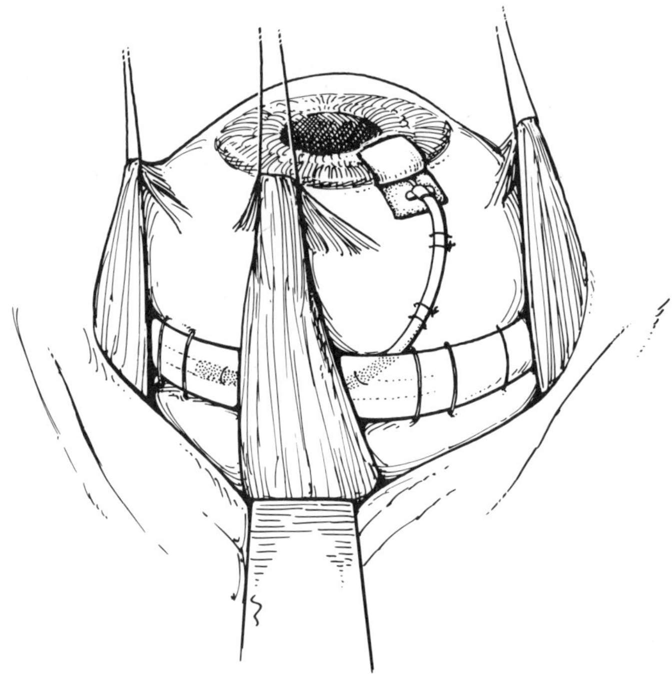

**Fig. 12-23** Krupin-Denver long-glaucoma valve implant.

long. The strap is attached to the sclera for approximately 180°.

V. These devices have been used in various subgroups of difficult glaucoma patients with success ranging from 50%–90%. While these results are encouraging, these devices should be reserved for eyes with an extremely poor surgical prognosis or prior filtration failure. Neovascular glaucoma in an only eye or in an eye with visual potential, and angle-closure glaucoma with anteriorly located synechiae are the only conditions for which we recommend these procedures as the primary operation. In all other types of glaucoma, conventional filtration surgery and procedures that do not require setons should be performed initially. However, these long implants are alternative surgical procedures that may be beneficial in controlling intraocular pressure in eyes with recalcitrant glaucoma.

## SURGICAL IRIDECTOMY

I. The indications for a surgical iridectomy are similar to those for laser iridotomy (see Chapter 11) and include elimination of pupillary block in acute, subacute, chronic, and secondary angle-closure glaucoma as well as in combined mechanism glaucoma.

II. Laser iridotomy has replaced surgical iridectomy in most patients with closed-angle glaucoma. However, surgical iridectomy may still be indicated in the following situations:
   A. Inability to produce a patent laser iridotomy
   B. When a laser iridotomy closes repeatedly, as in chronic uveitis
   C. Unavailability or nonfunctioning of a laser
   D. Media opacification preventing laser treatment, e.g., edema or scarring of

the cornea, striate keratopathy, or hyphema

E. During an acute attack of angle-closure glaucoma that cannot be terminated medically in which the anterior chamber is very shallow and the iris is inflamed and thickened

F. A patient who is unable to sit at the laser slit-lamp because of physical or mental disability

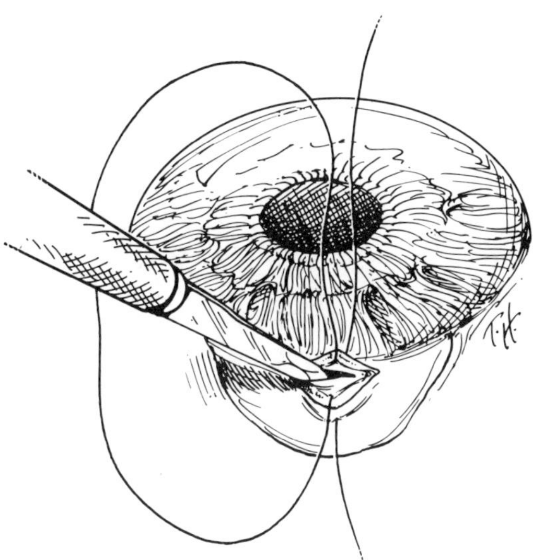

**Fig. 12-24** Peripheral iridectomy. Limbal incision with traction suture to expose the interior of the incision during deepening with a knife.

## Technique

Surgery is performed using local or general anesthesia. Some surgeons do an iridectomy with just topical anesthesia. Topical miotics are instilled prior to surgery to produce maximum miosis. This also increases pupillary block which aids in spontaneous iris prolapse during the surgery.

Steps

1. Anterior chamber incision. The anterior chamber incision can be made either through clear cornea or at the limbus using a conjunctival flap. Eyes with angle-closure have small anterior segments, therefore the incision must be anterior to avoid entry over the root of the iris or ciliary body. The incision is placed at 12 o'clock to retain both upper quadrants for future surgery and to place the iridectomy under the upper lid.

   A clear 3-mm corneal groove is made at the 12 o'clock position immediately anterior to the conjunctival reflection.

   Alternatively, a small peritomy or a limbus based conjunctival flap is prepared at the 12 o'clock position and the 3-mm incision is placed midlimbal.
2. A 7-0 to 9-0 suture is placed across the groove and looped out. The loops of the suture are used to spread the incision and to expose the interior of the groove (Fig. 12-24).
3. The entire length of the groove is deepened by an ab-externo scratch incision. Deepening should expose corneal tissue, which assures an anterior location of the incision. An incision perpendicular to the corneal surface favors spontaneous prolapse of iris tissue.
4. Deepening is continued until Descemet's membrane is reached. A sharp blade is used to slit Descemet's membrane under direct visualization.
5. Usually the iris spontaneously prolapses into the wound when the chamber is entered (Fig. 12-25). The prolapse is secondary to pupillary block forcing the iris into the wound.

   The main cause for failure of the iris to spontaneously prolapse is an incision which has a too small or an incomplete internal opening into the chamber. Using a sharp knife, the incision is enlarged.

   Failure of the iris to prolapse may relate to an incision which is too posterior over the ciliary body. In this situation the wound is closed and a new site chosen.

   An incision which is too anterior will not allow iris tissue to plug the incision resulting in failure of spontaneous iris prolapse.

   Failure of prolapse can occur in a properly located midlimbal incision due to a very soft eye with lack of a

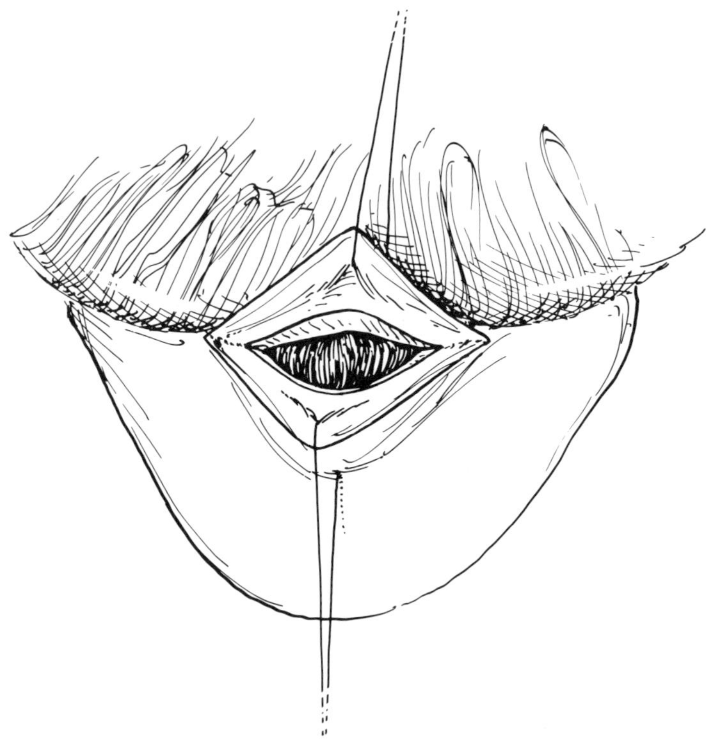

**Fig. 12-25** Prolapsed iris into the incision.

pupillary block. Additional pressure at the 6 o'clock limbus may be helpful in this situation. In addition, the surgeon can alternatively apply pressure to each loop of the preplaced suture, increasing pressure within the eye without opening the incision. An inadvertent puncture of the iris at the time of entry into the anterior chamber will eliminate pupillary block and prevent spontaneous iris prolapse. In this situation, the incision is enlarged with scissors, the iris grasped with a smooth iris forceps, and the iridectomy performed.

6. Once the iris is prolapsed into the wound, the iris is grasped with a toothed forceps and cut with a scissors held flush with the cornea (Fig. 12-26). The position of the iris sphincter is located prior to cutting the prolapsed iris. If a sector iridectomy is to be performed, the iris is removed from the anterior chamber by a hand-over-hand maneuver without posterior tension on the iris root, until the sphincter is removed from the eye. The iris is then excised.
7. The excised iris is examined to be sure pigment epithelium is present.
8. The iris usually springs back into the chamber after the iridectomy is completed. Pressure and massage of the cornea anterior to the incision with a muscle hook, tapping the wound, or depressing the posterior lip of the incision can assist in repositing iris into the chamber. Irrigation of the anterior chamber or repositing the iris with an instrument should be avoided if possible. The pupil should be round at the end of the procedure.
9. The preplaced suture is pulled up and tied. Additional sutures are placed as necessary. The conjunctiva is closed if it was incised. Subconjunctival antibiotics are administered and the eye is patched. We do not routinely use subconjunctival corticosteroids following a surgical iridectomy.

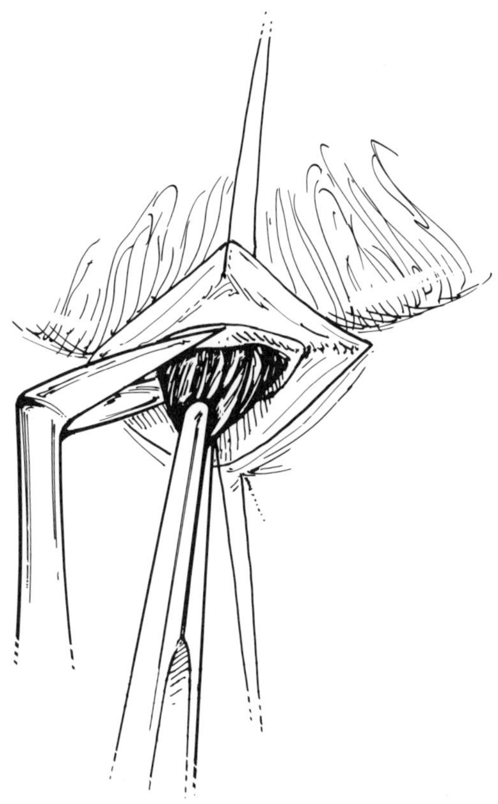

**Fig. 12-26** The iris is grasped with a toothed forceps and excised with a scissors.

10. Postoperatively topical corticosteroids and 2.5% phenylephrine are administered 2–3 times a day to reduce inflammation and to prevent the formation of posterior synechiae. Intraocular pressure is monitored.

## Operative Complications

I. Failure of the iris to prolapse spontaneously is a frequent operative complication.

II. Direct injury to the lens can occur if there is manipulation within the anterior chamber either to perform the iridectomy or to reposit the iris pillars after performing the procedure.

III. Small hyphemas are common after iridectomy but rarely cause a problem. Bleeding can be secondary to cutting iris vessels or ciliary processes which can be on the back surface of the iris.

IV. An incomplete excision of the iris can occur. This is more common if the prolapsed iris is grasped with a smooth iris forceps which can fixate only the anterior stroma of the iris. It is very dangerous to attempt to surgically complete the iridectomy by incising the remaining posterior pigment epithelium. A second iridectomy can be performed. However, the easiest method to manage this problem is to close the wound and take the patient to a laser where perforation of the pigment epithelium is safely performed (see Chapter 11).

## Postoperative Complications

I. Persistent pupillary block can occur postoperatively due to the following conditions:
   A. An incomplete iridectomy with an intact pigment epithelial layer. This is best managed using the laser as described above.
   B. Incarceration of the iridectomy into the wound or closure of the iridectomy by fibrous ingrowth or posterior synechiae. These conditions are managed by performing a new iridectomy.

II. Ciliary block (malignant) glaucoma is a rare but serious complication which is more common following surgery in eyes with chronic angle-closure glaucoma and uncontrolled intraocular pressure. In this condition, the iridectomy is patent, the anterior chamber is shallow to flat, and the intraocular pressure is increased. The medical and surgical management of ciliary block glaucoma is discussed on page 228.

III. A shallow or flat chamber with a low intraocular pressure is usually secondary to a wound leak. The wound should be explored and repaired immediately to prevent the formation of peripheral anterior synechiae.

### Plateau Iris

I. The diagnosis of plateau iris configuration is not made until a postoperative increase in intraocular pressure occurs following pupillary dilation in face of a patent iridectomy. The condition is recognized by noting a relatively deep central anterior chamber depth, and on goniscopy a flat iris plane. In plateau iris, the major factor contributing to angle closure is angle crowding, and pupillary block is a minor contributing factor.

II. An iridectomy is indicated in plateau iris to eliminate the pupillary block component. However, if the condition is suspected preoperatively, the postoperative use of mydriatics should be avoided.

III. Treatment of plateau iris, after an iridectomy has been performed, consists of avoiding dilating drugs and using a miotic to reduce angle crowding.

## CYCLOCRYOTHERAPY

Destruction of the ciliary body to reduce aqueous humor formation can be performed using cryotherapy or transscleral laser treatment (see page 190). While transscleral electrodiathermy was the first cyclodestructive procedure, the procedure is no longer performed due to extensive damage to the sclera overlying the ciliary body. Transscleral therapeutic ultrasound and direct endophotocoagulation are also used for cyclodestruction; however, because these techniques are not readily performed by the practicing ophthalmologist, they will not be covered in this manual.

### Mechanism of Action

I. Cyclocryotherapy lowers intraocular pressure by
   A. producing necrosis of the ciliary epithelium thereby reducing the active production of aqueous humor
   B. producing necrosis to the capillaries of the ciliary body thereby reducing blood flow to the ciliary processes, which acts to reduce aqueous humor formation.

II. The temperature attained within the eye is primarily dependent on ciliary body blood flow which resupplies heat to counteract the effect of the cryo application. There is currently no method to measure ciliary body blood flow. The effects of cryotherapy will be greater in eyes with underlying ischemia, e.g., neovascular glaucoma.

III. The destructive nature of cyclocryotherapy acts to reduce aqueous humor formed by active secretion. Aqueous humor will still be formed by ultrafiltration and entry of fluid into the eye across disrupted blood-aqueous barriers. This aqueous humor will have the characteristics of plasma and not that of active secretory processes, e.g., higher protein concentration and components similar to plasma.

### Indications

I. Cyclocryotherapy is rarely performed as the primary surgical procedure in an eye with a favorable prognosis. The procedure is usually reserved for conditions in which other glaucoma operations have repeatedly failed or in which the surgeon desires to avoid intraocular surgery.

II. Conditions in which cyclocryotherapy may be indicated include
   A. severe yet transient glaucoma such as that following blunt trauma.
   B. glaucoma after penetrating keratoplasty.
   C. chronic open-angle glaucoma in aphakia.
   D. managing pain in absolute glaucoma when the patient wishes to retain the eye.
   E. managing neovascular glaucoma. However, the technique is associated with complications (see below) and poor visual results in this con-

dition and is therefore recommended for the relief of pain in eyes with neovascular glaucoma and no visual potential.

## Technique

Many different techniques have been described. The following is our recommended procedure:

Steps
1. Topical and retrobulbar anesthesia without a lid block are used. If vision is not a goal of treatment, 1 ml of absolute alcohol can be added to the retrobulbar injection to reduce postoperative pain. The alcohol must be injected within the muscle cone to prevent anterior dissection of the drug into the eyelids which can result in postoperative ptosis. In addition, retrobulbar alcohol can result in extraocular muscle weakness.
2. A lid speculum is inserted and the surface of the globe is dried with applicators.
3. A nitrous oxide or carbon dioxide gas cryosurgical unit is used. A cryoprobe with a diameter of 3.5 or 4.0 mm is used. A modified probe with a curved 3 × 6 mm tip can be used to reduce the number of applications.
4. The tip of the probe is placed so the nearest edge is placed 2.5–3.0 mm from the limbus. This location maximizes treatment to the ciliary body and reduces an anterior freeze of the cornea, trabecular meshwork, or iris.
5. There are no precise parameters to serve as guidelines for the number of cryo applications which should be delivered. We perform six to eight applications either overlapping over one-half of the globe or six to eight applications evenly spaced over 360°.
6. The warm probe is placed against the globe to produce slight indentation. The cryo unit is activated to achieve a temperature of −60°C to −80°C at the tip. Treatment at each application is for 45–60 sec with the ice ball allowed to thaw before the probe is removed. We do not perform a freeze-thaw-refreeze technique because it does not appear to have any advantage over the freeze-thaw method.
7. Subconjunctival corticosteroids are given at the conclusion of the treatment. Postoperatively topical atropine (1%) is administered twice a day and topical corticosteroids (0.1% dexamethasone or 1% prednisolone) 4–6 times daily.

## Complications

I. Ocular pain can be severe and may last for days to weeks following cyclocryotherapy. Retrobulbar alcohol injection, in eyes with no visual potential, may reduce this complication. Systemic analgesics may be required.

II. Postoperative intraocular inflammation occurs in all eyes and may contribute to the ocular pain. Topical cycloplegics and corticosteroids are administered postoperatively. Occasionally periocular or systemic corticosteroids are required. Chronic anterior chamber flare usually follows cyclocryotherapy and does not necessarily indicate chronic iritis requiring treatment.

III. Marked elevations in intraocular pressure can occur within the first 24–48 h after surgery. Topical beta blockers, systemic carbonic anhydrase inhibitors, and occasionally systemic hyperosmotic agents are used to lower the pressure.

IV. Chronic hypotony occurs in 5%–10% of eyes treated with cyclocryotherapy. This complication increases with time following the treatment; many eyes develop phthisis bulbi. Hypotony is more frequent in eyes with preexisting ocular ischemia, e.g., neovascular glaucoma. Reports suggest that hypotony and phthisis bulbi may be decreased in frequency by both reducing the number of treatment spots and limiting the extent of treatment. For these reasons, we recommend that a limited amount of treatment be given, either a total of six to eight spots over 180° or 360° at any one treatment session. This recommendation is particularly important in neovascular glaucoma. However, there are no methods to determine the effect of treatment on ciliary body blood flow. The combination of cyclocryotherapy-induced ischemia and the preexisting ocular ischemia may not be tolerated by the eye.

V. Macular edema frequently follows cyclocryotherapy, but may not be recognized because of preexisting poor vision.

VI. Cataract formation is a common postoperative complication. Therefore, the procedure should not be performed in phakic eyes with visual potential.

VII. Other complications include vitreous hemorrhage, hyphema, suprachoroidal hemorrhage, persistent corneal epithelial defects, thinning of the sclera, and staphyloma formation.

## SUGGESTED READINGS

Cairns JE: Glaucoma, vol. 1. Grune & Stratton, London, 1986

Krupin T, Waltman SR: Complications in ophthalmic surgery. 2nd Ed. JB Lippincott Company, Philadelphia, 1984

Waltman SR, Keates RH, Hoyt CS, et al: Surgery of the eye. vol. 1. Churchill Livingstone, New York, 1988

# 13

# Congenital Glaucoma

Congenital glaucoma is a rare condition and therefore not frequently encountered by the general ophthalmologist. Unless the ophthalmologist has experience in the surgical management of this condition, these patients are best handled in centers where children with congenital glaucoma are regularly treated.

## CLINICAL PRESENTATION

I. The classic signs of congenital glaucoma consist of a triad of epiphora, photophobia, and blepharospasm. The condition may be present at birth or have its onset within the first year of life.

II. Changes in the cornea occur within the first 2 years of life and include

   A. increased corneal diameter. The normal neonatal horizontal diameter is 10.0–10.5 mm increasing to 11.0–12.0 mm by the end of the first year of life. Horizontal corneal diameter is markedly increased in congenital glaucoma.

   B. corneal edema due to the direct effect of elevated intraocular pressure or an acute tear in Descemet's membrane. The former clears as the intraocular pressure is lowered medically while the latter may not. An acute rupture in Descemet's membrane results in an acute onset of corneal edema (hydrops) which is usually associated with a lowering in intraocular pressure due to "decompression" of aqueous into the cornea.

   C. single or multiple tears in Descemet's membrane (Haab's striae) (Fig. 13-1) that occur either horizontally or concentric to the limbus in the peripheral cornea.

III. Intraocular pressure is elevated while outflow facility is reduced. Intraocular pressures are usually measured under general anesthesia which usually decreases aqueous humor formation. Therefore, intraocular pressure should be measured as early as possible after the administration of the inhalation anesthetic. This requires coordination with the anesthesiologist. We prefer to have the anesthesiologist administer anesthesia by face mask; this allows early pressure measurements with a portable Perkins applanation tonometer or the pneumatonometer (see Chapter 2). While intraocular pressure can be reduced by the anesthetic agent, outflow facility is unaltered. Therefore, tonography may be useful in the evaluation of these patients. Tonography can be done manually by holding a Schiotz tonometer on the eye for 4 min and noting the scale reading at the beginning and every minute for the 4 min (see Chapter 3). Following the measurement of intraocular pressure, intubation anesthesia can be administered to complete the examination or to perform surgery if necessary.

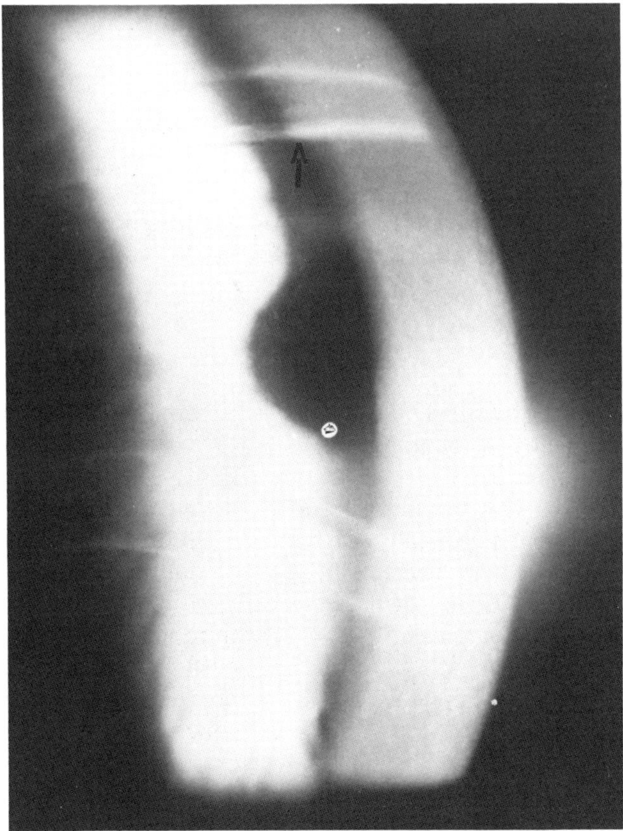

**Fig. 13-1** Congential glaucoma. Haab's striae representing tears in Descemet's membrane (arrow).

IV. Gonioscopy in primary congenital glaucoma (see Chapter 4) often shows the iridocorneal angle to be open with a high insertion of the iris root which forms a scalloped line. Loops of iris vessels from the major arterial circle may be seen above the iris root. The peripheral iris may be covered by a fine, fluffy tissue. These observations are not necessarily diagnostic because the normal anterior chamber angle in childhood may have many of these characteristics.

V. Glaucomatous cupping of the optic nerve head is present.

VI. The size of the globe is enlarged. Axial length as determined by A-scan ultrasonography may be useful as a diagnostic method and for following progression of the disease. The increased size of the globe is associated with axial myopia.

## DIFFERENTIAL DIAGNOSIS

I. Excessive tearing is most commonly due to obstruction of the lacrimal system. However, congenital glaucoma should be ruled out in all children undergoing nasolacrimal probing.

II. A large cornea occurs in the condition of congenital megalocornea, a sex-linked recessive condition in which the anterior segment is enlarged with a normal intraocular pressure. In this condition the cornea may be 14–16 mm in diameter and iridodonesis may be present. Intraocular pressure may be elevated later in life.

III. A large globe is associated with high myopia with normal intraocular pressures.
IV. Birth trauma can cause tears in Descemet's membrane. In contrast to Haab's striae, tears from birth trauma usually occur in a vertical or oblique direction.
V. Opacification of the cornea results from other nonglaucomatous causes (i.e., birth trauma, intraocular inflammation, congenital corneal dystrophies, and inborn errors of metabolism).

## SECONDARY CONGENITAL GLAUCOMA

Numerous ocular and systemic conditions can be associated with congenital glaucoma. In some of these conditions the glaucoma appears identical to primary congenital glaucoma. A partial listing with clinical findings of the more common associated conditions are as follows:

I. Aniridia
   Sporadic cases require general medical evaluation to rule out an associated Wilm's tumor.
II. Congenital rubella
   The glaucoma may be transient and secondary to intraocular inflammation, or developmental and not unlike primary congenital glaucoma.
III. Phakomatoses
   A. Sturge-Weber (encephalotrigeminal angiomatosis) syndrome
      The presence of nevus flammeus of the upper eyelid is associated with a high frequency of glaucoma. The glaucoma may be indistinguishable from primary congenital glaucoma, a secondary open-angle glaucoma, or secondary glaucoma due to elevated episcleral venous pressure.
   B. Neurofibromatosis (von Recklinghausen syndrome)
      Involvement of the upper eyelid is usually present in eyes with associated glaucoma which may be similar to congenital glaucoma. However, malformation or absence of Schlemm's canal has been reported in this condition. Systemic involvement is widespread including the cutaneous café au lait spots and neurofibromas, glial neoplasms or meningoblastomas of the optic nerve, and orbital neurofibromas.
   C. Angiomatosis retinae (von Hippel Lindau syndrome)
   D. Oculodermal melanocytosis (Nevus of Ota)
IV. Chromosomal abnormalities including
   A. trisomy 13.
   B. chromosome 18 deletion syndrome.
   C. trisomy 18 (Edwards syndrome).
   D. trisomy 21 (Down's syndrome).
   E. Turner's syndrome.
V. Oculocerebrorenal (Lowe's) syndrome
VI. Rubinstein-Taybi syndrome consisting of congenital glaucoma with large, broad thumbs and toes, hypertelorism, and mental retardation.
VII. Pierre Robin syndrome
VIII. Microphthalmos
   Various conditions can have an associated microphthalmic eye with glaucoma including trisomy 13, congenital rubella, Hallermann-Streiff syndrome, Goldenhar's syndrome, oculodentodigital syndrome, Pierre Robin syndrome, and oculocerebrorenal syndrome.

## MANAGEMENT

The management of primary congenital glaucoma consists of surgery. Medical therapy is used temporarily before surgery. The various secondary types of congenital glaucoma may be managed medically prior to resorting to filtration surgery. Adequate management requires a detailed ocular examination which is usually performed under anesthesia with the special precautions as noted above.

## Examination under Anesthesia

Steps 1. Measure intraocular pressure shortly after the induction of inhalation anesthesia by face mask.
2. Instill dilating drops if they were not administered preoperatively.
3. Record horizontal and vertical corneal diameters.
4. Examine the anterior segment with a portable slit-lamp or operating microscope.
5. Gonioscopy.
6. Retinoscopy.
7. Examine of the fundi with optic disc photographs if possible.
8. Axial length measurement.

## Medical Management

Medical management utilizes topical beta blockers and systemic carbonic anhydrase inhibitors (see Chapter 7). Acetazolamide is administered orally in 5–10 mg/kg body weight every 6 or 8 hours.

## Trabeculotomy Technique

While we perform goniotomy in the surgical management of congenital glaucoma, trabeculotomy, which is as successful as goniotomy when employed as the primary procedure for congenital glaucoma, is preferred by many surgeons since the technique is more similar to standard microsurgical procedures. Goniotomy, which will not be covered in this manual, is preferred by some surgeons as the primary procedure because it is less destructive to ocular tissues. Goniotomy requires specialized skills and an excellent visualization of the anterior chamber angle. If prior goniotomies have failed, trabeculotomy is useful. In addition, trabeculotomy may also be useful for the treatment of juvenile open-angle glaucoma.

Steps 1. A small limbus- or fornix-based conjunctival flap is prepared in an oblique meridian. Excessive conjunctival manipulation and dissection is avoided.

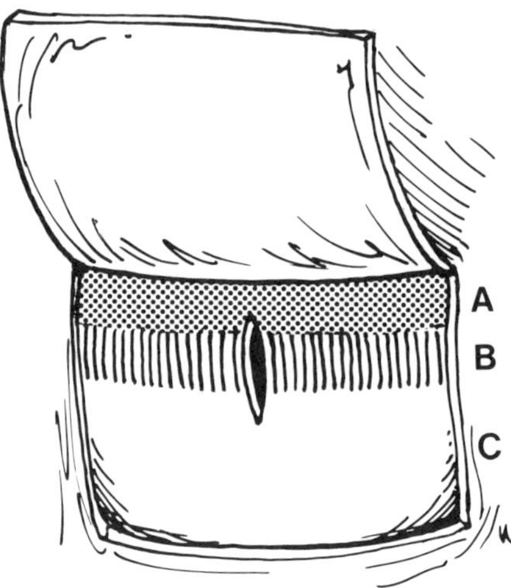


**Fig. 13-2** Scleral flap dissection bed for trabeculotomy: Peripheral cornea **(A)** is characterized by a translucent blue color. Transition zone **(B)** includes the scleral spur and Schlemm's canal, Sclera **(C)** is opaque.

2. A scleral flap, two-thirds of the scleral thickness, is prepared. This can be a 3-mm triangular or a rectangular flap with a 3-mm long base at the limbus and extends 2 mm posterior from the limbus. The dissection is carried into clear cornea.
3. The scleral spur is located within the dissection bed (Fig. 13-2). This is a critical step because Schlemm's canal lies adjacent to the scleral spur, in the transition zone between the white of the sclera and the blue of the peripheral cornea. Identification is made easier by transilluminating through the cornea. The light source is placed on the center of the cornea, with the room and operating microscope lights off. This will demonstrate the iris insertion with the scleral spur "lighting up" as a posterior white limit with clear cornea anteriorly.
4. Using 16 to 25 × magnification, a radial scratch incision is made over the area of the scleral spur; 1 mm anterior and 1–2 mm posterior to the center of the transition zone. The area is kept dry as the incision is deepened. The scleral fi-

bers are pushed to the side with the knife blade after each cutting stroke until Schlemm's canal is reached and unroofed.

5. It is critical not to enter the anterior chamber during this dissection. If this occurs, it is very difficult to probe Schlemm's canal and the procedure is best converted into a trabeculectomy procedure.
6. Identification of the canal is performed after it is unroofed by passing a 5-0 or 6-0 monofilament nylon suture into the canal. The suture should pass without resistance in both directions. If the suture is within the canal, flexion of the external part produces no movement of the suture in the canal (Fig. 13-3). If the suture is in the anterior chamber, it will be visible when its exterior portion is rotated posteriorly. If the suture is in the suprachoroidal space, it will move posteriorly when its exterior portion is rotated anteriorly (Fig. 13-4).
7. An angled McPherson or Harms trabeculotome is placed within the lumen of Schlemm's canal for 5–10 mm to one side. The probe is kept parallel to the iris and midway between the iris and cornea as the tip is gently rotated into the anterior chamber (Fig. 13-5). The probe is pulled back toward the incision. Minimal resistance should be encountered during these maneuvers.
8. The probe is removed and the procedure repeated in the opposite direction with the paired trabeculotome.
9. The scleral flap is sutured tightly with 10-0 nylon sutures.
10. The conjunctival flap is closed with absorbable sutures.
11. Subconjunctival injections of an antibiotic and a short-acting corticosteroid are made and the eye is patched.

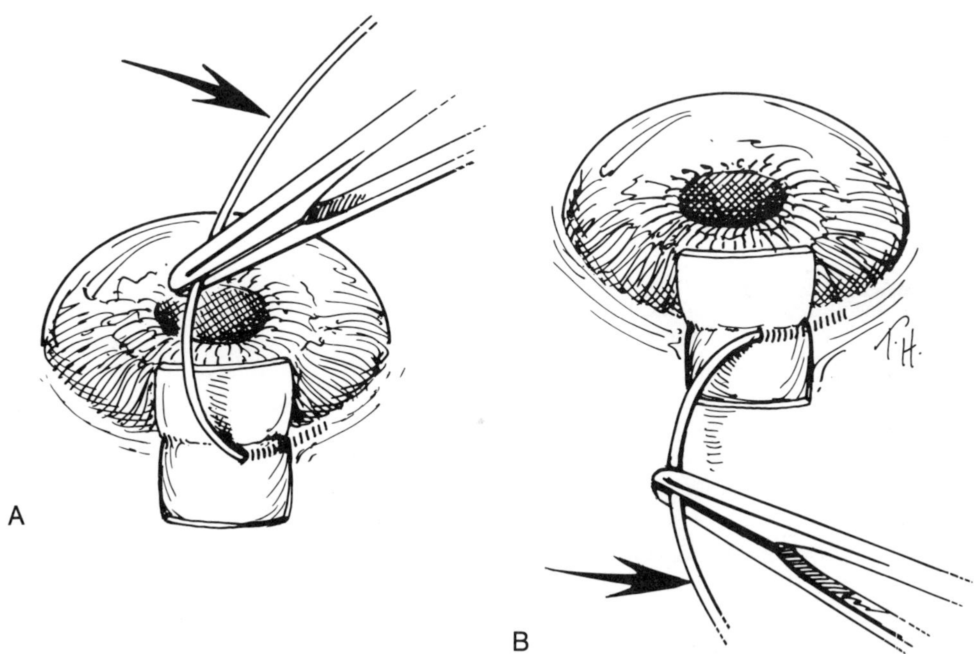


**Fig. 13-3** Suture within Schlemm's canal. If the suture is in the canal, anterior flexion **(A)** or posterior flexion **(B)** of the external segment produces no movement of the intercanalicular portion. After release of the external portion, the suture springs back into place parallel to Schlemm's canal.

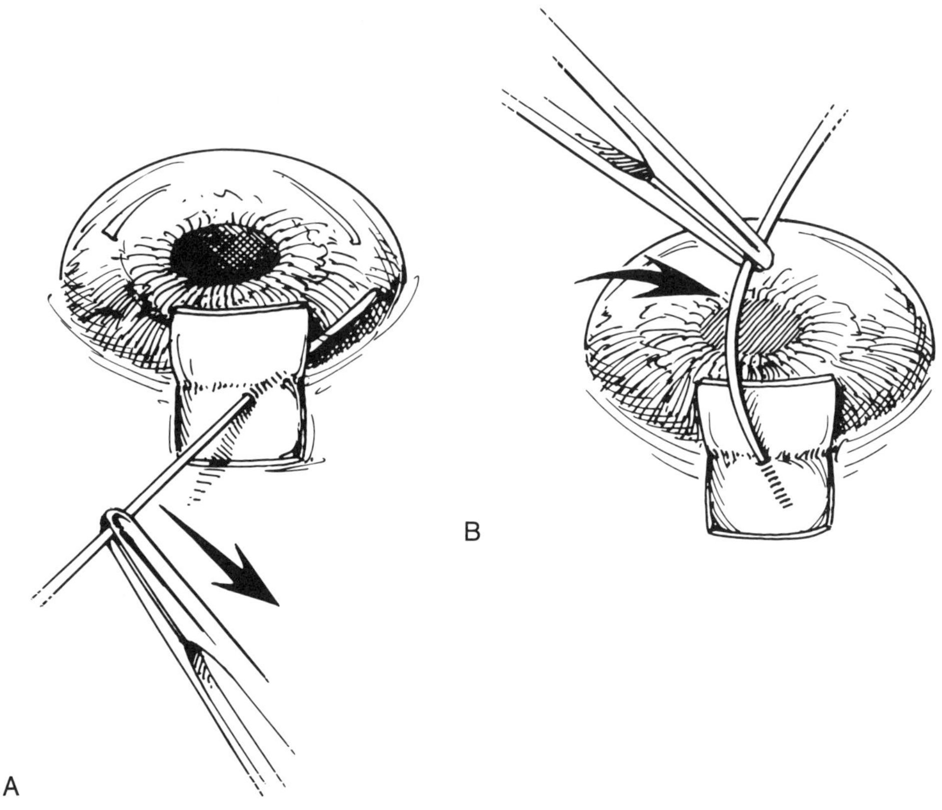


**Fig. 13-4** Suture outside Schlemm's canal. If the suture is in the anterior chamber (**A**), posterior flexion allows visualization of the tip of the suture in the chamber. If the suture is in the supraciliary space (**B**), anterior flexion allows the tip to pass posteriorly. In both conditions, after release of the external portion, the suture does not spring back to its previous position.

12. Topical corticosteroids and atropine are administered postoperatively.

## Operative Complications

I. Small hyphemas are common following trabeculotomy. They usually resolve spontaneously and only rarely require surgical evacuation.

II. An inadvertent cyclodialysis can be produced during the procedure. This usually closes spontaneously.

III. A postoperative filtration bleb occurs in approximately 10%–15% of cases. While not an aim of the surgery, this is helpful in lowering intraocular pressure.

IV. Detachment of Descemet's membrane, an iridodialysis, an iridotomy, or dislocation of the lens can occur during rotation of the trabeculotomy probe.

## Follow-up Treatment

I. In bilateral cases, we only rarely perform surgery on both eyes at the same operating room session. The major concern is the potential complication of bilateral endophthalmitis. Therefore, we prefer to operate on the second eye 3–7 days after the first. A postoperative examination of the first operated eye is performed at this time. The disadvantage of separating the days of surgery is increased anesthetic exposure and as-

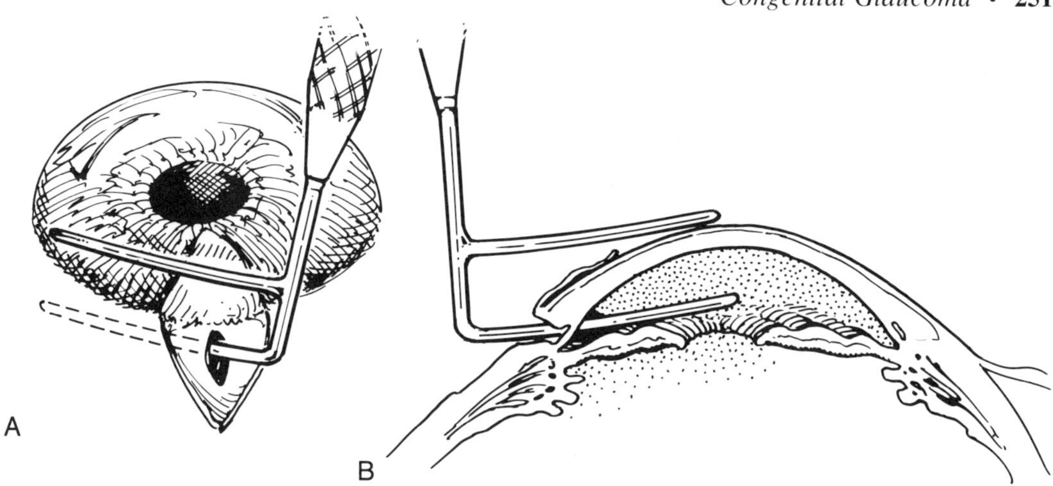


**Fig. 13-5** Trabeculotomy. Angled Harms trabeculotome in Schlemm's canal (**A**) is rotated into the anterior chamber (**B**).

sociated risks. Therefore, if the child is a very high anesthetic risk, we will consider doing surgery on both eyes at the same session. In this case, surgery is performed on each eye "separately": after completion of the first operation, the second eye is re-drapped, the surgical team rescrubs and regowns, and a new surgical set-up is used.

II. A postoperative examination under anesthesia is repeated 3–5 weeks after surgery. Adequacy of treatment is determined by a normalized intraocular pressure, a stable or smaller degree of optic disc cupping, stable corneal diameters, stable or decreasing myopia, and stable or decreasing axial length by ultrasonography, if performed.

III. If the initial surgical procedure is unsuccessful, a repeat trabeculotomy is performed. We will do this procedure three separate times and use topical beta blockers to control the glaucoma. If this is unsuccessful, filtering surgery is attempted. We prefer full-thickness filtration surgery over trabeculectomy. Seton procedures are not recommended before this stage of the management. Cyclocryotherapy is the last resort in recalcitrant cases.

IV. It is important to detect and treat possible amblyopia after the intraocular pressure is successfully treated. These eyes are usually moderately to highly myopic and require careful refraction and treatment. This is especially important in unilateral cases.

## SUGGESTED READINGS

Harms H, Dannheim R: Trabeculotomy results and problems. In Mackensen G (ed): Microsurgery in Glaucomas, Basel, S Karger, 1970

Kwitko ML: Glaucoma in infants and children. Appleton-Century-Crofts, East Norwalk, CT, 1973

Quigley HA: Childhood glaucoma. Results with trabeculotomy and study of reversible cupping. Ophthalmology 89:219, 1982

Ritch R, Shields MB: The Secondary Glaucomas. CV Mosby, St Louis, 1982

# INDEX

*Page numbers followed by* f *indicate figures; those followed by* t *indicate tables.*